Instrumentation
for the Operating Room

A Photographic Manual

Instrumentation
for the Operating Room

A Photographic Manual

SEVENTH EDITION

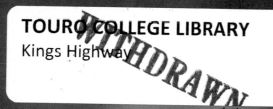

Shirley M. Tighe, RN, BA

AD in Applied Science in Photography

Consultant for the Operating Room

Lake Havasu City, Arizona

with over 800 color digital photographs

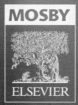

MOSBY

ELSEVIER

**ELSEVIER
MOSBY**

11830 Westline Industrial Drive
St. Louis, Missouri 63146

INSTRUMENTATION FOR THE OPERATING ROOM

ISBN: 978-0-323-04310-6

NOTICE

Nursing is an ever-changing field. Standard safety precautions must be followed, but as new research and clinical experience broaden our knowledge, changes in treatment and drug therapy may become necessary or appropriate. Readers are advised to check the most current product information provided by the manufacturer of each drug to be administered to verify the recommended dose, the method and duration of administration, and contraindications. It is the responsibility of the licensed prescriber, relying on experience and knowledge of the patient, to determine dosages and the best treatment for each individual patient. Neither the publisher nor the author assumes any liability for any injury and/or damage to persons or property arising from this publication.

Previous editions copyrighted 1978, 1983, 1989, 1994, 1999
International Standard Book Number: 978-0-323-04310-6

Executive Publisher: Darlene Como
Managing Editor: Tamara Myers
Developmental Editor: Laura Selkirk
Publishing Services Manager: Jeff Patterson
Project Manager: Jeanne Genz
Designer: Jyotika Shroff

Printed in Canada

Last digit is the print number: 9 8 7 6 5 4 3 2 1

Instrumentation for the Operating Room, A Photographic Manual,
seventh edition, is dedicated to **Cynthia Spry, Pauline Vorderstrasse,**
and my husband, **Glen E. Tighe.** It is not until one attempts to create a book
that one realizes how important family, friends, and consultants really are.
I couldn't have completed this book without their dedication to teaching
and to the project. Three of us have been perioperative nursing instructors,
and Glen taught in the U.S. Navy. The completion of this book has also required
many dedicated consultants whom I will always remember and be indebted to for
all their hard work. Perioperative nursing and the people who are in that field
are very important to all of us.

Thank you so much, Cynthia, Pauline, and Glen.

Love, Shirley

Contributors/Consultants

NURSE/CONSULTANTS

Cynthia C. Spry, RN, MA, MSN, CNOR
New York City, New York
International Clinical Consultant,
Advanced Sterilization Products
Division of Johnson & Johnson
 Medical, Inc.
Irvine, California

Arlene Carlo, RN, BSN, FCSP
Clinical Specialist/Educator
Carlo Consulting Company, Inc.
Miromar Lakes, Florida

Pauline E. Vorderstrasse, RN, BSN
Director/Instructor Surgical
 Technology
Mt. Hood Community College,
 Retired
West Linn, Oregon

CLINICAL CONSULTANTS

Bill Allison, Surgical Technologist
Urology
Legacy Emanuel Hospital &
 Medical Center
Portland, Oregon

Julie A. Beeber, Certified Surgical Technologist
Lead Technologist, Clinical
 Instructor, MIS and General
 Surgery
Legacy Good Samaritan
 Hospital & Medical Center
Portland, Oregon

Wendi Blevins, RN
Patient Care Director
Havasu Surgery Center
Lake Havasu City, Arizona

Cheryl Boyer, RN, CNOR
Operating Room Manager
Legacy Emanuel Hospital &
 Medical Center
Portland, Oregon

Sheryl Bundy, RN
Pediatric Surgical Coordinator
Legacy Emanuel Childrens'
 Hospital
Portland, Oregon

Beverly I. Burns, RN, CNOR
Portland, Oregon
Perioperative Nurse Consultant
AchieveMentors, Inc.
Cleburne, Texas

Myrna H. Butler, RN, BA, CNOR
Wilsonville, Oregon
Perioperative Nurse Consultant
AchieveMentors, Inc.
Cleburne, Texas

Candace Carson, RN
Central Service Manager
Legacy Emanuel Hospital &
 Medical Center
Portland, Oregon

Gerry J. Casale, RN
Perioperative Nurse, Retired
Tualatin, Oregon

Aloa L. Day, RN
ENT and Plastic Surgery
  Coordinator
St. Vincent Hospital & Medical
  Center, Retired
Portland, Oregon

Beverly J. Eagle, RN, CNOR
EENT/Plastic, Ambulatory
  Surgery
Legacy Good Samaritan
  Hospital & Medical Center
Portland, Oregon

Meseret Eichman, RN
General, MIS, and Bariatric
  Surgery Coordinator
Legacy Good Samaritan
  Hospital & Medical Center
Portland, Oregon

Beckie Elton, RN
Open Heart Preceptor
  Coordinator
Legacy Good Samaritan
  Hospital & Medical Center
Portland, Oregon

Michael Johnson, RN
Neuro/Orthopedic Coordinator
Legacy Good Samaritan
  Hospital & Medical Center
Portland, Oregon

Sherry Labavinch, RN, MPA/HA
Operating Room and Central
  Service Supervisor
Shriners Hospital for Children
Portland, Oregon

**Ronnie Mills, Certified Surgical
Technologist**
Pediatric Orthopedics and
  Plastics
Shriners Hospital for Children
Portland, Oregon

Wendi A. Moore, RN
Gynecology, Urology, and
  Kidney Transplant, Specialty
  Coordinator
Legacy Good Samaritan
  Hospital & Medical Center
Portland, Oregon

Adriana Morera Moss, RN, BSN
Neurosurgical Clinical
  Coordinator
Legacy Emanuel Hospital &
  Medical Center
Portland, Oregon

Teresa Ochsner, RN
Central Service Manager
Legacy Good Samaritan
  Hospital & Medical Center
Portland, Oregon

Sharon B. Ramos, RN
MIS Coordinator
Legacy Emanuel Hospital &
  Medical Center
Portland, Oregon

Carol L. Ritzheimer, RN
Day Charge Nurse, Operating
  Rooms
Legacy Good Samaritan
  Hospital & Medical Center
Portland, Oregon

Greg Selivonchick, RN
Orthopedic Surgical Coordinator
Legacy Emanuel Hospital &
  Medical Center
Portland, Oregon

Dawn M. Sloss, RN, AD
Open Heart, Vascular, and
  Trauma Specialty Coordinator
Legacy Emanuel Hospital &
  Medical Center
Portland, Oregon

Julie Stamper, RN
EENT and Plastic Surgery,
   Ambulatory Surgery
Legacy Good Samaritan
   Hospital & Medical Center
Portland, Oregon

Karen M. Underwood, RN,
CNOR
Operating Room Supervisor
Legacy Emanuel Hospital &
   Medical Center
Portland, Oregon

Helen Worcester, RN
EENT, Oral, Maxillary, and
   Facial Surgery Coordinator
Legacy Good Samaritan
   Hospital & Medical Center
Portland, Oregon

Sandy Zarosinski, RN
Open Heart/Vascular
   Coordinator
Legacy Good Samaritan
   Hospital & Medical Center
Portland, Oregon

**Consultant to Chapter 1, Care
and Handling of Surgical
Instruments**

Nancy Chobin, RN
CS/SPD Educator
Saint Barnabas Health Care System
Lebanon, New Jersey

**CONTRIBUTORS/
CONSULTANTS**
Sharry Fassett, RN, CRNA, MS
Mayo Clinic Hospital
Phoenix, Arizona

Marcia Frieze, owner
Arlene Carlo, Kia Holmes
Case Medical, Inc.
Ridgefield, New Jersey

Jack W. Sanders, BA
Medical Photography/
   Videographer
Southwest Washington Medical
   Center
Vancouver, Washington

Tamara A. Schuman, RN, MS
Illustrator
Portland, Oregon

Rose Seavey, RN, MBA, CNOR
ACSP
Director, Sterile Processing
   Department
The Children's Hospital
Denver, Colorado

Glen E. Tighe
Photography & Computer
   Consultant
Lake Havasu City, Arizona

Dr. Blayne Standage, Dr. Earl
Schuman, and staff
Oregon Surgical Consultants
Portland, Oregon

Legacy Emanuel Hospital &
Medical Center
Portland, Oregon

Legacy Good Samaritan
Hospital & Medical Center
Portland, Oregon

Shriners Hospital for Children
Portland, Oregon

Arizona Heart Institute
Dr. Edward B. Diethrich
Christine Seibert, RN, BA,
   MEd.
Educational Coordinator
Phoenix, Arizona

Intuitive Surgical, Inc.
Sachin Sankholkar, Marketing
Bill Britt
Sunnyvale, California

Intuitive Surgical, Inc.
Daren LeCrone
Scottsdale, Arizona

V.A.S. Communications
Yvonne Smith
Phoenix, Arizona

V. Mueller Specialty Armamentarium & Cardinal Health
Scott Fitzwilson, Sales
  Representative
Janice Trapp
McGaw Park, Illinois

Preface

The organization of the seventh edition of *Instrumentation for the Operating Room: A Photographic Manual* has been changed and updated in an effort to expand the information concerning the various surgical procedures. The layout of the book follows a logical path from the basic to the advanced, just as you would progress when working in the perioperative arena.

Knowing the history of the instruments and understanding their care and handling, their classification, and the correct type of sterilization to be used for each instrument will assist you in any perioperative role, whether you are working in the central service, the ambulatory surgery, or the operating room. In addition, it is important to know the types of sterilization-container systems in which instruments can be sterilized and transported among departments while maintaining their sterility.

Instrumentation for more than 135 surgical procedures is shown according to the body systems involved. Each unit begins with a basic set of instruments or most of the instruments required to perform that surgery. Most of the basic units begin with a description of how the instruments are used in those procedures and then continue with photographs of the sets of instruments. The sets are photographed in groups, showing instruments that are normally placed in a sterilizing container together. Then some instruments are shown individually, with a close-up photograph of their tips if the tips are not visually clear in the group photograph. Once an instrument is shown individually, it will not be shown again as an individual instrument. If you are interested in a specific type of surgery and wish to learn about or review the instruments for that surgery, check the table of contents. If you are searching for an individual instrument, check the index, which provides you with the page on which the individual instrument and the close-up of its tip or tips are found.

The perioperative role has continued to expand, and each procedure requires that you understand the importance of your position in the health care arena. Your position in caring for patients while they are undergoing surgery, whether they are receiving local, block, or general anesthesia, holds a wide spectrum of responsibilities that cannot be taken lightly. If instruments are not cleaned properly, do not work correctly, or are not sterilized, it is the patient who will suffer the many consequences.

We listened to your requests to add definitions of the procedures, to explain why and where the instruments are used, and to include more close-up photographs of instruments to assist you in identifying them. We have also included a CD that allows you to learn via your computer. The photographs have been taken with a high-resolution digital camera so as to portray the instruments as clearly as possible. My consultants and I have reviewed the entire book, and we have attempted to meet most of your requests.

Many thanks to the variety of outstanding perioperative nurses (international and national clinical consultants, directors, managers, coordinators, and staff), surgeons, experienced surgical technologists, illustrators, central service staff, hospitals, and instrument companies that have contributed to this book because they believe it is important to aspiring perioperative staff members.

I must give special recognition to the retired nurses who contributed their time to this project and rediscovered how valuable they and their knowledge really are! It has been my pleasure to know and work with all of you. I am proud to be a member of your group and pleased to have been a perioperative nurse.

Last, but not least, I thank Mosby. I have been an author for Mosby since 1972 and have worked with many vice presidents, executive editors, editors, project managers, designers, and staff members over the years. I am pleased to say that I have been impressed with their willingness to assist me in past projects (a total of nine books). Yes, sometimes I was hard to work with, but the staff was willing to help with the problems that occur in completing books like these. I send sincere thanks to all of you who assisted me in the past and to all who have been working with me in the present.

Sincerely,

Shirley M. Tighe
RN, BSN, AD in Applied Science of Photography

Contents

UNIT FOUR: GENITOURINARY SURGERY

UNIT FIVE: ORTHOPEDIC SURGERY

UNIT NINE: PERIPHERAL VASCULAR, CARDIOVASCULAR, AND THORACIC SURGERY

UNIT TEN: PEDIATRIC SURGERY

UNIT ELEVEN: NEUROSURGERY

Care and Handling of Surgical Instruments*

Although evidence exists that stone knives were used to perform surgery as early as 10,000 BC, modern surgical instrumentation began with the introduction of stainless steel in the early 1900s. Approximately 85% of all surgical instrumentation is now made of stainless steel. Although stainless steel continues to compose the bulk of instrumentation used in surgery today, there have been dramatic changes over the past several decades. One has been the addition of new materials. In addition to stainless steel, titanium, Vitalium, and various polymers are also used. The introduction of minimally invasive surgery coupled with the availability of space-age materials have wrought instrumentation once only dreamed of. Cameras, flexible and rigid endoscopes, minimally invasive surgery techniques, and advanced imaging technology now make it possible to explore almost every crevice within the human body without having to perform open surgery and without requiring a hospital stay. Instrument design has focused on enhancing the surgeon's ability to visualize, maneuver, diagnose, and manipulate tissue with increasingly smaller instrumentation. In particular, the working channel of a flexible endoscope can be as small in diameter as 0.15 mm and as long as 2200 mm. It is possible to repair an aortic aneurysm, perform a coronary artery bypass, operate on a fetus, and so forth, without making a major incision. Advances in instrumentation design have contributed significantly to improved patient outcomes, early discharge, reduced recuperation time, and less physical trauma and pain. The consequence of improved instrument design, however, is higher cost, less inventory of like instrumentation, greater challenge to clean and sterilize, and an even more critical need to handle and care for instrumentation properly.

In addition to improvements in instrument design, several new sterilization and instrument processing technologies are now widely used. As a result, the required knowledge base of the person responsible for the care and handling of instruments has expanded significantly. The person caring for instruments must know the instruments' intended uses, their functions, and their compatibility with various cleaning, disinfecting, and sterilizing methods and must have an understanding of the disinfecting and sterilizing technologies. In recognition of the skill required to process surgical instruments properly, certification of processing personnel is required in many facilities, and certification is a requirement for employment in at least one state. Although the care and handling of surgical instrumentation is not revenue producing, appropriate and meticulous care and handling can result in lower overall costs for a surgical department by preventing damage and consequently reducing expenditures for repair and replacement. However, the primary concern should be that the instrument be truly patient ready—that is, safe and free of microorganisms. Instruments must be in excellent working condition and adequately cleaned and processed in preparation for surgery. Instrumentation that malfunctions or is not appropriately cleaned and sterilized or disinfected can result in extended surgery time, poor technical results, patient infection, patient injury, and even death. The November 1999 report issued by the Institute of Medicine stated that as many as 98,000 injuries to patients occur each year in hospitals. The report has been a wake-up call to healthcare providers to institute mechanisms that prevent errors. As a

*This chapter was written by Cynthia C. Spry. The author thanks Nancy Chobin for her review of the text and contributions to this chapter.

result, there is intense focus on patient safety throughout the healthcare industry. Proper care and handling of instrumentation is a critical component of patient safety.

In summary, the proper care and handling of surgical instrumentation is not a simple rote task; it requires specialized knowledge, competence, judgment, and a commitment to excellent patient care.

EVOLUTION OF SURGERY AND SURGICAL INSTRUMENTATION

Surgery was practiced long before the development of sophisticated surgical instruments. Stone knives and sharpened flints and animal teeth were the instruments of choice for trephination, circumcision, and bloodletting in prehistoric times. In *Corpus Hippocraticum,* Hippocrates (460-377 BC) wrote of the use of iron and steel in instrument making; however, there are no existing examples of surgical instruments before the early Roman period. Excavations begun in 1771 in the city of Pompeii reveal surgical instruments that bear amazing resemblances to contemporary instrumentation. Among the instruments found were a foreign-body remover, a speculum, retractors, probes, a periosteal elevator, forceps, and hooks. Metal analysis indicates three materials—copper, bronze, and iron.

Until the 1790s, surgery was not a strict discipline, and surgeons were not afforded equal status with physicians. Instruments were made by blacksmiths, cutlers, and armorers. However, as surgery evolved into a scientific discipline and achieved a measure of status, the specialty of instrument making also emerged. Surgeons employed coppersmiths, steelworkers, silversmiths, wood turners and other artisans who handcrafted instruments to individual specifications. Instruments often had ornate ivory or carved wooden handles and were cased in velvet.

The introduction of anesthesia in the 1840s and the adoption of Lister's antiseptic technique in the 1880s greatly influenced the making of surgical instruments. The use of anesthesia enabled the surgeon to work more slowly and accurately and to perform longer, more complex procedures. The variety of surgeries performed increased, as did the demand for specialized instruments. The ability to sterilize instruments also had an impact on instrument design. When steam sterilization became a standard process, carved wood or ivory handles were replaced with all-metal instruments made of silver, brass, or steel. Velvet-lined boxes were replaced by trays that could be lowered into steam sterilizers.

MANUFACTURE OF STAINLESS STEEL INSTRUMENTATION

The development of stainless steel in the 1900s provided a superior material for the manufacture of surgical instruments. Subsequently, instrument making evolved into a highly skilled occupation. Shortly thereafter, crafters from Germany, France, and England were brought to the United States to instruct apprentices in their craft. Even today, many of the delicate, high-quality, stainless steel instruments are manufactured in Europe. Germany is often considered the home of high-quality surgical instruments. Other metals like Vitallium and titanium are used today, but the bulk of surgical instrumentation is made of stainless steel and is manufactured in the United States.

Stainless steel is a compound of varying amounts of carbon, chromium, and iron. Small amounts of nickel, magnesium, and silicone may also be incorporated. Varying the amount of these materials produces a variety of qualities, such as flexibility, temper, malleability, and corrosion resistance. There are more than 80 different types of stainless steel. The American Iron and Steel Institute uses three-digit numbers to grade steel based on its various qualities and composition. The most commonly used steel alloys for the manufacture of heat-stable, reusable surgical instruments are stainless steel series 300 and 400, with 400 being the most common. The 300 series is generally used for noncutting surgical instruments requiring high strength, such as speculums and large retractors. The 400 series is used for both cutting and noncutting. Both series resist rust and corrosion, have good tensile strength, and will retain a sharp edge through repeated use. The chromium content in stainless steel provides the stainless quality. Stainless steel is really a misnomer. The degree to which the steel is "stainless" is also determined by the chemical composition of the metal, the heat treatment, and the final rinsing process.

The first step in the manufacture of stainless steel instruments is the conversion of raw steel into sheets that are milled, ground, or lathed into instrument blanks. These blanks are then die-forged into specific pieces and, where appropriate, male and female halves. Excess metal is trimmed away and the pieces are milled and hand-assembled. Jaw serration and ratchet, and shank alignment are achieved, after which the instrument is hand-assembled and then ground and buffed. It is then heat-treated to reach its proper size, weight, spring, temper, and balance. Following testing for desired hardness, jaw closure, and ratchet and locking action, a finish is applied.

The final two processes are passivation and polishing. Passivation is the immersion of the instrument in a dilute solution of nitric acid that removes carbon steel particles and promotes the formation of a coating of chromium oxide on the surface. Chromium oxide is important because it produces corrosion resistance. When carbon particles are removed, tiny pits are left behind. These are removed by polishing that creates a smooth surface upon which a continuous layer of chromium oxide may form. Passivation and polishing effectively close the instrument's pores and prevent corrosion.

There are three types of instrument finishes: highly polished, satin or dull, and ebony. The highly polished finish is the most common, but it does reflect light and can cause glare that may interfere with the surgeon's vision. The satin finish does not reflect light and eliminates glare. The ebony finish is black and also eliminates glare. The ebony finish is suitable for laser surgery, in which it is critical that the laser not be accidentally reflected, creating the potential for burn or fire.

QUALITY OF STAINLESS STEEL INSTRUMENTS

Stainless steel instruments may appear to be of uniform quality when they are new. However, there are various grades of quality, ranging from high quality and premium grade to OR and floor grade. Some instruments appearing to be stainless steel are of such poor quality that they are sold as single-use instruments. In the United States there is no agency that sets standards for instrument quality. Quality is determined by the manufacturer. In addition, an instrument labeled "Germany" may have been forged in Germany but actually assembled in a country where quality standards are minimal or nonexistent. Because instruments represent a substantial portion of a surgical suite's budget, it is important to be knowledgeable about buying and selecting products with the desired quality. Many factors affect quality. Two major factors are a balanced carbon-chrome ratio and the process of passivation. A balanced carbon-chrome ratio is important for instrument strength and long life. Instruments that are classified as premium have the correct balance. The passivation process is important to create a protective coat on the outer layer of an instrument to prevent corrosion and extend its life. Electropolishing is sometimes substituted for passivation. The result is a less expensive instrument but one that will not last as long. When purchasing stainless steel instruments it is best to deal with a reputable manufacturer who will explain the variation in quality of the products available.

It is important to verify that an instrument manufacturer has clearance from the U.S. Food and Drug Administration (FDA) to market its products. Instruments manufactured in countries such as Pakistan, Russia, or Malaysia have been known to enter the American market without this clearance and without adequate instructions for use and processing. Another reason to deal with a reputable instrument manufacturer is authenticity. In recent years counterfeit products have found their way into hospitals in the United States. When an instrument that usually sells for $150 is being offered for $50, the buyer should beware and should check for FDA clearance before considering purchase.

Instruments manufactured of materials other than stainless steel present an additional set of factors to consider before purchasing. These include their ability to be disassembled, cleaned, and reassembled; their life expectancy; and their compatibility with the existing cleaning, disinfecting, and sterilizing capabilities of the institution.

CARE AND HANDLING OF BASIC SURGICAL INSTRUMENTS: OVERVIEW

A well-made, properly cared for instrument can be expected to last 10 years. The most important considerations in extending the life of an instrument are appropriate use, careful handling, and proper cleaning and sterilization. Other considerations are disinfection, packaging, and storage. Every instrument is designed for a specific purpose. Using it for an unintended purpose is a sure method of damaging an instrument. Examples of misuse include securing surgical drapes or opening a medicine vial with an instrument designed to grasp tissue.

The proper cleaning of instruments during and after surgery can help to prevent stiff joints, malfunctions, and deterioration of the instruments' material, including stainless steel. During surgery, instruments contaminated by blood or tissue should be properly wiped and rinsed in the sterile distilled water in the sterile field. Thorough rinsing is important to ensure removal of blood and other contaminants from hinges, joints, and crevices. Blood and foreign matter that are not removed or are allowed to dry and harden may become trapped in jaw serrations, between scissor blades, or in box locks, making final cleaning more difficult and the sterilization or disinfection process ineffective. It can cause instruments to become stiff and eventually break. Channels, or lumens, within instruments such as suction tips should be irrigated periodically to prevent blood from drying and adhering to the inside of the lumen. Neglecting this action can cause blood and other debris to remain in lumens throughout the postoperative cleaning, decontamination, and sterilization processes. A syringe should be present in the sterile field for the purpose of flushing lumens with water throughout the procedure. Flushing the lumen should be done below the surface of the water to prevent the aerosolization of debris. Instruments should be rinsed in distilled water. Saline should not be used for this purpose. Prolonged exposure to saline can result in corrosion and can eventually lead to the pitting of stainless steel. Pitting can permit entrapment of debris, interfere with sterilization, and result in the destruction of an instrument.

Instruments should be handled carefully and gently, either individually or in small lots, to avoid possible damage caused by their becoming tangled, dented, and misaligned. During and after surgery they should be placed, not tossed, into the basin. Heavy instruments should be on the bottom, with the lighter, more delicate and fragile ones on top. Rigid endoscopes and fiberoptic cables should also be placed on top or separated. Fiberoptic cables should be loosely coiled, never wound tightly. When the procedure is complete, instruments that can be immersed are disassembled and all box locks are opened. Care should be taken to ensure that they are not tangled or piled high. Instruments should be returned to their respective containers or baskets to prevent sets from becoming incomplete, and they should be covered for transport to the decontamination area. All disposable blades and sharps should be removed and placed in a designated sharps container. Delicate instruments, endoscopes, and other specialty instruments may have to be separated and transported to the decontamination area in containers specifically designed to prevent damage to these devices. Instruments with cutting edges, pointed tips, or other sharp components should be placed in such a manner that sharp edges are protected and personnel responsible for cleaning and decontamination are not injured when reaching into the container.

AFTER SURGERY: CLEANING

Whenever possible, instruments should be taken apart at the point of use. Anything that can be disassembled must be disassembled before cleaning. After surgery, instruments are transported in leak-proof containers or trays encased in plastic bags to a designated area for cleaning and decontamination. Instruments should not be transported in basins containing water because the water may spill. The decontamination area may be within the operating suite or, more commonly, in the central processing department. Instruments that cannot be cleaned immediately should be treated with an enzymatic foam or gel to prevent formation of biofilm. All instrumentation should be cleaned according to the instructions of the devices' manufacturers. Generally, instruments should be placed horizontally beneath the water; however, some types of lumened laparoscopic instruments may have to be soaked vertically, with the entire shaft submerged. Horizontal soaking of lumens can cause air bubbles to form and prevent the solution from traveling the length of the inner lumen.

All instruments placed in the sterile field for use in a surgical procedure are considered contaminated and should be cleaned whether or not they were actually used. Blood, saline, or debris can be splashed or inadvertently deposited on any of the instruments; therefore, they all require decontamination and processing.

There are several methods of decontaminating instruments, but all begin with thorough cleaning. The usual steps in the decontamination process include sorting, soaking, washing, rinsing, drying, and lubricating.

Cleaning is the removal of adherent visible soil from the surfaces, crevices, serrations, joints, and lumens of instruments. Cleaning may be manual or automated and is accomplished with detergent, water, and friction. Proper use of the detergent is essential. Detergents should always be mixed according to the proportions indicated on the label or in the manufacturer's instructions for use. If enzymatic detergents are over- or underconcentrated or have been improperly rinsed off the instruments, interference with subsequent disinfection and sterilization can occur (Hutchisson and LeBlanc). Regardless of how heavily soiled instruments appear to be after use, adding more detergent to the water is inappropriate. To ensure proper detergent concentration it is advisable to obtain an exact measuring device for the detergent and to mark the sink with a piece of tape or a nontoxic, permanent marker to indicate the correct water level. For example, if the instructions call for a mix of 1 ounce of detergent to 1 gallon of water, a 1-ounce container should be obtained and kept next to the detergent bottle or sink. A 1-gallon container should be filled with water and poured into the sink in which instruments are washed manually, and the water level marked. The presence of the 1-ounce container and the mark in the sink should help to ensure the correct preparation of the detergent solution. Instructions for rinsing are also important. Some products call for multiple rinses. When a choice is made to switch to an alternative detergent, it is important to ensure that all personnel responsible for instrument processing receive the appropriate notification and information.

When possible, mechanical cleaning is preferred. However, some specialty instruments and those that cannot tolerate immersion or mechanical processing require manual washing. Some instruments, because of their design, require manual as well as mechanical cleaning. Examples are laparoscopic instruments and bone reamers. Debris and tissue can easily become trapped in these devices, and mechanical cleaning alone may not be sufficient to remove the debris. Soaking in an enzymatic detergent can help to break down organic soil. Reamers with many crevices tend to trap debris and may have to be soaked and manually brushed before automatic cleaning. Much will depend upon the capability of the automatic cleaners in the decontamination area. Laparoscopic and other lumened instruments should be flushed and brushed. Flushing can be achieved by attaching a Luer-Lok syringe filled with an enzymatic detergent solution to one of the instrument's ports. Brushing must be carried out using a brush that is long enough to exit the distal end of the shaft and wide enough in diameter to cause friction on the walls of the lumen so soil is loosened. Mechanical washers and ultrasonic irrigators designed for laparoscopic and lumened devices do an excellent job of cleaning and are preferable. When instruments cannot tolerate immersion, high temperatures, or the pressures of mechanical cleaning units, or if no such unit is available, the instruments must be cleaned manually. Instruments that are washed manually should always be completely immersed and allowed to soak in a cleaning agent intended for manual cleaning of surgical instruments. Instruments should be disassembled and box locks, hinges, and joints should be opened.

Serrations, box locks, crevices, and lumens must be brushed to remove imbedded particles. Scouring pads, stiff brushes, abrasive powders and soaps, and sharp implements should not be used to remove debris because they can destroy the protective coating on surgical instruments.

Instruments that are washed manually should always be washed one at a time beneath the surface of the water to prevent the aerosolization and splashing of debris.

Personnel responsible for cleaning must wear personal protective attire to prevent contact with blood or with fluid that might contain blood and or other body fluids. Protective attire consists of a head cover, face shield, heavy-duty cuffed decontamination gloves, and a waterproof gown that covers the scrub suit underneath. Masks are recommended when cleaning items that can create aerosols (e.g., lumened devices). Aprons are not acceptable. Fluid-resistant shoe coverings or waterproof boots are appropriate when fluid may be expected to pool on the floor.

Ultrasonic cleaning is another component of instrument cleaning. Ultrasonic cleaners should be used only on devices that can tolerate this process and only after gross debris has been removed. Ultrasonic washers use a process called cavitation to remove fine soil from difficult-to-reach areas of a device that manual cleaning may not remove. High-frequency sound waves are captured and converted into mechanical vibrations in the solution. The sound waves generate microscopic bubbles that form on the surfaces of the instruments. These bubbles expand until they become unstable and collapse or implode (collapse inwardly), creating minute vacuums that rapidly disrupt the bonds that hold debris to instrument surfaces. The tiniest particles are rapidly drawn from every crevice in the instrument. Ultrasonic cleaning is especially effective for box locks and instruments with serrations and interstices that are not easily accessible.

Ultrasonic cleaning does not kill pathogens; it only removes them and deposits them in the ultrasonic bath. The energy created in an ultrasonic cleaner is not biocidal, and unless the solution is changed frequently the bioburden on instruments can actually increase. The cover of the ultrasonic cleaner should be closed during operation to prevent the spread of microorganism-containing aerosols that are created during the cleaning process and that may be harmful to personnel.

Instruments made of dissimilar metals can be damaged if cleaned together in the ultrasonic cleaner. The electroplating of the more active metal onto the less active metal can result in permanent discoloration of the less active metal (for example, brass plating on stainless steel turns the steel a golden color) and will eventually weaken the instrument from which the metal is being removed. In addition, some instruments cannot tolerate the energy waves of the ultrasonic cleaning process, and manufacturers of delicate instruments do not always recommend ultrasonic cleaning.

Personnel responsible for processing instruments should check with the manufacturers of both the instrument and the ultrasonic cleaner before employing this process.

At the completion of the ultrasonic cycle, the instruments are placed in a mechanical washer or rinsed and dried.

The most common automated cleaning machine in use is the washer-decontaminator/disinfector. Washer-sterilizers are also available. These machines offer a variety of cycles, including cool-water rinse, enzyme soaking, washing, sonication (ultrasonic cleaning), hot-water rinse, germicide rinse, and drying. Washer-decontaminators have, to a great extent, replaced manual cleaning and the use of washer-sterilizers.

In a washer-sterilizer the instruments are washed and rinsed and then subjected to a short flash-sterilization process. Debris that may not have been removed during the wash phase may become hardened onto the instrument during the sterilization phase. For this reason, washer-decontaminators/disinfectors are generally preferred.

Detergent should be selected according to the type of debris and the tolerance of the instrument. The manufacturer of both the instrument and the mechanical cleaner should be consulted. A detergent's pH can be alkaline, neutral, or acidic. Acidic and heavily alkaline detergents should not be used routinely because they can destroy the passivation layer and promote corrosion. There are many enzymatic detergents on the market. Some formulations contain only one enzyme; others contain multiple enzymes.

There are enzymatic detergent products suitable for ultrasonic cleaners, automated washers, and manual cleaning. Some can be used for manual and automated cleaning. Some are intended for specialties, such as orthopedic procedures or endoscopies, or for specific instruments such as those used in laparoscopic surgery or cholecystectomies. Some target blood, fat, or organic soil. As a general rule, a low foaming detergent with a neutral pH is preferable. High foaming detergents may not be completely rinsed off and can leave spots and stains on instruments. In areas where the water is hard, a water-softener should be used to minimize scum and scale formation.

As a final step before inspection and packaging for sterilization, instruments should be lubricated with a nonsilicone, water-soluble lubricant. The manufacturer's instructions for dilution of the lubricant should be followed and the expiration date after mixing should be noted and indicated on the instrument milk bath.

SPECIALTY INSTRUMENTS

Specialty instruments require exceptional handling. Instruments used in microscopic surgery should be handled separately from those used for general surgery. They easily become tangled or misaligned when the heavier instruments used in general surgery are placed on top of them. Other specialty instruments, such as powered hand pieces and telescopes, will be destroyed if subjected to ultrasonic cleaning or to a washer-decontaminator or washer-sterilizer cycle and should be meticulously cleaned by hand. Manufacturers' instructions for their care and handling should always be followed.

Powered Instruments

Powered instruments, such as saws and drills, should never be immersed in solutions or come into contact with saline solutions, detergents with high or low pH levels, or chemical disinfectants.

As an initial step, a powered instrument should be disassembled according to the manufacturer's instructions. If an air hose is one of the components, it should be inspected for damage and washed with a mild detergent under lukewarm running water. A cloth or brush may be used to clean it. If a brush is used, the bristles should be soft. Hoses should be held coiled in a manner that prevents water from entering the open ends. Electrical cords should be inspected for damage such as insulation defects and wiped with a cloth soaked in mild detergent. All components should be rinsed with distilled or deionized water and wiped dry.

Flexible Endoscopes

Flexible endoscopes contain long narrow lumens and are inherently difficult to clean. A number of infections have been reported in patients as a direct result of inadequate cleaning and processing of endoscopes. Instructions for cleaning flexible endoscopes are quite detailed and specific and are beyond the scope of this review. The Society of Gastroenterology Nurses and Associates has developed detailed cleaning and disinfecting protocols for flexible endoscopes and their accessories. In 2003 the *Multi-society for Reprocessing Flexible Gastroenteroscopes* was released. This guideline was endorsed by 11 agencies, including the Joint Commission on Accreditation of Healthcare Organizations, professional nurse and physician endoscopic societies, and the Association of Practitioners in Infection Control and Epidemiology. In 2005 the American College of Chest Physicians and the American Association of Chest Bronchology published *Recommendations for the Cleaning, Disinfection, and Post Processing of the Flexible Bronchoscope.*

Adherence to these guidelines is critical to proper processing. The endoscope manufacturers' guidelines should always be consulted for design features specific to the scope in question. Manufacturers usually provide in-service education in the cleaning and sterilization of these devices. Personnel responsible for cleaning and processing these devices must have thorough knowledge of the process and must have demonstrated competence as well.

Proper cleaning of flexible scopes should begin immediately after their use. The lumen should be flushed with an enzymatic detergent solution and the outside wiped to remove gross soil. Debris must not be allowed to dry within the lumen, and the scope should be delivered to the decontamination area as soon as possible after use. Meticulous cleaning must precede exposure to disinfection or sterilizing agents. The lumens and internal channels should be cleaned using an appropriately sized brush and then rinsed. It is important that endoscope cleaning agents be mixed and used precisely according to the label. Following manual cleaning, the scope may then be processed in an automated scope reprocessor designed specifically for this purpose. The compatibility of the endoscope with the endoscope reprocessor must be determined. In the absence of an automated system, additional meticulous manual cleaning according to the manufacturer's recommendations is required. Strict adherence to manufacturers' instructions concerning use of disinfectants and automatic endoscope reprocessors is critical to achieve adequate cleaning and disinfection. As a final step, all channels should be flushed with 70% alcohol to facilitate drying. Storage in an appropriate drying cabinet that has humidity and temperature control is an additional method of facilitating drying. Pathogenic microorganisms found in rinse water can colonize in a relatively short time (overnight) in an endoscope that has not been adequately dried. In addition, it is possible for a biofilm to form in a lumen that has not been sufficiently dried. A biofilm is an assemblage of microbial cells that forms when bacteria attach themselves to a surface and then exude an extracellular polysaccharide that acts as a glue and as a protective layer of slime in which the bacteria proliferate. The extracellular polysaccharide film prevents antibiotic penetration. Biofilms can be removed only by mechanical action. If a biofilm breaks from the surface and enters a patient, the consequences can be deadly because of the especially large number of bacteria in a biofilm. It can require more than 100 times the normal dose of an antibiotic to treat an infection caused by a biofilm. Biofilms have been found to form in moist endoscope lumens as a result of inadequate drying and have been implicated in patient mortality. An alcohol flush can prevent the growth of water-borne microorganisms and biofilms.

CONSIDERATIONS FOR INSTRUMENTS CONTAMINATED WITH PRIONS

A prion is an infectious proteinaceous particle that is responsible for causing Creutzfeldt-Jakob disease and several other fatal degenerative neurological diseases. Because prions are resistant to routine disinfection and sterilization processes, instruments that have come in contact with prions require treatment according to special processing protocols. Information about appropriate processing protocols is not consistent and continues to evolve. The Centers for Disease Control and Prevention and the World Health Organization are two organizations with recognized processing guidelines. The Association of periOperative Registered Nurses Recommended Practice on Care of Instruments includes recommendations concerning the care of instruments exposed to prions. The protocols are based on the presence or suspected presence of a prion disease in a surgical patient, the type of tissue that comes into contact with the instruments used during the surgery, and the design of the instrument. Each healthcare facility should have policies and procedures for screening patients to determine the presence or possible presence of a prion disease, for identifying and tracking the instruments used in these patients, and for establishing protocols for processing these instruments. Current research supports the importance of cleaning and the use of an alkaline cleaner and an extended steam-sterilization cycle.

SPOTTING, STAINING, AND CORROSION

Although stainless steel is highly resistant to spotting, staining, rusting, and pitting, these conditions can occur for many reasons. Understanding the cause of the specific problem usually provides an effective solution.

Minerals in the water may cause light and dark spots. Instruments processed in healthcare facilities in which the water supply has a high concentration of minerals may show spotting.

When water droplets condense on the instruments and evaporate slowly, mineral deposits in the water can remain and leave spots. Sodium, calcium, and magnesium minerals are particularly problematic. Using demineralized water for rinsing and pure steam for sterilizing may solve the problem. After the sterilization cycle, the door to the autoclave should remain closed until all the steam in the chamber has been allowed to escape. This reduces the amount of condensate remaining on the instruments. Vigorous rubbing with a cloth or cleaning with a soft brush may be sufficient to remove mineral-deposit spotting. If spotting remains a problem, the autoclave may need servicing. Leaky or faulty gaskets can be the cause of the problem.

A rust-colored film on instruments may be the result of a high iron content in the water or foreign material within steam pipes. Yellow-brown to dark-brown spots are sometimes mistaken for rust; the eraser test can be used to determine whether it is rust. If the stain disappears when it is rubbed with a pencil eraser, is not rust. In some instances the installation of a steam filter may help prevent this type of stain.

Brownish staining can occur when the detergent used for cleaning contains poly-phosphates that dissolve copper elements in the sterilizer. The result is that a layer of copper is deposited on the instruments by electrolytic action. If this happens, a different detergent should be used and the manufacturer's instructions followed.

Brownish-orange stains can be caused by a high pH level in the detergent used to clean the instruments.

Black spots are the result of exposure to ammonia, which is found in many cleaning agents. The problem can be resolved by using a different detergent and rinsing thoroughly. Black stains can also be caused by amine deposits that can be traced to the autoclave steam. Amines are used in the boiler to prevent mineral salt deposits on the walls of the boiler and steam pipes. Some of the amines are carried with the steam into the autoclave and by means of electroplating are deposited on the instruments, causing staining to occur. Adding amines to the boiler must be done in a controlled and gradual manner to minimize the risk of concentrations high enough to cause spotting on items to be sterilized.

A blue-gray stain can result when cold liquid sterilants are used beyond their recommended time limit.

Rusting of stainless steel is unlikely, and what often appears to be rust may actually be organic residue in box locks or mineral deposits baked onto the instrument surface. Unless the cause is remedied, corrosion may occur.

Actual corrosion is a physical deterioration of the stainless steel. Pitting is a severe form of corrosion in which small pits form on the surface of the instrument. Corrosion and pitting can occur when instruments are exposed to saline for extended periods of time and when organic debris such as blood and tissue is left in difficult-to-clean areas such as box locks, serrations, and ratchets. Detergents that are either too alkaline or too acidic can also cause corrosion and pitting. Detergents with a chlorine base or an acid pH should be avoided. Exposure to carbolic acid, calcium chloride, ferrous chloride, potassium permanganate, and sodium hypochlorite can cause severe pitting. To avoid electrolysis, stainless steel instruments should not be mixed with instruments containing aluminum or copper. Improperly cleaned wraps can also create a corrosive environment. The detergent can leach from the wrap during exposure to heat and steam and remain on the instrument.

Measures that can be taken to avoid instrument corrosion and pitting include soaking or spraying instruments with an enzymatic foam or spray after use to prevent debris from drying and hardening; scrubbing hard-to-clean areas; using a neutral-pH detergent; thoroughly rinsing with distilled water; and routinely cleaning the sterilizer with water and vinegar to remove impurities.

It is sometimes difficult to identify the cause of stains. Both the instrument manufacturer and the sterilizer manufacturer should be consulted when the cause is unclear.

In summary, the following steps should be taken to prevent spotting, staining, and corrosion:

1. Clean well, remove all soil.
2. Rinse well. When water contains high mineral content, rinse with demineralized water.
3. Do not place instruments of dissimilar metal in the ultrasonic cleaner.
4. Select only detergents and disinfecting solutions that are recommended for instruments. Check with the instrument and washer-decontaminator/disinfector or washer-sterilizer manufacturer.
5. Mix and use detergent solutions exactly as indicated by the manufacturer's instructions for use.
6. Dry instruments before wrapping. Ensure adequate drying following exposure to sterilization. Check autoclaves for proper functioning to ensure drying of packs.
7. Have the steam lines and boiler periodically inspected to prevent boiler additives from being discharged into the steam.

INSPECTION AND TESTING

Prior to packaging, instruments should be inspected for cleanliness, proper functioning, and absence of defects. An inadequately cleaned, improperly functioning, or damaged instrument is a source of frustration to the surgeon, can cause critical delays in surgery, and can contribute to patient infection or serious injury.

Box locks, serrations, crevices, and other hard-to-clean areas should be examined for cleanliness. Deposits left on instruments may prevent sterilization from being achieved and may dislodge in the patient.

Box locks should be inspected for minute cracks. Cracks are an indication that breakage is imminent. Other common areas where cracks may appear include hinges, lumens, and the base of needle jaws. Jaw movement, jaw alignment, and ratchet function should be checked on all hinged instruments. Joints should work smoothly, and jaws should be in perfect alignment and not overlap. Ratchets should close easily and hold securely. Joint movement can be tested by opening and closing the instrument several times. The instrument should close and release with ease. Stiff joints can be caused by inadequate cleaning, resulting in minute particles remaining in the joint. Stiffness can also result when water used to clean instruments contains impurities that collect in the joint. Joints that are stiff should be recleaned if necessary and lubricated with a water-soluble lubricant before they are packaged for processing.

Jaw alignment can be tested by lightly closing the instrument and inspecting the jaws. Any overlap indicates lack of alignment and need for repair. If there are serrations or teeth on the jaws, they should meet and mesh perfectly. This can be tested by closing the instrument and holding it up to the light. Light should not be visible through the jaws. Instruments with misaligned jaws can damage tissue and will not effectively occlude bleeders. Misalignment of hemostatic clamps is a common problem most commonly caused by improper use of the instrument. Hemostatic clamps should not be used as towel clips, needle holders, or pliers or for purposes other than those for which they were designed.

Ratchets may be tested by clamping the instrument on the first ratchet, holding it at the box lock, and lightly tapping the ratchet portion against a solid object. The instrument should remain closed. Instruments that spring open are faulty and require repair.

The edges of cutting instruments should be inspected for nicks, burrs, and broken tips. Dull, nicked, or dented cutting edges can cause trauma to tissue. Delicate knives, keratomes, needles, and rongeurs can be tested for burrs and rough edges by passing them through kidskin. The sensation of a slight drag is an indication of a burr or a rough edge. Scissors should be tested for cutting ability. Heavy scissors such as Mayo scissors should cut easily through four layers of gauze. Metzenbaum and other more delicate scissors should cut easily through two layers of gauze. One of the most frequent complaints regarding instruments is that scissors are not sharp. One solution is to create a preventive maintenance schedule for sharpening scissors before edges become dull and problematic. Scissors are most often damaged when used to cut material other than that for which they were designed. One example is the use of Metzenbaum scissors to cut suture material.

A needle holder must hold a needle securely without permitting it to slide or slip during suturing. Needle holders can be tested by grasping a needle in the jaws and locking on the second ratchet. If the needle can be turned easily by hand, the instrument should be tagged for repair or replacement. Inappropriate use is a common cause of damage. Needle holders should be selected to match needle size. Using a large needle with a delicate needle holder can spring the jaws of the holder and reduce its holding ability. If the needle holder has tungsten jaws, identified by gold handles, the jaws can be replaced when worn, thus extending the overall life of the instrument.

Fiberoptic light cords are checked by holding one end up to a light and looking through the other. Broken glass fibers will appear as black dots. The cord should be replaced if more than 20% of the area is affected.

Rigid endoscopes, once used only for diagnostic purposes in gynecology, are now used routinely in every surgical specialty. A rigid endoscope is one of the most expensive instruments used in the operating room. It is also easily damaged, and costly repair can be a frequent occurrence. Many operating rooms spend more annually for the repair of rigid endoscopes than for the purchase of new ones. Rigid endoscopes may be damaged in many ways: during surgery, such as during an arthroscopy procedure when the distal tip is nicked by an intraarticular shaver; placement under heavy instruments, which can cause a dent or bend in the shaft and subsequent damage to one or more of the glass rods inside the shaft; sterilization using an incorrect cycle; and careless handling of or dropping of the scope. Many companies offer scope repair services. It is important to ensure that only original parts are used during repair. Some third-party repair companies use replacement parts that can cause the endoscope to fail shortly after repair. The best assurance that the original parts will be used for repair is to use the original manufacturer's repair services. Rigid endoscopes should be checked to ensure that the lens is not cloudy or otherwise occluded. Telescopes are checked by holding the scope up to the light and observing the lens image at the distal end. The image should be clear and easily visualized. The light source used in the operating room should not be used for this test because the high-powered light can cause eye damage.

A more precise test of optical resolution is to use a resolution chart. These can be obtained at low cost from an optical imaging company or can be downloaded free of charge at http://lighthouseoptics.com/chart/. A resolution chart consists of identical sets of increasingly small bars printed on a circular chart. A set is printed at 5 locations on the chart—in the center and at the circumference edges to the left, right, top, and bottom of the center. The bar sets are numbered. For example, a set of the largest bars is numbered 75 and a set of the smallest bars is labeled 450. The number represents the number of bars that can be seen if they were lined up across the image. The user should look through the scope and line up the chart so that it fills the field of view. The number in each of the five locations should be recorded. The lower the number is, the poorer the resolution. An optical resolution chart is useful in determining the quality of repair. Measurements should be taken when new, that is, before the first use, between each use, and after each repair. If the resolution is lower after repair than before damage, the quality of the repair should be questioned. This is one way to hold repair companies accountable.

Each time they are processed, insulated instruments should be inspected for breaks in the insulation and for areas where the insulation has separated from the instrument shaft and appears loose. Both are indications that the insulation is not intact. Reusable and single-use insulation testers are available. If either defect is observed, the instrument should be removed from service. Loose or nonintact insulation is a serious defect and can result in an unintended burn inside the patient at the point where the insulation is not intact. Insulated instruments are used in endoscopic surgery where there is a limited field of vision. The site of the burn may not be in the surgeon's field of vision and can go unnoticed. The patient may even be discharged before a complication is noted. In the case of a burn that causes bowel perforation, the patient can develop peritonitis which in turn can lead to additional surgery, extended recovery, and even death caused by infection.

Microscopic instrumentation should be examined under a microscope to check for burrs or nicks on tips and to check alignment. Some of the teeth on microscopic forceps are very difficult to see with the naked eye and forceps alignment should be inspected under a microscope.

PREPARATION FOR STERILIZATION OR DISINFECTION
Classification of Surgical Instruments

In 1972, Dr. E. Spaulding classified medical devices and instruments into three categories, based on the risk of infection involved in their use. The categories are critical, semicritical, and noncritical. This classification was accepted by the Centers for Disease Control and Prevention and is used today to determine the processing strategy for surgical instruments. Critical devices are the devices that penetrate mucous membranes and enter normally sterile areas of the body. Examples of critical devices are instruments used in surgery, needles, and scalpels. Critical devices must be sterile. Semicritical devices contact intact mucous membranes and must be disinfected at the high level, at a minimum. Examples of semicritical devices are bronchoscopes, thermometers, and endotracheal tubes. Noncritical items contact intact skin and require low-level disinfection or cleaning with soap and water. Examples of noncritical devices are crutches and blood pressure cuffs.

Packaging

In preparation for sterilization, instruments should be carefully arranged in containers or baskets with wire mesh or perforated bottoms or in other trays that are compatible with the intended sterilization method and that may be wrapped in reusable or single-use wrapping material. Alternatively, instruments can be arranged within rigid instrument containers made of plastic or metal that are compatible with the intended sterilization method. Rigid containers do not require outer wraps. They offer the advantage of greater protection to the instruments during handling and transport and can be stacked for efficient storage after sterilization. Containers should not be stacked within the sterilizer unless indicated in writing by the containers' manufacturer. Stacking can interfere with sterilization and drying. Always follow the container manufacturer's written instructions for cleaning, replacement of filters and valves, sterilization methodologies, and sterilization exposure times.

Whenever practical, contents of instrument sets should be standardized. Standardization reduces the need for inventory, facilitates instrument replacement, and makes it easier to identify and locate sets needed for a surgical procedure.

Placement

Instruments should be placed so that joints and hinges are in the open position. Instruments with multiple parts should be disassembled. Retractors and other heavy instruments should be placed on the bottom or at one end of the basket, with lighter instruments strung open and placed alongside or on top. Sharp edges should be protected. Delicate, fragile, and lensed instruments should be protected from collision with other instruments in the set. Fingered mats, foam pockets, scope holders, and tip protectors are examples of items that protect instruments. Some instrument sets are supplied in specialized containers either to secure and protect the instruments, as in the case of fine microsurgical instruments, or to facilitate their location within the set, as with some orthopedic joint replacement sets.

Loading and operating any sterilizer should be carried out in accordance with the sterilizer manufacturer's written instructions.

Sterilization

Steam sterilization is the most commonly used method for sterilizing instruments. Instruments that can tolerate repeated exposure to the moisture and high temperature of steam should be steam sterilized. Steam sterilization is an economical and reliable method available in almost every healthcare facility. Items sensitive to heat and moisture are sterilized using alternative methods, such as ethylene oxide and hydrogen peroxide gas plasma. Cutting instruments and other instruments with sharp edges, although they can be processed in steam, will hold their edges longer if sterilized in low-temperature sterilization systems.

Instruments, pans, containers, and any packaging material, as well as any padding or protective material used in the pan, must be compatible with the sterilization method. For example, placing a cotton surgical towel in the bottom of a pan or container is useful in steam sterilization to absorb condensate and facilitate drying. However, cotton or other cellulose-containing materials cannot be used in hydrogen peroxide gas plasma sterilization. Cellulose absorbs the hydrogen peroxide, causing the sterilization cycle to cancel.

Although one sterilization cycle may be appropriate for the majority of instruments, there are many instrument sets that require extended or unusual cycles. In addition, some manufacturers' instructions concerning recommendations and instructions for flash sterilization of devices have been omitted. Sterilization cycles should be selected according the device-manufacturer's instructions for use and the sterilizer manufacturer's instructions for use. Any discrepancy between the two should be resolved prior to sterilization.

Instruments should be dry prior to sterilization. Processing wet instruments by steam sterilization may cause difficulties in obtaining a dry set. Sterile items that are not completely dry at the end of the cycle are considered contaminated because the moisture inside the package can breach the sterile barrier and create a pathway for microorganisms to enter the package. An exception to this occurs when instruments with small lumens are to be steam-sterilized. In these cases it may be necessary to place a few drops of distilled water in the lumen to create steam that will force air out of the lumen during the heat-up phase of the sterilization cycle. Placing wet instruments into ethylene oxide can lead to the formation of ethylene glycol (antifreeze), a byproduct of water and ethylene oxide. This chemical byproduct is not removed during the aeration process and can harm patients. Wet instruments processed in hydrogen peroxide gas plasma will cause the sterilization cycle to cancel because the hydrogen peroxide vapor dissolves in water, lowering the concentration of the hydrogen peroxide below effective levels.

Some facilities may choose an automated sterilization system that uses a liquid chemical sterilant such as peracetic acid. These systems are commonly used to process flexible gastrointestinal endoscopes that cannot tolerate steam or that have lumens too long for hydrogen peroxide gas plasma and that require faster turnaround than is possible with ethylene oxide sterilization.

Disinfection

Common liquid chemicals used to disinfect surgical instruments include glutaraldehyde, hydrogen peroxide, peracetic acid, and ortho-phthalaldehyde. Each has unique characteristics and should be chosen in accordance with department needs and instrument compatibility.

Instruments to be disinfected should be clean and dry before placement into the disinfectant. Moisture from instruments that are not dry can dilute the disinfectant, causing it to lose its effectiveness. The disinfectant solution should be tested for minimum effective concentration according to the manufacturer's instructions. This is usually done on a daily basis using test strips specific to the product selected. The immersion time required for high-level disinfection is indicated on the product's label and should be strictly adhered to. Following disinfection, items should be rinsed with copious amounts of water according to the manufacturer's instructions. Disinfected instruments should be allowed to dry and should be stored in a clean dry area.

IDENTIFICATION SYSTEMS

Instrument identification and related instrument-tracking systems are becoming commonplace in healthcare facilities. Instrument identification is used for inventory control, for reordering, and as a deterrent to theft. Color coding and etching are two methods of coding. Color coding may be adapted for a specific instrument set, specialty, department, or surgeon. Most systems use a hard color coating that is permanently fused to the instrument's ring handle. For example, a set with green ring handles may indicate that the set belongs within a specific specialty. Marking tape may be used to color code instruments manually. It is important to follow the manufacturer's instructions for proper tape application and to obtain written verification of tape compatibility with the intended sterilization method. It is important to inspect the condition of the tape before packaging the instrument. Tapes may peel or flake over time and harbor microorganisms. Loose, cracked, or flaking tape must be removed and new tape applied.

Another method of instrument identification is etching or engraving the shaft with the desired information. Vibrating mechanical engravers that scratch the surface should not be used because they break down the rust-resistant protective coating of the instrument, potentially allowing corrosion to begin. When a mechanical engraver is used in the area of the box lock, minute fault lines can be created and can result in premature breakage of the lock. Newer acid or laser etching processes are preferred because they do not harm the instruments.

It is important to check with the instrument's manufacturer to ensure that the instrument can withstand the desired coding system. Many instrument companies offer engraving at the time of purchase.

CLASSIFICATION OF INSTRUMENTS

The three broad categories of instruments are handheld, nonpowered surgical instruments; powered tools or devices; and endoscopic equipment and instrumentation. Handheld, nonpowered instruments are used for cutting, clamping, grasping, retracting, chiseling, and manipulating tissue and bone. Powered instruments are used for drilling, sawing, or cutting bone and cauterizing tissue. Drills, oscillating and sagittal saws, and wire drivers are examples of powered devices. They may be powered by electricity, compressed gas, or battery. Endoscopic equipment and instruments are used to perform minimally invasive surgery and to examine internal organs through very small incisions. Examples of endoscopic instruments are rigid and flexible endoscopes along with cameras and light cords.

The following information describes the general classifications of handheld, nonpowered instruments. Descriptions and examples are included. The names of the instruments may vary with the manufacturer, the geographic location within the country, the surgeon's preference, and the healthcare facility in which they are used.

Handheld, Nonpowered Instruments

Clamps

Hemostats are used to control the flow of blood. The jaws of a hemostat contain horizontal serrations designed to close the severed edge of a blood vessel, allowing for minimal tissue damage. There are several sizes of hemostats, for example, mosquito, Crile, Halsted, and Mayo-Péan. The larger hemostats are also used to clamp tissue.

Occluding clamps are used to clamp bowel or vessels that will be reanastomosed. The jaws of occluding clamps used on bowel contain vertical serrations. Occluding clamps used on blood vessels contain multiple longitudinal rows of finely meshed teeth. Both are designed to prevent leakage while minimizing trauma to the tissue.

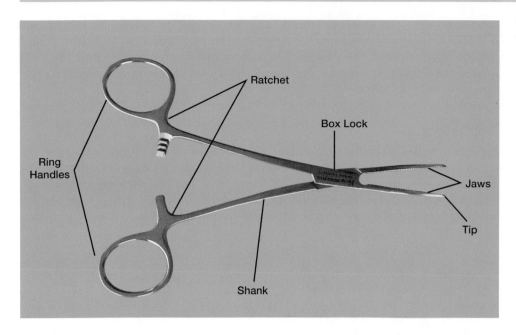

1-1 Components of a typical clamping instrument.

Cutting Instruments

Knife handles are usually straight handles that hold knife blades of various shapes that are used for incision and dissection. Examples of knife handles are Bard-Parker and Beaver. Other knives, such as fisher tonsil, Smillie cartilage, and myringotomy knives, incorporate the blade into the structure of the handle.

Scissors exist in many different forms; the two basic types are dissection and suture scissors. Dissection scissors are manufactured according to their intended purpose. Small,

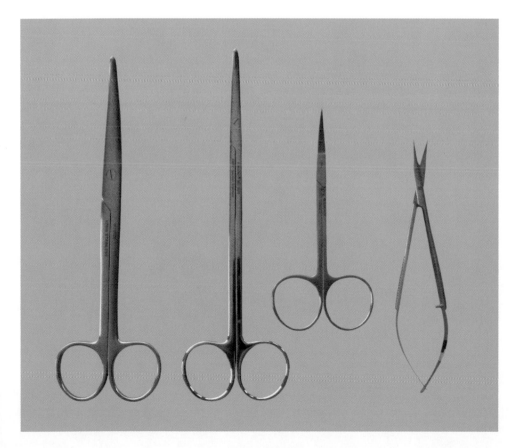

1-2 Scissors. *Left to right:* Mayo dissecting scissors, straight; Metzenbaum dissecting scissors; iris scissors, straight; and Westcott tenotomy scissors, straight.

delicate scissors, such as iris or Westcott scissors, are used in ophthalmic, plastic, and microscopic surgery. Metzenbaum scissors are used in intraabdominal and other general surgeries. More sturdy scissors such as Mayo scissors are appropriate for cutting fascia or sutures. Metzenbaum and Mayo dissecting scissors are found in most general surgery sets. Curvature, weight, size, and flexibility vary according to intended use.

Retractors

Retractors are used to hold back the edges of a wound to permit visualization of the operative site. A handheld retractor consists of a shaft to hold and an end piece for retracting. The end piece may be a hook, a blade, or a rake. Examples of handheld retractors are skin hook, Senn, Army Navy, Parker, and rake. Self-retaining retractors do not require that someone hold them in place. Some self-retaining retractors consist of two blades that are held apart

1-3 Hand-held retractors. *Top to bottom:* skin hook and double-ended Richardson retractor.

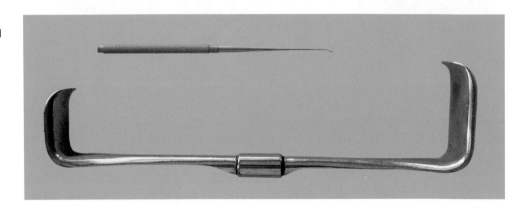

1-4 Self-retaining retractors. *Top to bottom:* Weitlaner retractor and unassembled O'Sullivan-O'Connor retractor.

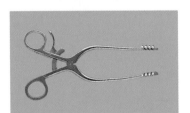

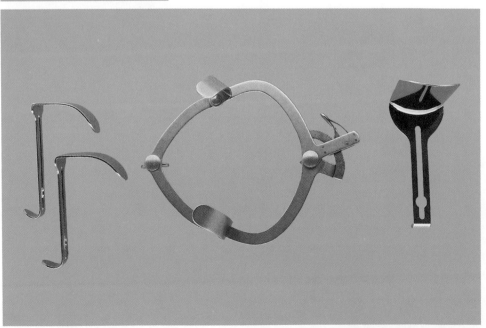

by a ratchet, such as the Weitlaner, Jansen, and Gelpi. Larger self-retaining retractors consist of a series of blades that attach to bars that are held in place by a screw or similar device. The bars that hold the blades may be attached to the operating table itself. Examples of larger self-retaining retractors are the O'Sullivan-O'Connor, Thompson, and Balfour.

Grasping and Holding Instruments

Forceps, also referred to as pickups, are shaped like tweezers and are used to grasp and hold tissue. The tips of forceps vary according to their intended uses. The tips may be smooth or serrated or have single or multiple teeth that interlock.

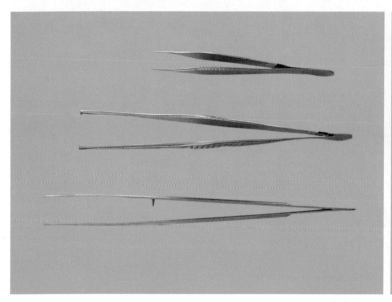
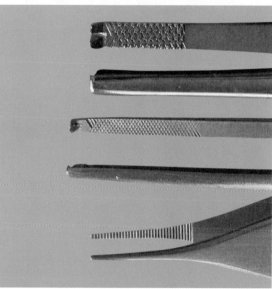

1-5 Grasping and holding instruments. *Top to bottom, left to right:* Adson tissue forceps without teeth; Ferris-Smith tissue forceps (1 × 2); tissue forceps with teeth (1 × 2). *Tips on the right, top to bottom:* Ferris Smith tissue forceps (1 × 2); tissue forceps with teeth (1 × 2); and Adson tissue forceps without teeth.

Examples of common clamp-shaped grasping instruments (also called forceps) include the Ochsner, Allis, and Babcock. The Ochsner forceps (Kocher forceps have wider jaw) has a heavy tooth at the jaw tip and is used to grasp and hold tissue without concern for trauma. The Allis tissue forceps has multiple noncrushing teeth and is used to grasp tissue without crushing. The Babcock tissue forceps has a curved, fenestrated tip without teeth. It is useful for grasping structures such as the fallopian tube or ureter.

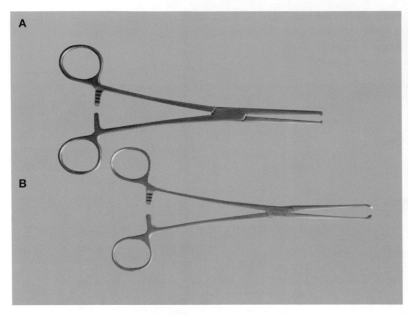 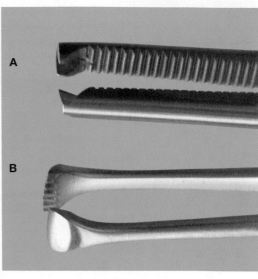

1-6 Grasping instruments. *Top to bottom:* **(A)** Oschner forceps and tip; **(B)** Allis tissue forceps and tip.

A needle holder is a grasping instrument designed to secure a suture needle in its jaws. A needle holder may be a clamp type with a ratchet handle or may be a spring-action type. Size and jaw surface vary and are selected with regard to the procedure and the size of the needle being used.

A towel forceps is a holding instrument that is used to secure towels and drapes in place. The tip may be pointed and designed to penetrate or the tip may be blunt.

A sponge holder is a clamplike instrument with rounded jaws that is used to hold a folded 4 × 4 sponge.

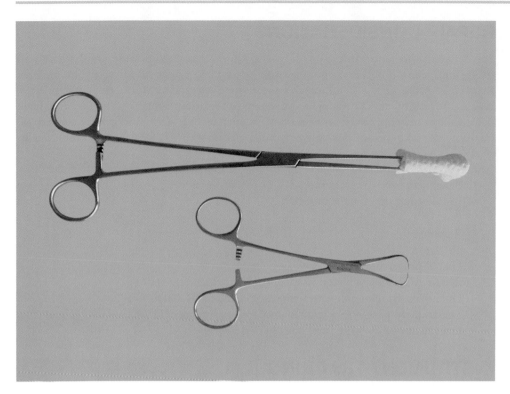

1-7 Grasping instruments. *Top to bottom:* Foerster sponge forceps with sponge in the jaws and Backhaus towel forceps.

Accessory Instruments

Suction tubes vary in length, curvature, and lumen diameter and are selected according to the type of surgery and the amount and depth of fluid to be suctioned. Minor, delicate surgery and surgery on small vessels require small-diameter suction. Two examples of small-diameter suction tubes are Frazier and antrum. Abdominal, deep-joint, and other general surgery usually require a Yankauer or Poole suction tube. Poole suction tubes are used in areas where the fluid is deep. Yankauer suction tubes are curved, and the suction opening is on the tip. Poole suction tubes are straight and have multiple holes along the length of the shaft.

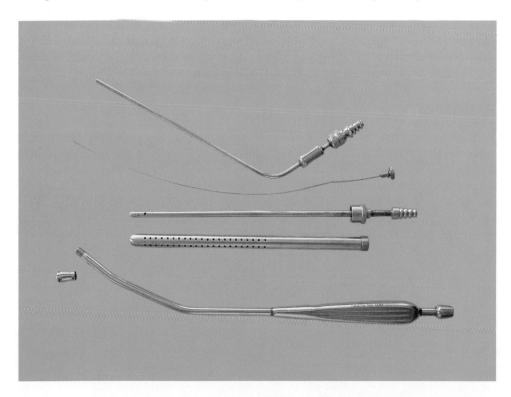

1-8 Accessory instruments. *Top to bottom:* Frazier suction tube with stylet below; Poole abdominal suction tube with shield below; and Yankauer suction tube with tip off.

REPAIR CONSIDERATIONS

Preventive maintenance coupled with careful handling and proper use are the best ways to prevent deterioration and equipment failure and to extend the lives of instruments. Regardless of the care in handling and use, some instruments will need replacement or repair. The facility may choose to send the item to the original manufacturer or an outside contractor or may utilize the services of an independent service manufacturer that repairs instruments and performs preventive maintenance on site. When selecting a repair facility or service the following should be considered:

- Company reputation
- References from other users
- Liability and shipping insurance
- Cost
- Response time
- Turnaround time
- Loaner program
- Repair exchanges: will your original equipment be returned?
- Quality measures: quality measured according to ISO 9000?
- Replacement parts: are original manufacturer parts provided?
- On-site inspection visits: are they unrestricted?

INSTRUMENT TRACKING

Several companies offer instrument-tracking software that allows the facility to monitor the productivity of processing personnel and track the use and inventory of surgical instrument sets. These programs make it possible to know where any set is within the system at any time. Instruments can be tracked by serial number, where appropriate, according to the patient, surgeon, and procedure. This information would be particularly helpful, for example, in tracking sets used in neurosurgery when the patient is known, or suspected, to have Creutzfeldt-Jakob disease and the set has to be quarantined until a definitive diagnosis is made. Bar coding can be used to identify whether a set is complete and what needs to be ordered when a replacement is necessary. Replacement orders can be made via an automated procurement system that interfaces with the tracking program. Data from a tracking system can be used to identify the costs of acquisition and repair. Information about repair rates, reasons for repair, and costs is useful when determining where to focus quality-improvement efforts. Tracking systems also facilitate the optimization of instrument-set inventory based on actual use.

SUMMARY

Surgical instruments are a major financial investment in every surgical facility, and processes should be in place to protect this investment. The life of a surgical instrument is dependent upon the way it is used and the care it receives. It is the responsibility of the surgical team and the personnel who process the instruments to handle them carefully, use them for the purpose for which they were designed, and process and maintain them appropriately. The extra time it takes to care for instruments properly is well worth the investment and is always in the patients' best interests.

Sterilization Container Systems*

Reusable rigid container systems provide an efficient and cost-effective way to package and protect instruments for sterilization, transportation, storage, and aseptic presentation of the contents. They are an alternative to disposable and reusable flat packaging wrap.

Containers are most typically constructed of anodized aluminum and have a boxlike structure composed of a lid and base, carrying handles, and a locking mechanism. They are designed with either a perforated or a solid base, have a lid with a gasket to ensure a tight seal, and include a filter or valve system to allow the sterilant to enter and leave the container. The container's material composition, rigid construction, and design features combine to provide a sterilization packaging method that offers a high degree of sterility assurance, prevents instrument damage, and provides an optimum barrier to protect the sterilized contents until they are used.

The Food and Drug Administration (FDA) regulates sterilization containers as Class 11 medical devices. Container systems require an FDA 51-0(k) clearance for their intended use, that is, a prevacuum or gravity steam, ethylene oxide, hydrogen peroxide gas plasma, ozone, or sealed flash. Manufacturers must provide documentation of the testing and validation studies performed, special labeling, and complete written instructions.

Containers are available in a variety of sizes and can accommodate a wide range of instrument sets, from simple delicate sets to full complex sets that can be standardized and customized. Accessories include nameplates or tags to identify the sets and disposable items such as filters, tamper-evident seals/locks, and load cards/external chemical indicators. Inner baskets, trays, inserts, and ancillary products are available for organizing and protecting the instruments within the container.

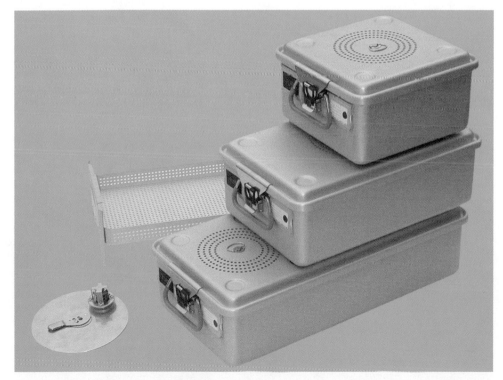

2-1 Flash Tite group. *Left to right:* disk, inside tray, and 3 sizes of instrument containers. (Courtesy Case Medical, Inc., Ridgefield, New Jersey.)

---

*This chapter was written by Arlene Como., Clinical Specialist/Educator, Case Medical, Inc. Additional images are available on the Companion CD.

2-2 Five sizes of Meditray insert boxes for the special and smaller instruments (scissors, scopes, needles, etc.). (Courtesy Case Medical, Inc., Ridgefield, New Jersey.)

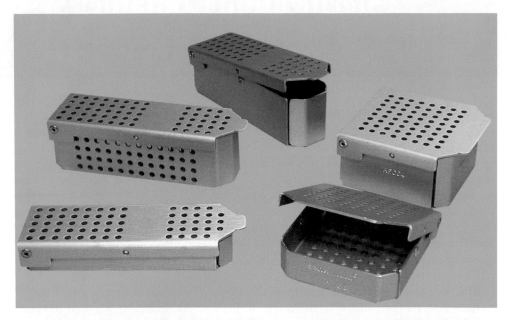

2-3 Steri Tite container and insert tray containing a Stryker camera set. (Courtesy Case Medical, Inc., Ridgefield, New Jersey.)

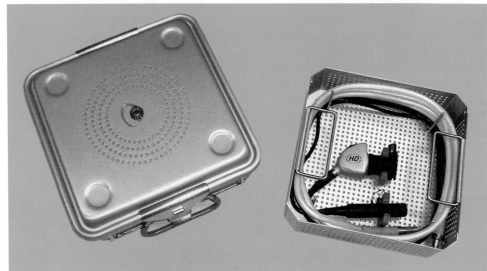

2-4 Steri Tite container and insert tray containing a Thompson retractor set with multiple blades. (Courtesy Case Medical, Inc., Ridgefield, New Jersey.)

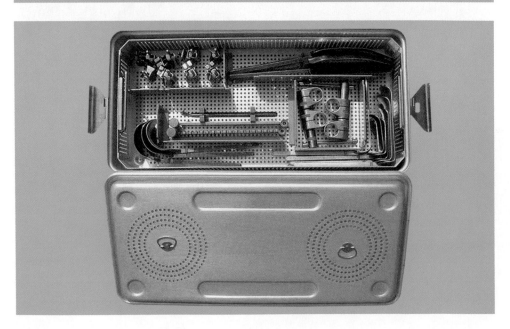

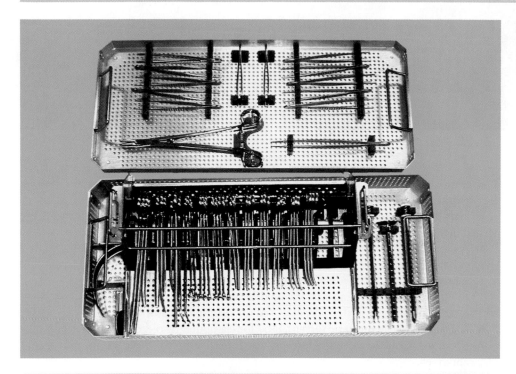

2-5 Insert trays containing instruments for a suprapubic procedure. (Courtesy Case Medical, Inc., Ridgefield, New Jersey.)

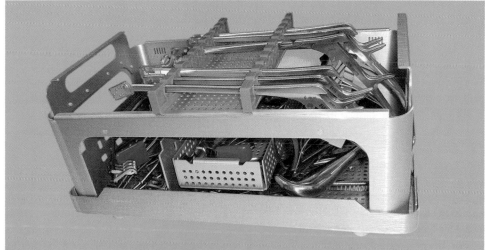

2-6 Double-layer insert trays containing instruments for a major disk procedure. (Courtesy Case Medical, Inc., Ridgefield, New Jersey.)

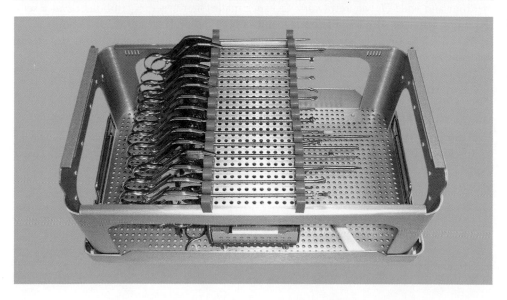

2-7 Double-layer insert trays containing instruments for an arthroscopic procedure. (Courtesy Case Medical, Inc., Ridgefield, New Jersey.)

Chapter

3

Basic Laparotomy*

A laparotomy is an incision into the abdominal cavity for the purpose of exploration or the performance of an operative procedure on organs or structures within.

To start the procedure, a dissection set is placed on the Mayo stand. Possible instruments needed include:

1. A Bard-Parker scalpel handle #4 with a #20 blade, used for the skin incision.
2. A Bard-Parker scalpel handle #3 with a #10 blade, used for the abdominal layers.
3. 2 Ferris Smith tissue forceps, used for grasping the abdominal layers.
4. A curved Mayo dissecting scissors, used for the dissection.
5. A straight Mayo dissecting scissors, used for cutting the suture.
6. 6 straight Crile hemostatic forceps, used for clamping the bleeders.
7. 6 curved Crile hemostatic forceps, used for clamping bleeders in the deeper abdomen.
8. 2 Army Navy retractors, used for retracting the abdominal layers.
9. 2 small Richardson retractors, used for retracting the abdominal layers.

During the exploration, longer and heavier instruments may be needed. Add the following instruments to the Mayo stand:

1. A Bard-Parker scalpel handle #7 with a #10 blade, used for the deeper dissection.
2. A Bard-Parker scalpel handle long #3 with a #10 blade, used for the deeper dissection.
3. A Mayo-Péan hemostatic forceps, used for clamping the deeper bleeders.
4. A Babcock tissue forceps, used for "running the bowel" and retracting structures without injury to tissue.
5. A tonsil hemostatic forceps, used for clamping the deeper bleeders.

If heavy graspers are needed, add the following instruments: Kocher clamps, regular and long, used for grasping structures that may be removed; Ochsner hemostatic forceps; and Allis tissue forceps, regular and long.

For deeper retraction, add the following instruments: a large Richardson retractor; medium and wide Deaver retractors; Ochsner malleable retractors (ribbons); and a self-retraining retractor such as a Balfour, O'Sullivan-O'Connor, Harrington, or Thompson.

After the exploration has been completed, remove the instruments from the sterile field, and bring up the following incision-closing instruments:

1. 4 curved Crile hemostatic forceps, used to grasp the peritoneum.
2. An Army Navy retractor, used to retract the abdominal layers.
3. A Ferris Smith tissue forceps, used to hold the layer being closed.
4. A 7-inch Mayo needle holder with suture and needle, used for suturing the tissue.
5. Straight Mayo dissecting scissors, used for cutting suture.

To close the skin, possible instruments include Adson tissue forceps with teeth, used to grasp the tissue and a skin stapler.

---

*Additional images are available on the Companion CD.

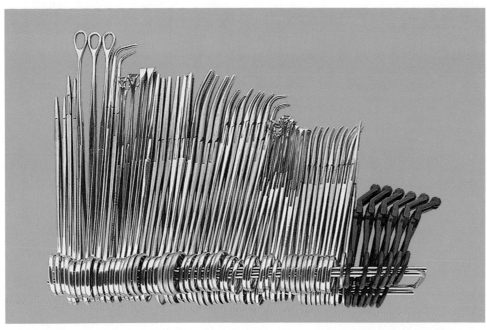

3-1 *Left to right:* 2 Mayo-Hegar needle holders, 7 inch; 2 Ayers needle holders, 8 inch; 3 Foerster sponge forceps; 2 Mixter hemostatic forceps, long, fine-point; 2 Babcock tissue forceps, long; 2 Allis tissue forceps, long; 6 Ochsner hemostatic forceps, long, straight; 4 Mayo-Péan hemostatic forceps, long, curved; 6 hemostatic tonsil forceps; 2 Westphal hemostatic forceps; 4 Babcock tissue forceps, short; 4 Allis tissue forceps, short; 8 Crile hemostatic forceps, curved, 6½ inch; 1 Halstead mosquito hemostatic forceps, straight; 6 paper drape clips.

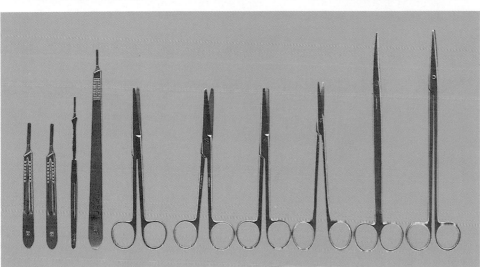

3-2 *Left to right:* 2 Bard-Parker knife handles #4; 1 Bard-Parker knife handle #7; 1 Bard-Parker knife handle #3, long; 1 Mayo dissecting scissors, curved; 2 Mayo dissecting scissors, straight; 1 Metzenbaum dissecting scissors, 7 inch; 1 Snowden-Pencer dissecting scissors, curved; 1 Snowden-Pencer dissecting scissors, straight.

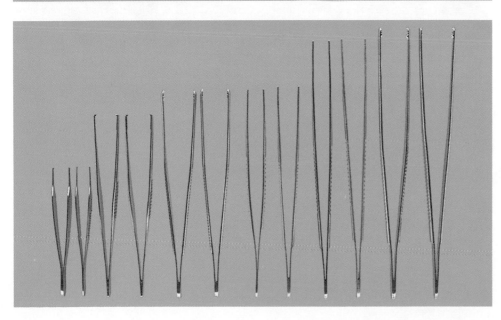

3-3 *Left to right:* 2 Adson tissue forceps with teeth (1 × 2 teeth); 2 Ferris Smith tissue forceps; 2 Russian tissue forceps, medium; 2 DeBakey vascular Autraugrip tissue forceps, medium; 2 DeBakey vascular Autraugrip tissue forceps, long; 2 Russian tissue forceps, long.

3-4 *Left to right:* 2 Goelet retractors; 2 Army Navy retractors; 1 Richardson retractor, medium; 1 Richardson retractor, large; 1 Yankauer suction tube and tip; 1 Poole abdominal shield and suction tube.

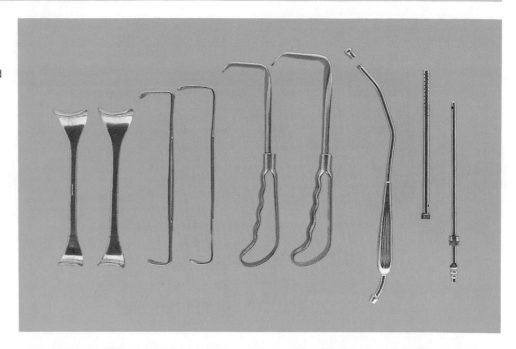

3-5 *Left to right:* Deaver retractors, small, medium, and large; Oschsner malleable retractors, narrow, medium, wide.

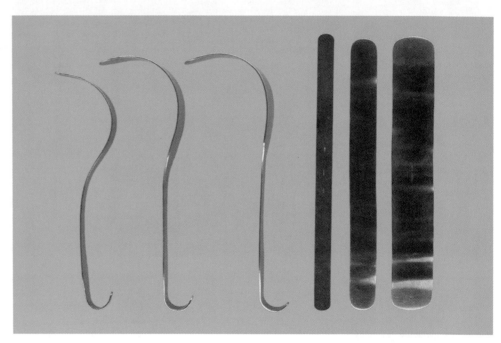

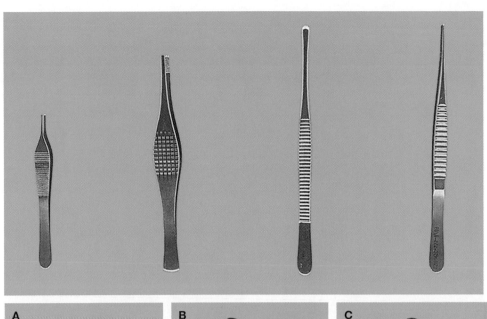

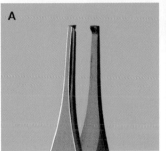
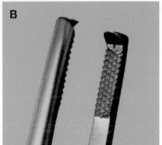
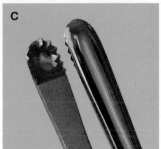
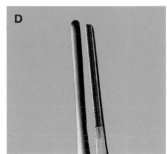

3-6 *Left to right:* **A**, Adson tissue forceps and tip; **B**, Ferris Smith tissue forceps and tip; **C**, Russian tissue forceps and tip; **D**, DeBakey vascular Autraugrip tissue forceps and tip.

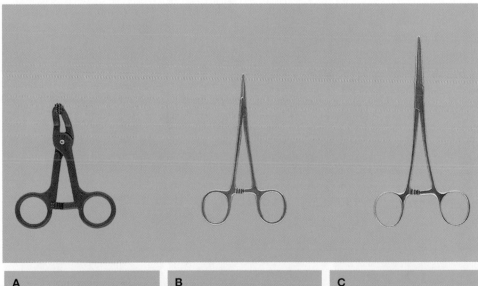

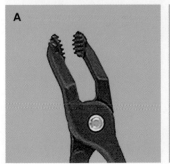
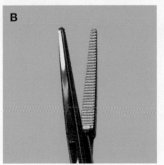
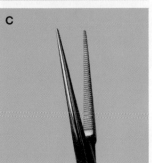

3-7 *Left to right:* **A**, Paper drape clip and tip; **B**, Halstead mosquito hemostatic forceps, straight, and tip; **C**, Halstead hemostatic forceps and tip.

3-8 *Left to right:* **A**, Crile hemostatic forceps and tip; **B**, Allis tissue forceps and tip; **C**, Babcock tissue forceps and tip.

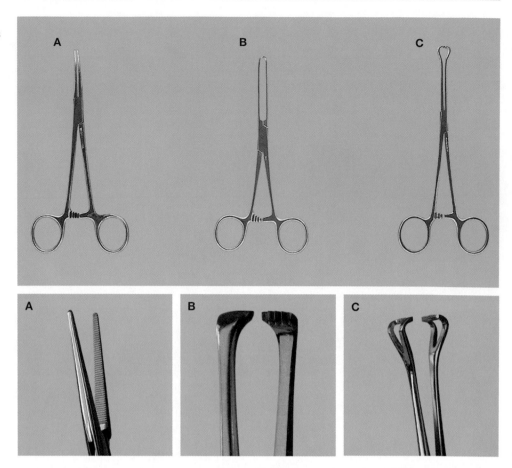

3-9 *Left to right:* **A**, Tonsil hemostatic forceps and tip; **B**, Westphal hemostatic forceps and tip; **C**, Mayo-Péan hemostatic forceps, curved, and tip; **D**, Mixter hemostatic forceps, fine-point tip.

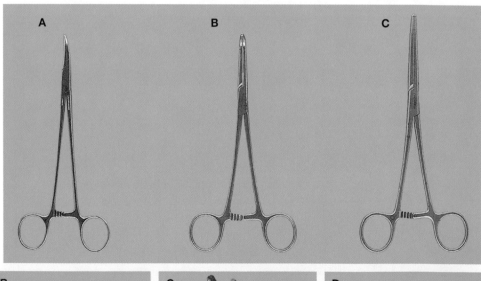

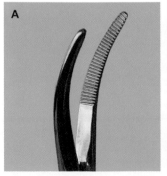
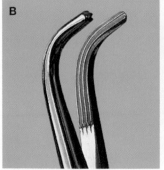
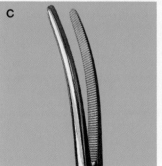
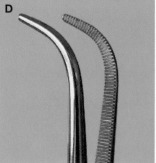

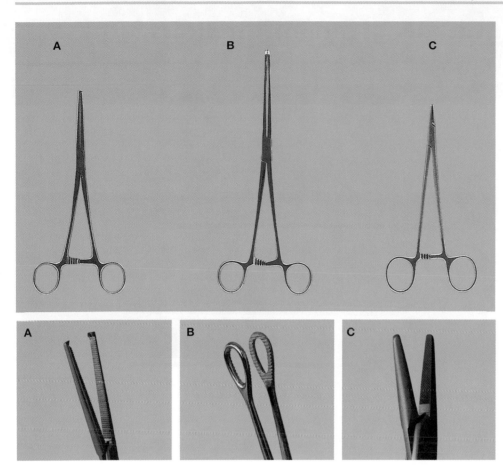

3-10 *Left to right:* **A**, Ochsner hemostatic forceps and tip; **B**, Foerster sponge forceps and tip; **C**, Mayo-Hegar needle holder and tip.

Abdominal Self-Retaining Retractors

4-1 *Top to bottom:* Bookwalter retractor table post; Bookwalter retractor horizontal bar; Bookwalter retractor horizontal flex bar.

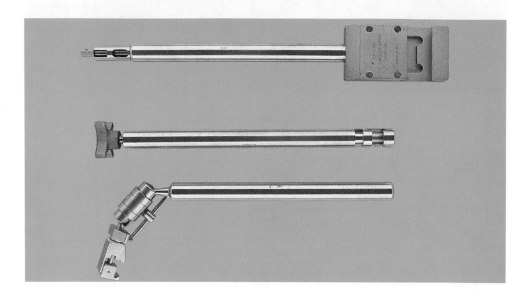

4-2 *Top to bottom:* Bookwalter retractor oval ring, medium; Bookwalter retractor: Balfour blades, second blade, side view.

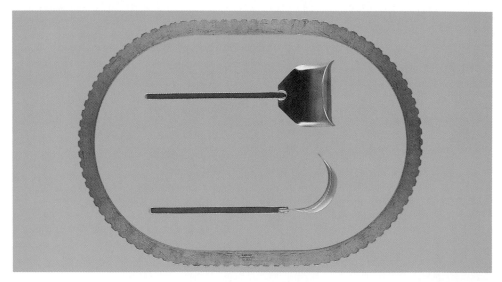

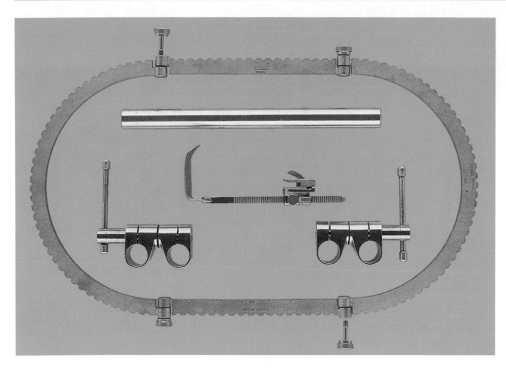

4-3 *Top to bottom:* Bookwalter retractor: segmented parts (2 segmented half circles, medium; 2 segmented straight extensions) placed together with 4 locking screws; 1 vertical extension bar; 1 Kelly retractor blade with ratchet mechanism attached; 2 post couplings.

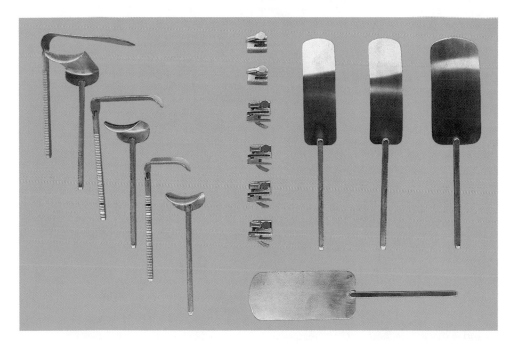

4-4 *Left to right:* 1 Harrington retractor blade; 1 Kelly retractor blade (2 × 6 inch); 1 Kelly retractor blade (2 × 4 inch); 1 Kelly retractor blade (2 × 3 inch); 2 Kelly retractor blades (2 × 2½ inch); 6 ratchet mechanisms; 2 malleable retractor blades (2 × 6 inch); 2 malleable retractor blades (3 × 6 inch).

4-5 O'Sullivan-O'Connor retractor with 3 blades.

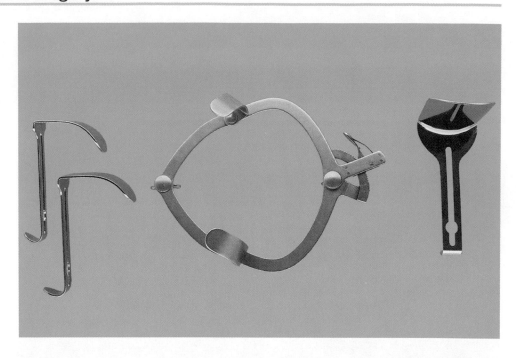

4-6 *Top to bottom:* Upper hand retractor: 1 horizontal bar with 3 blade supports; 2 vertical arms; and 2 table attachments.

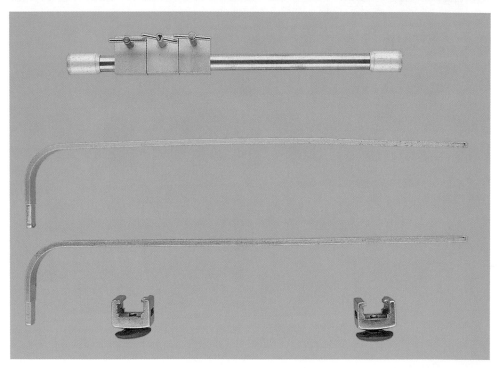

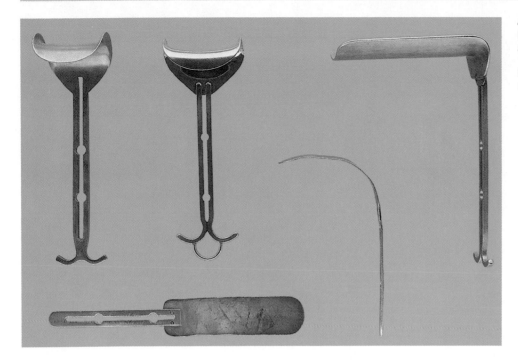

4-7 *Top to bottom, left to right:* Upper hand retractor: 2 Balfour abdominal blades, deep and shallow; 1 Deaver blade, side view; 1 Weinberg blade (modified Joe's Hoe); and 1 malleable blade.

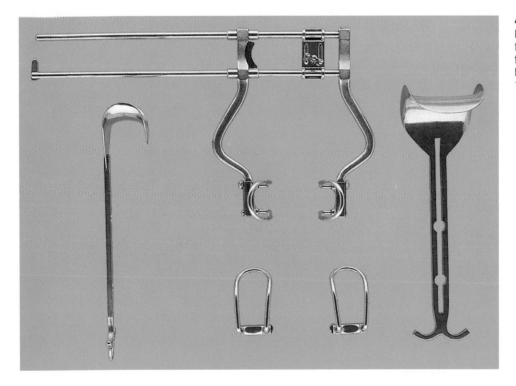

4-8 *Top to bottom, left to right:* Balfour abdominal retractor: retractor frame with 2 detachable shallow fenestrated blades; 1 shallow center blade; 2 deep fenestrated blades; and 1 deep center blade.

4-9 *Top to bottom:* Thompson retractor arms: 3 crossbar Thompson elite, angular; 1 Thompson extension, straight, 20 inch; and 1 rail clamp Thompson elite with 2 joints.

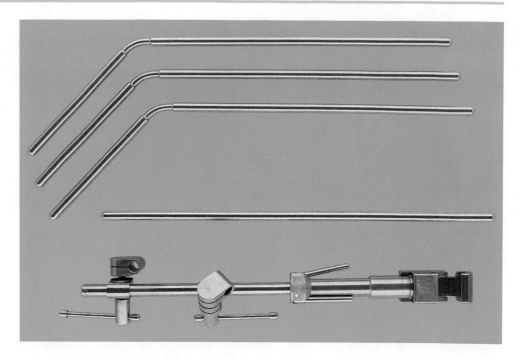

4-10 *Left to right:* Thompson retractor rotatable blades: 1 Deaver, medium, side view; 1 Harrington, side view; 1 Deaver, medium (2½ × 5 inch), side view; and 1 Deaver, large, front view.

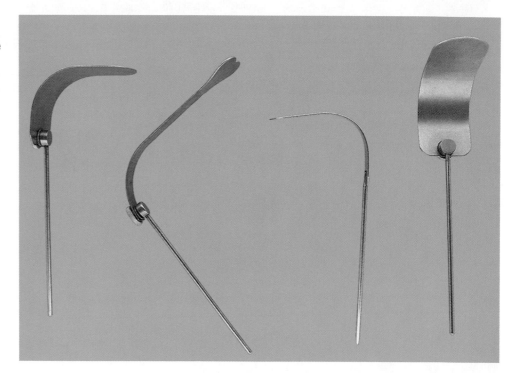

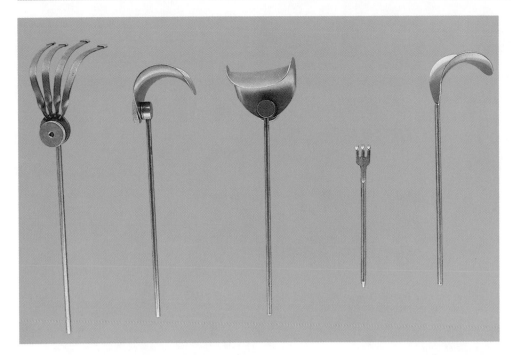

4-11 *Left to right:* Thompson retractor rotatable blades: 1 finger malleable; 2 Balfour, side view and back view; 1 rake Murphy, sharp, 3 prong; and 1 Balfour-Mayo center (2¾ × 5 inch), side view.

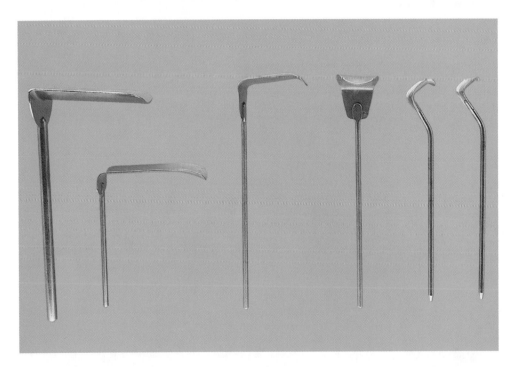

4-12 *Left to right:* Thompson retractor rotatable blades: Welnberg (3¼ × 5¼ inch), side view; Richardson (2 × 5 inch), side view; Kelly (2½ × 3 inch), side view; Kelly (2 × 2½ inch), front view; and 2 Richardson carotid (1 × ¼ inch and ¾ × 1 inch), side view.

4-13 *Top to bottom:* Thompson retractor. Various sizes of malleable rotatable blades.

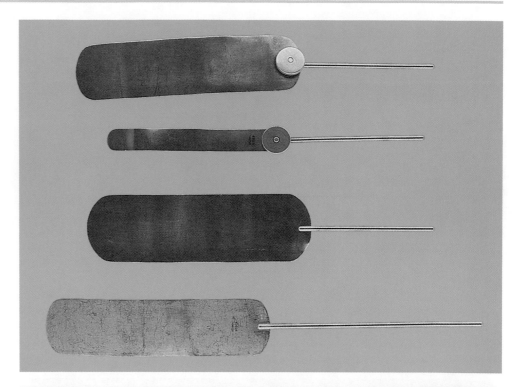

4-14 *Top to bottom, left to right:* Thompson retractor joints: 1 extension arm, angular, 12 inch; 1 wrench, universal; 1 adaptor blade universal; 2 universal (½ × ¼ inch); 2 universal split (½ × ¼ inch); 2 universal (½ × ½ inch); and 2 universal (½ × ½ inch), large.

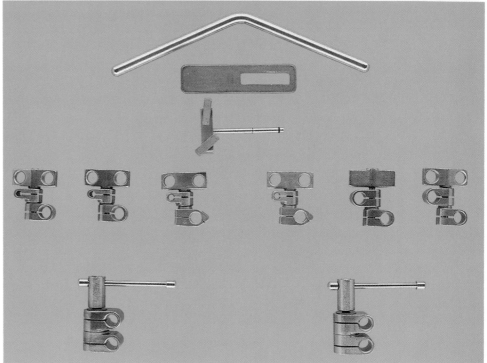

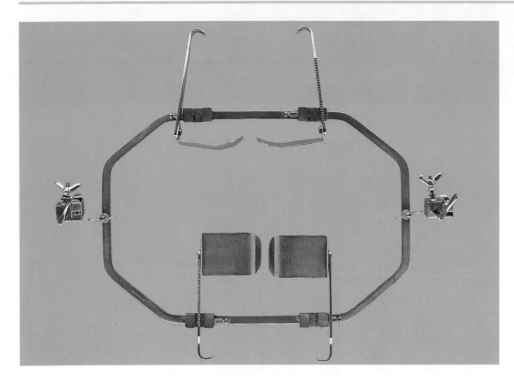

4-15 Wexler retractor: 1 octagon frame; 2 universal joints at each end; and 4 lateral blades: *top*, side view, and *bottom*, top view.

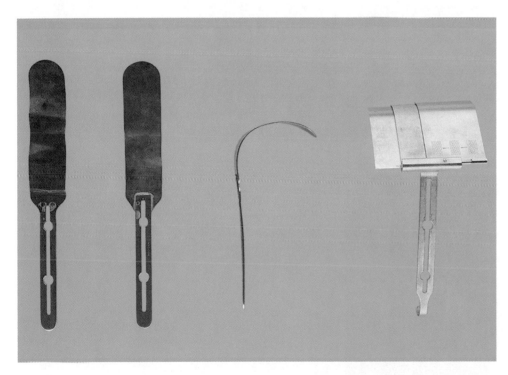

4-16 *Left to right:* Wexler retractor blades: 2 malleable; 1 Deaver; and 1 expandable.

Extra Long Instruments

Instruments needed for the procedure include a basic laparotomy set.

5-1 *Left to right:* 1 Bard-Parker knife handle #4; 1 Bard-Parker knife handle #3, long; 4 tonsil hemostatic forceps, long; 2 Allis tissue forceps, extra long; 2 Babcock tissue forceps, long; 2 Mixter hemostatic forceps, fine tip, extra long; 2 Crile-Wood needle holders, 11 inch.

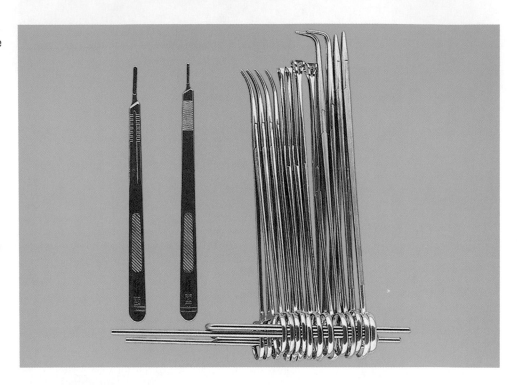

5-2 Crile-Wood needle holder, 7 inch, and tip.

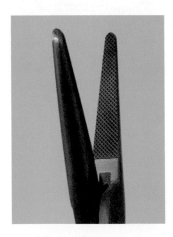

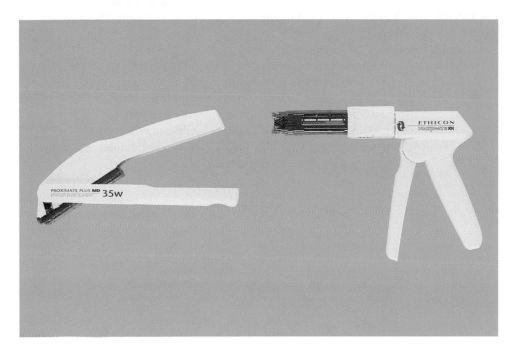

6-1 *Left to right:* Skin staplers; disposable, fixed head, and rotating head.

Small Laparotomy Set

A smaller number of instruments may be used for less involved procedures, such as an appendectomy or an inguinal herniorrhaphy. An appendectomy is the removal of the vermiform appendix of the bowel. An inguinal herniorrhaphy is the repair of an outpouching of the abdominal wall in the lower right or left quadrant of the abdomen. These procedures may also be done through a laparoscope.

A brief description of the instruments follows:

1. Adson tissue forceps without teeth, used for the handling of delicate tissue.
2. Adson tissue forceps with teeth, used for grasping the skin edges.
3. Halstead mosquito hemostatic forceps, used for clamping the bleeders.
4. Babcock tissue forceps, used for handling the appendix or hernia sac.
5. Short Allis forceps, used for grasping the tissue when closing the incision.
6. A Weitlaner self-retaining retractor, used for the retraction of the abdominal layers.
7. Farr spring retractors, used for retracting the skin edges.

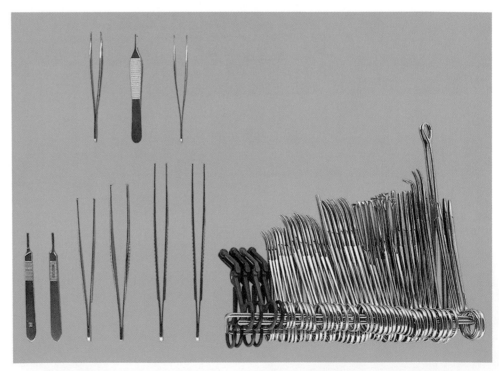

7-1 *Top, left to right:* 1 Brown-Adson tissue forceps (9 × 9 teeth); 2 Adson tissue forceps with teeth (1 × 2). *Bottom, left to right:* 2 Bard-Parker knife handles, #3; 1 Cushing forceps with teeth (1 × 2); 1 Ferris Smith tissue forceps (1 × 2); 2 DeBakey vascular Autraugrip tissue forceps, medium; 4 paper drape clips; 6 Halstead mosquito hemostatic forceps, curved; 1 Halstead mosquito hemostatic forceps, straight; 8 Crile hemostatic forceps, curved, 5½ inch; 1 Halstead hemostatic forceps, straight; 6 Crile hemostatic forceps, curved, 6½ inch; 4 Allis tissue forceps, short; 4 Babcock tissue forceps, short; 4 Ochsner hemostatic forceps, short; 1 Westphal hemostatic forceps; 2 hemostatic tonsil forceps; 1 Foerster sponge forceps; 2 Mayo-Hegar needle holders, 6 inch; 1 Crile-Wood needle holder, 6 inch.

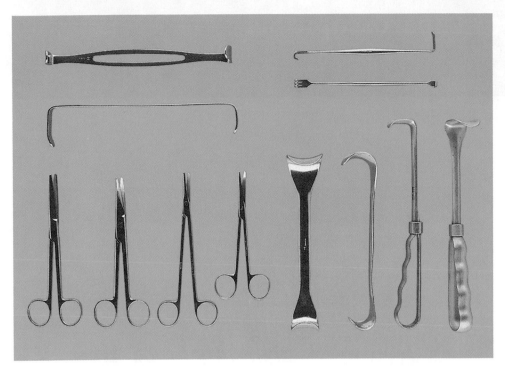

7-2 *Top pairs, left to right:* 2 Army Navy retractors, front view and side view; 2 Miller-Senn retractors, side view and front view. *Bottom, left to right:* 1 Mayo dissecting scissors, straight; 1 Mayo dissecting scissors, curved; 1 Metzenbaum dissecting scissors, 7 inch; 1 Metzenbaum dissecting scissors, 5 inch; 2 Goelet retractors, front view and side view; 2 Richardson retractors, small, side view and front view.

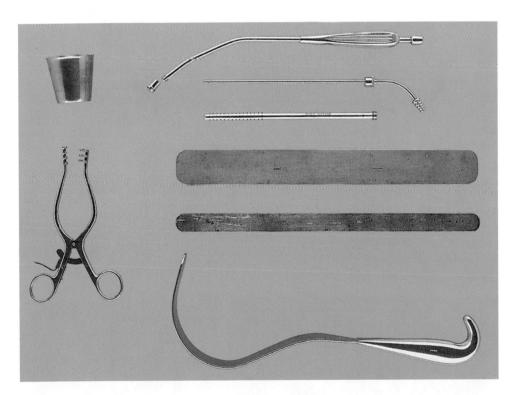

7-3 *Left, top to bottom:* 1 metal medicine cup; 1 Weitlaner retractor, medium. *Right, top to bottom:* 1 Yankauer suction tube with tip; 1 Poole abdominal suction tube with shield; 1 Ochsner malleable retractor, medium; 1 Ochsner malleable retractor, narrow; 1 Deaver retractor, medium.

8-1 *Left to right:* 6 Halsted mosquito hemostatic forceps, curved; 2 Halsted mosquito hemostatic forceps, straight; 8 Crile hemostatic forceps, curved; 2 Mayo-Péan hemostatic forceps, curved; 2 Mayo-Péan hemostatic forceps, long, curved; 1 tonsil hemostatic forceps; 1 Westphal hemostatic forceps; 1 Randall stone forceps, ¼ curved; 2 Halstead hemostatic forceps, straight; 4 Allis tissue forceps, short; 2 Babcock tissue forceps, short; 1 Foerster sponge forceps; 2 Crile-Wood needle holders, 7 inch; 2 Crile-Wood needle holders, 6 inch; 2 Johnson needle holders, 5 inch; 1 bandage scissors; 1 Mayo dissecting scissors, straight; 1 Metzenbaum dissecting scissors; 1 Mayo dissecting scissors, curved; 4 Backhaus towel clips; and 4 paper drape clips.

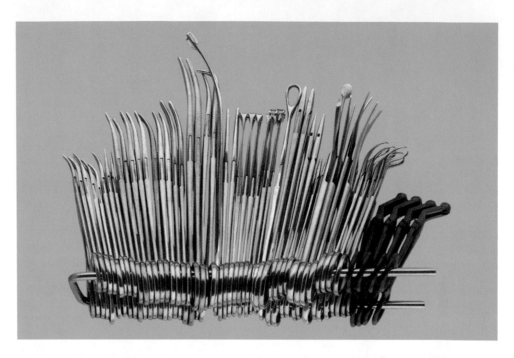

8-2 *Top to bottom, left to right:* 2 skin hooks, single; 1 News tracheal hook; 2 skin hooks, double; 1 Frazier suction tube; 1 Poole abdominal suction shield and tube. *Bottom, left to right:* 1 Bard-Parker knife handle #7; 1 Bard-Parker knife handle #3; 1 Bard-Parker knife handle #7; 1 Bard-Parker knife handle #3; 1 Metzenbaum dissecting scissors, curved, 5 inch; 2 Adson tissue forceps without teeth; 2 Adson tissue forceps with teeth, 1 × 2; 2 Brown-Adson tissue forceps with multiteeth, 9 × 9; 2 Russian tissue forceps; 2 DeBakey vascular Autraugrip tissue forceps, short; 2 DeBakey vascular Autraugrip tissue forceps, medium; and 2 DeBakey vascular Autraugrip tissue forceps, long.

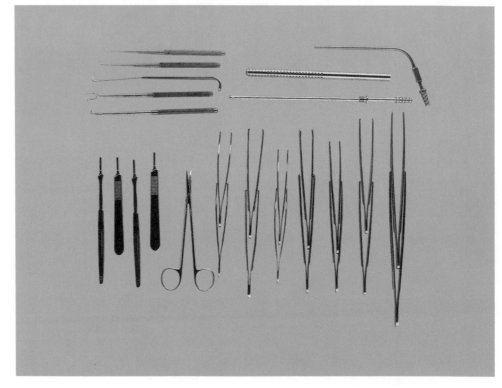

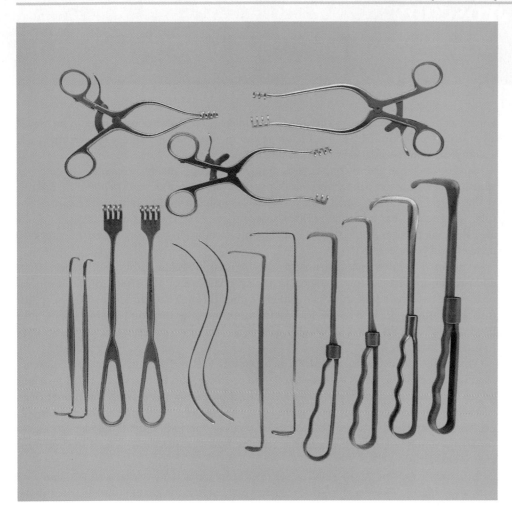

8-3 *Top, left to right:* 3 Weitlaner retractors, closed to open. *Bottom, left to right:* 2 Senn retractors; 2 Volkmann retractors, 4 prong sharps; 2 S retractors, side view; 2 Army Navy retractors, side view; and 4 Richardson retractors, 2 small, 2 medium.

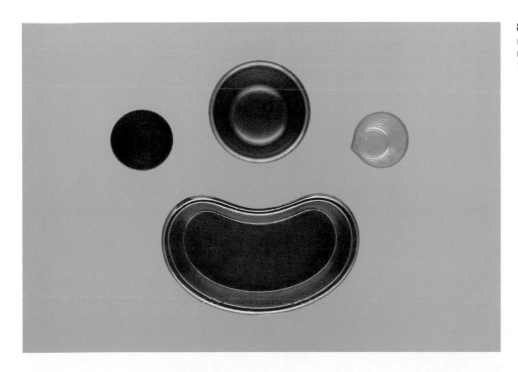

8-4 *Top to bottom, left to right:* 1 medicine cup, metal; 1 small basin, metal; 1 medicine cup, glass. *Bottom:* 1 emesis basin.

Laparoscopy*

Laparoscopy is visualization within the abdominal cavity. The structures have to be moved away from the abdominal wall so the scope can be inserted safely. Pneumoperitoneum is accomplished by insufflation of carbon dioxide.

Laparoscopes, like arthroscopes, cystoscopes, hysteroscopes, nephroscopes, sigmoidoscopes, sinusoscopes, thoracoscopes, and urethroscopes, are types of endoscopes. Endoscopy is the introduction of a small tube to visualize inside a body cavity or structure. The tube (endoscope) has a lens and a light source for vision. The lens angle determines the area that will be seen inside the patient. The most common lens angles are 0 degrees, 30 degrees, and 70 degrees.

Many of the endoscopic instruments can be used interchangeably within the various endoscopic specialties. Interchangeable terms include obturator/trocar and cannula/port or sleeve. The addition of instruments either through attachments to the scope or through another port into the cavity or structure allows the surgeon to perform operative procedures. The light source is usually a fiberoptic cable, or cold light, that prevents injury to internal structures.

Minimally invasive surgery (MIS) incorporates all the fields of endoscopic surgery (orthopedic; genitourinary; gynecological; and ear, nose, and throat) using small incisions or no incisions, such as when using an endoscope rather than using traditional open methods. The advantages of MIS include: (1) decreased size of the incision sites; (2) decreased postoperative pain; (3) decreased recovery period; and (4) quicker return to work and family. Almost all surgical specialties now perform MIS procedures on most anatomical areas.

In laparoscopy, the Mayo stand is set up to include a Bard-Parker scalpel handle #3 with a #11 blade; 2 Backhaus towel forceps; a Verres needle for insufflation; Silastic tubing; trocars with sleeves; a laparoscope; and a fiberoptic light cable.

A brief description of the laparoscopic procedure follows:

1. The abdominal wall is elevated with 2 Backhaus towel clips.
2. A stab wound is made near the umbilicus with a Bard-Parker scalpel.
3. The Verres needle is inserted at a 45-degree angle.
4. The Silastic tubing is attached to the needle and the CO_2 is insufflated to create the pneumoperitoneum. At 12 to 15 mm Hg pressure, the needle is removed.
5. A trocar with sleeve is introduced.
6. The trocar is removed and laparoscope is inserted.
7. The fiberoptic cable is attached.

---

*Additional images are available on the Companion CD.

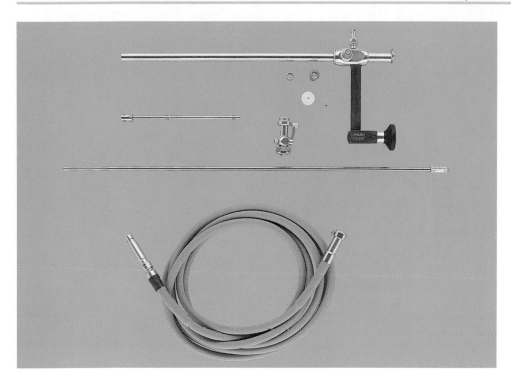

9-1 *Top to bottom:* Laparoscope and fiberoptic light cord.

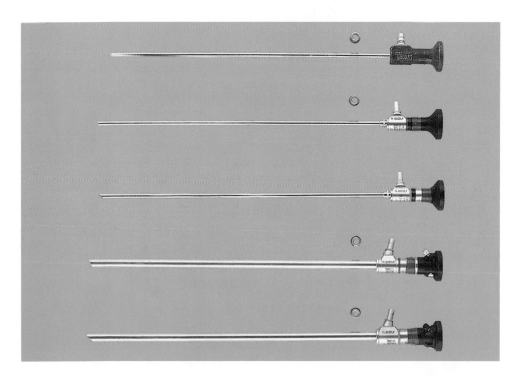

9-2 *Top to bottom:* Nondisposable laparoscopic lens: 0 degree, 5 mm; 25 degree, 5 mm; 50 degree, 5 mm; 25 degree, 10 mm; and 50 degree, 10 mm.

9-3 *Left to right:* Camera and light cord.

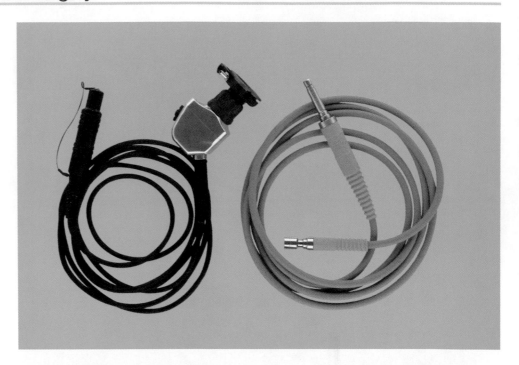

9-4 *Left to right:* 1 port and 1 trocar, 5 mm × 100 mm, separated, then together; port and trocar together and then separated, 11 mm × 100 mm; 1 Hasson trocar 12 mm.

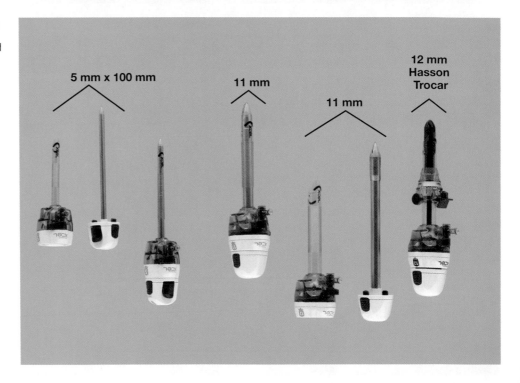

5 mm x 100 mm

11 mm

11 mm

12 mm Hasson Trocar

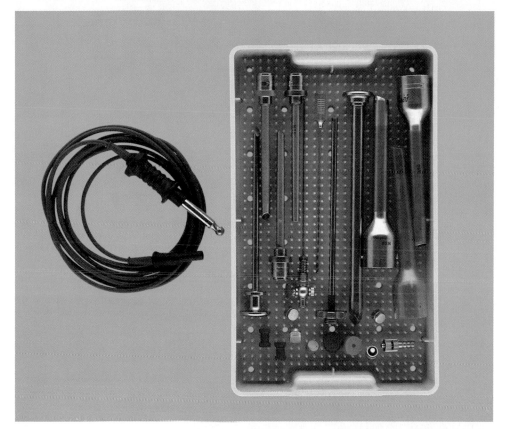

10-1 *Left to right:* Nondisposable cautery cord; instrument pan with 1 applied obturator 5 mm × 100 mm; 3 applied cannulas, 5 mm; 1 Verres needle stylet; 1 Verres needle, medium; 1 Nezhat dorsal plug; 1 applied obturator 10 mm × 100 mm; 3 applied cannulas, 10 mm. *Bottom, in pan:* 2 red port caps; 5 gray port caps; 1 red cap with pinhole; 1 gray cap with 3-mm hole; 1 male Luer-Lok adaptor.

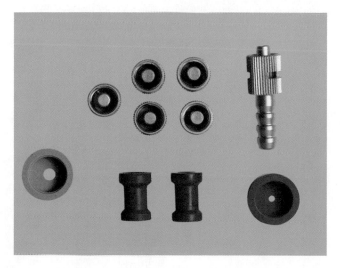

10-2 *Top, left to right:* 5 grcy port caps; I male Luer-Lok adapter. *Bottom, left to right:* 1 gray rubber cap with 3-mm hole; 2 red port caps; 1 red rubber cap with pinhole.

10-3 First rack, with laparoscopic instruments that fit inside a sterilization container.

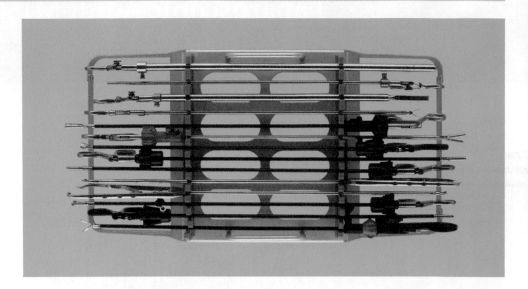

10-4 *Top to bottom:* **A**, Nezhat-Dorsey L-shaped cautery with sheath below, tip (note **A** below has protective cover); **B**, needle-tip suction, tip; **C**, spatula cautery, tip; **D**, spatula suction, tip; **E**, L-hook cautery, tip; **F**, Marlow knot pusher, tip; **G**, Ranfac knot pusher, tip; **H**, 10-mm and 5-mm Nezhat-Dorsey suction, tips. (Tips shown are enlarged.)

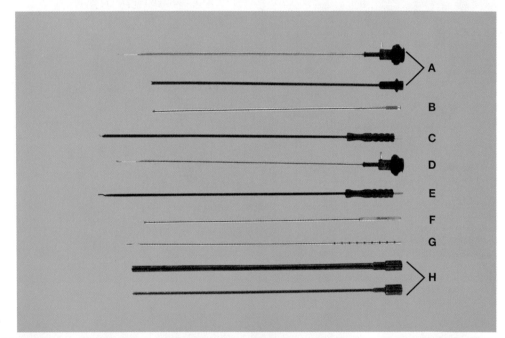

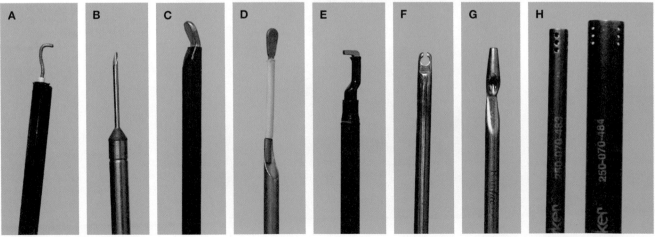

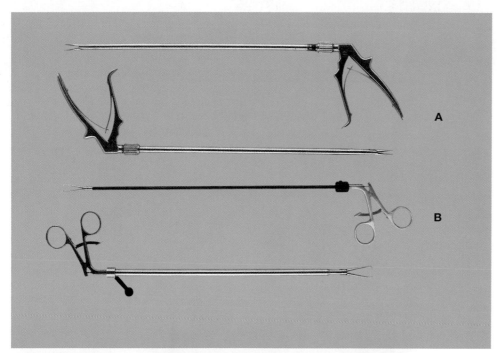

10-5 *Top to bottom:* **A**, 2 Ligaclip appliers, tip; **B**, 2 tenaculums, 1 small with cautery, 1 large on nondisposable handle, tips.

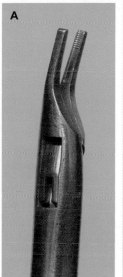

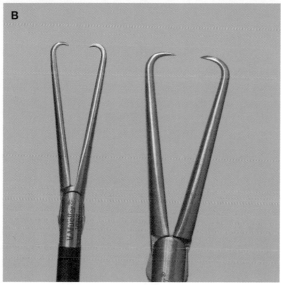

10-6 *Top to bottom:* 2 Hunter bowel graspers, 5 mm (Glassman type). *Bottom, left to right:* 1 Everest bipolar cord; 1 monopolar cord.

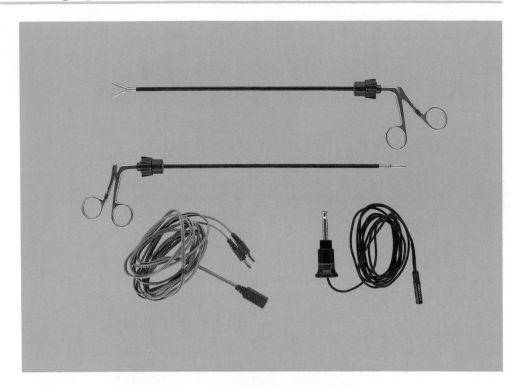

10-7 Tips of Hunter bowel grasper (Glassman type), 5 mm: **A**, closed; **B**, open.

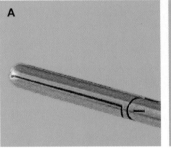
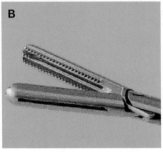

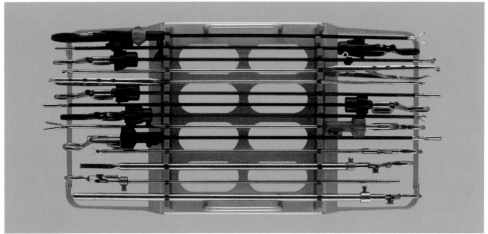

10-8 Second rack, with laparoscopic instruments that fit inside a sterilization container. The laparoscopic instruments in this rack are: **A**, 10-mm cup forceps; **B**, 5-mm grasper with teeth; **C**, 10-mm grasper with teeth; **D**, Olsen clamp; **E**, double-action grasper; **F**, hook scissors; **G**, 5-mm Apple needle holder with left curve; **H**, 5-mm Babcock grasping forceps; **I**, monopolar scissors 5 mm × 32 mm; and **J**, Maryland dissector.

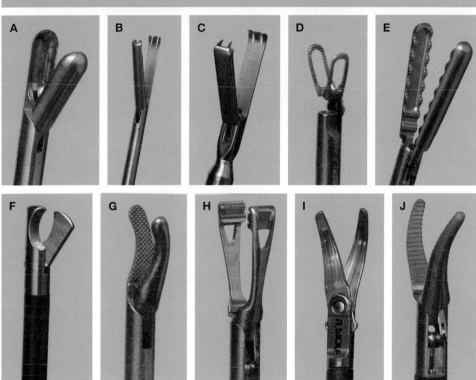

10-9 *Left to right:* insufflation tubing
and insufflation tubing with battery-
operated suction/irrigator system.

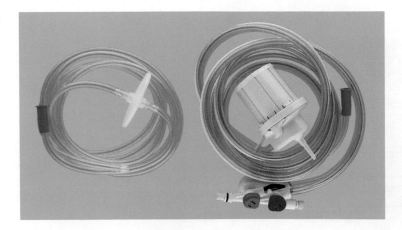

10-10 Position for laparoscopic
appendectomy and herniorrhaphy.

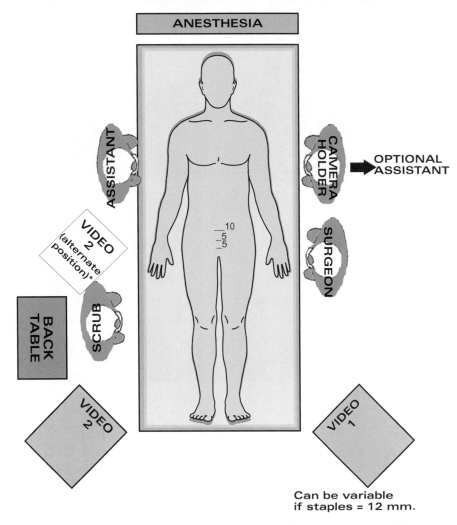

ANESTHESIA

ASSISTANT

CAMERA HOLDER

OPTIONAL ASSISTANT

SURGEON

VIDEO 2 (alternate position)*

BACK TABLE

SCRUB

VIDEO 2

VIDEO 1

Can be variable
if staples = 12 mm.

* Change per physician
preference

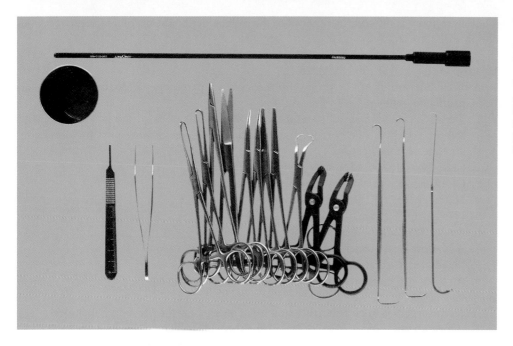

11-1 *Top to bottom:* 1 suction tip; 1 medicine cup, metal. *Bottom:* 1 Bard-Parker knife handle #3; 1 Adson tissue forceps with teeth, 1 × 2; 2 Allis tissue forceps; 1 Crile-Wood needle holder, 7 inch; 1 Mayo dissecting scissors, straight; 2 Crile hemostatic forceps, curved; 2 Kocher clamps; 1 Backhaus towel clip; 2 paper drape clips; 2 Senn retractors; and 1 News tracheal hook.

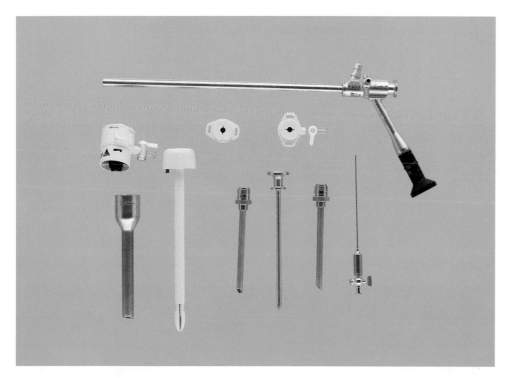

11-2 *Top to bottom:* Laser laparoscope; 3 disposable ports, 2 with adapter on side. *Bottom:* 1 applied cannula, 10 mm; disposable trocar; 1 applied cannula, 5 mm; 1 obturator, 5 mm; 1 applied cannula, 5 mm; and a 1 Verres needle stylet.

Laparoscopic Cholecystectomy

Cholecystectomy is the surgical removal of the gallbladder by means of a laparoscope or an abdominal incision.

Possible equipment needed for the procedure includes a minor laparoscopic set, a laparoscope set, and an adult MIS set.

A brief description of the procedure through a laparoscope, after the abdomen has been insufflated, follows:

1. 3 or 4 trocars with sheaths are needed. There is one port for the laparoscope, with camera attached; one port for the retraction instruments; one port for dissection; and one port for ligation.
2. Claw forceps are used to stabilize the gallbladder.
3. Olsen clamp is used to stabilize the cystic duct.
4. Hook scissors are used for dissection.
5. Ligaclip appliers are used for hemostasis.
6. An Apple needle holder is used for suture ligation.
7. A Marlow knot pusher is used for suture tightening.
8. Ligature scissors are used for cutting suture.
9. An Endo catch retriever is used for removing the specimen.

If electrosurgery is to be done, the equipment needed for the procedure includes:

1. A Swanstrom forceps, used for stabilizing the gallbladder.
2. A spatula electrode, used for hemostasis.
3. A monopolar Metzenbaum scissors, used for dissection.
4. A Maryland dissector, used to remove the specimen.

12-1 A, Endo catch with the tip closed; **B**, Endo catch with the tip expanded.

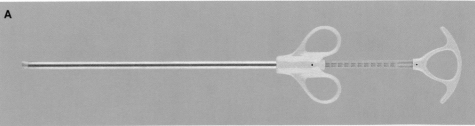

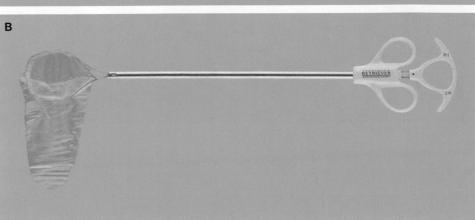

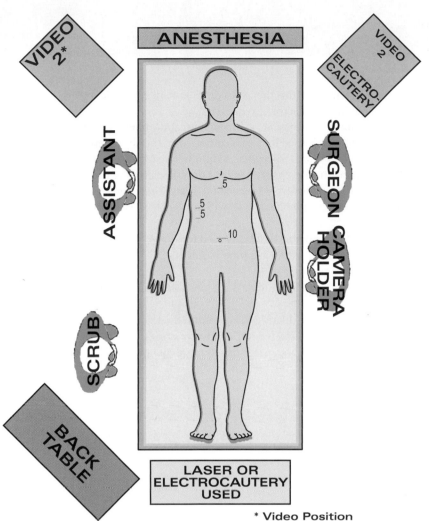

12-2 Position for laparoscopic cholecystectomy.

Cholecystectomy

Possible equipment needed for the procedure includes a basic laparotomy set and a Thompson self-retaining retractor, if requested.

A brief description of the procedure through an abdominal incision includes:

1. A Balfour retractor is used for visualization after the abdomen is opened.
2. A Mayo-Péan hemostatic forceps is used for hemostasis and grasping the gallbladder.
3. 2 Mixter hemostatic forceps are used for double-clamping the cystic duct.
4. A Westphal hemostatic forceps is used for blunt dissection of the gallbladder.
5. A long Bard-Parker knife handle #3 with a #10 blade is used for bisecting the cystic duct.
6. Long curved Metzenbaum scissors is used for dissection.
7. Ligaclip appliers are used for clipping bleeders.

If a common duct exploration is to be done, possible equipment needed for the procedure includes:

1. Bakes dilators, used for dilating the common duct.
2. Randall stone forceps, used for retrieving any stones.
3. A Ferguson gallstone scoop, used for scooping out any small, gravel-like stones.

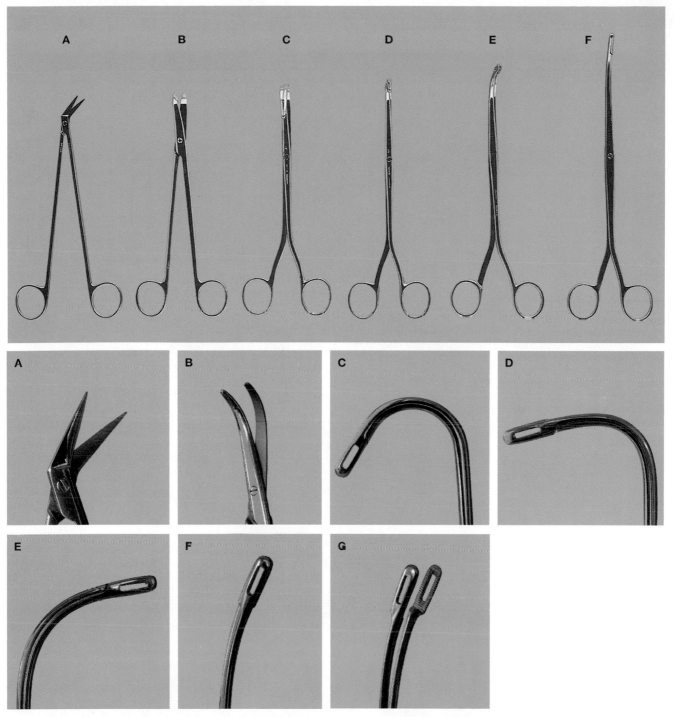

13-1 *Left to right:* **A**, 1 Potts-Smith cardiovascular scissors, 45-degree angle and tip; **B**, 1 Thorek scissors and tip; **C-G**, 4 Randall stone forceps and tips: **C**, full curved; **D**, ¾ curved; **E**, ½ curved; **F**, ¼ curved, closed; and **G**, ¼ curved, open.

13-2 *Top, left:* 1 grooved director; 1 probe dilator. *Bottom, left to right:* 3 gallbladder trocars with inserts, small, medium, and large; 9 Bakes common duct dilators, #3 through #11; 3 Ferguson gallstone scoops, small, medium, and large.

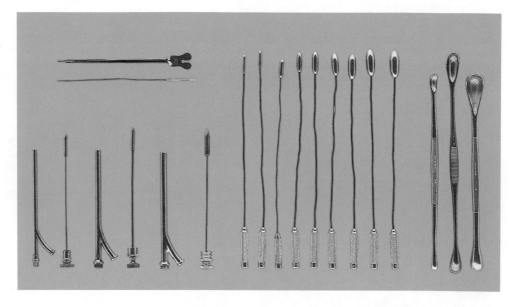

13-3 *Top, left to right:* 2 Adson hemostatic forceps, fine curved; 4 Westphal hemostatic forceps, short; 1 Borge cystic duct catheter clamp, 4 Fr; 1 Borge cystic duct catheter clamp, 6 Fr; 1 Mixter hemostatic forceps, fine point, 8½ inch. *Bottom:* 2 Mixter hemostatic forceps, fine point, extra long.

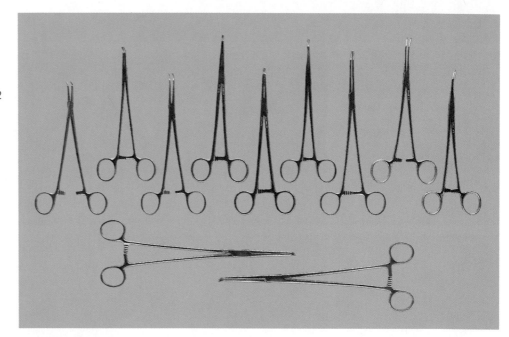

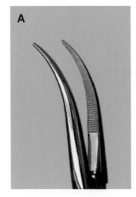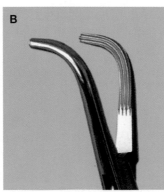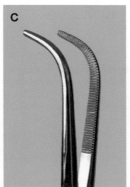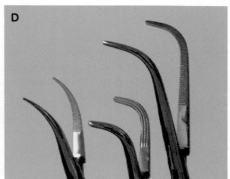

13-4 *Left to right:* Tips: **A**, Adson hemostatic forceps, fine curved; **B**, Westphal hemostatic forceps; **C**, Mixter hemostatic forceps, fine point; **D**, comparison of the three above tips.

Laparoscopic Bowel Resection

Chapter

14

A bowel resection is the excision of a portion of the small or large intestine and the reanastomosis of it through a laparoscope or through an abdominal incision.

Possible equipment needed for the procedure includes a minor laparoscopic set, a laparoscope set, and a laparoscopic adult MIS set.

A brief description of the procedure through a laparoscope, after the abdomen is insufflated, follows:

1. An Endoflex retractor is used for visualization.
2. A Hunter (Glassman) grasper is used for handling the bowel.
3. A Maryland dissector is used for freeing up the bowel.
4. A Nezhat suction/irrigator is used for lubrication and removal of fluid.
5. A linear stapling device is used for transecting the bowel.
6. A Ligaclip applier is used for hemostasis.
7. A needlepoint suture passer is used in suturing.
8. A Marlow knot pusher is used for suture tightening.
9. A linear stapling device is used for reanastomosis of the bowel.

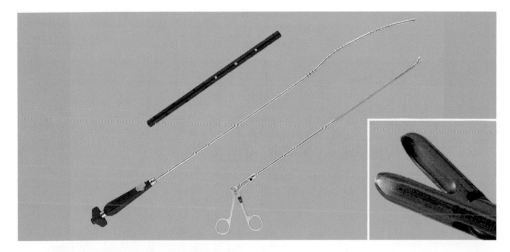

14-1 *Top to bottom:* 1 Endoflex protective cover; 1 Endoflex retractor, triangle, 5 mm, 80-mm length; 1 biopsy forceps, 5 mm, and tip.

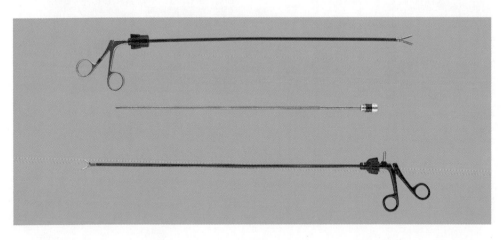

14-2 *Top to bottom:* These are extra-long instruments; 1 Glassman (Hunter bowel grasper), 5 mm, 45-cm length; 1 Nezhat suction irrigator, 5 mm, 45-cm length; 1 Maryland dissector, monopolar, 5 mm, 45-cm length.

14-3 *Left to right:* Tips: **A**, Hunter bowel grasper (Glassman type), 5 mm, 45-cm length; **B**, Nezhat suction irrigator, 5 mm, 45-cm length; **C**, Maryland dissector, monopolar, 5 mm, 45-cm length.

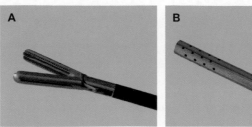
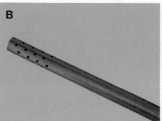
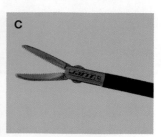

14-4 *Left to right:* 1 Verres needle, disposable; 3 dilating-tipped trocars, disposable, 5 mm, 10/11 mm, and 12 mm; 1 optical trocar, disposable, 10 mm; 1 blunt-tipped trocar (Hasson type), disposable, 10 mm.

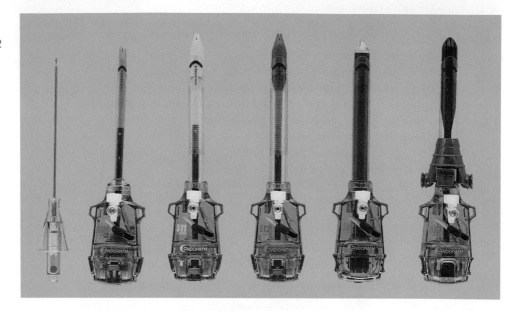

14-5 *Top to bottom:* Medium/large ligating and dividing Ligaclip applier; linear cutter with reloadable head.

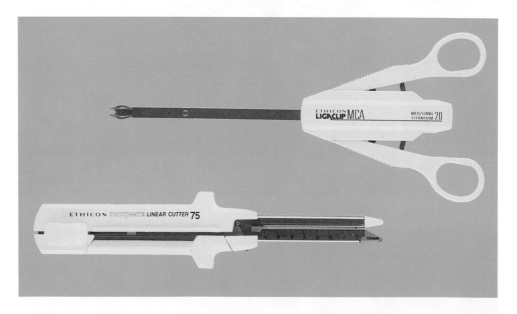

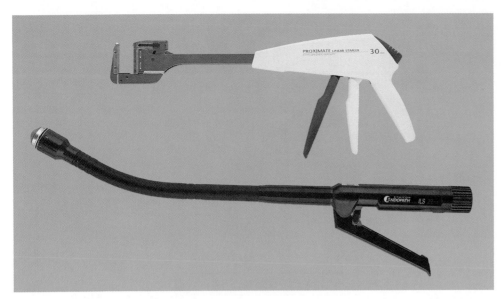

14-6 *Top to bottom:* Linear stapler, 30 mm; endoscopic circular stapler.

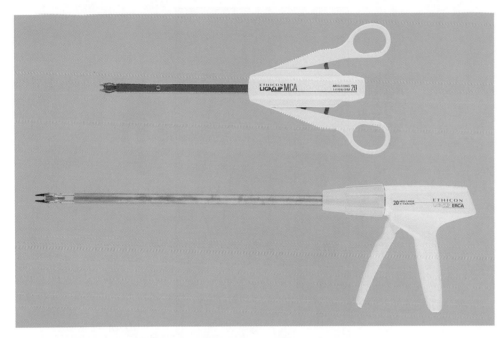

14-7 *Top to bottom:* 2 medium/large ligating and dividing Ligaclip appliers.

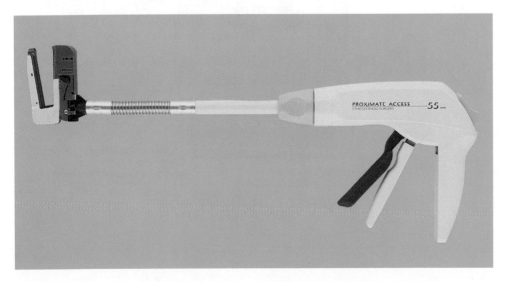

14-8 Linear stapler, 55 mm.

14-9 Endo GI stapler with universal handle and tip with staples.

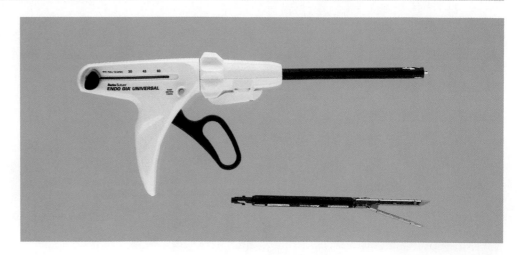

14-10 Position for laparoscopic bowel resection.

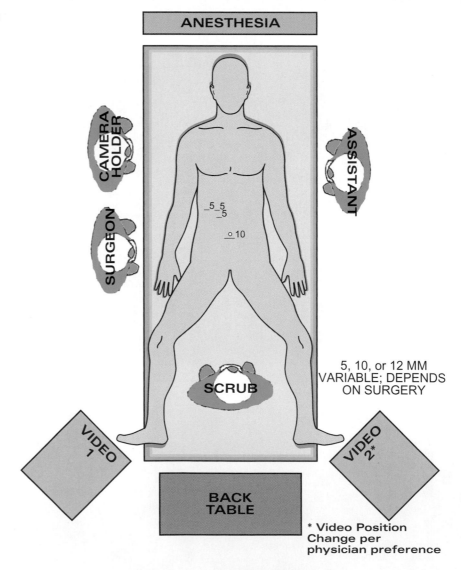

ANESTHESIA

CAMERA HOLDER

ASSISTANT

SURGEON

_5_5
_5

o 10

5, 10, or 12 MM
VARIABLE; DEPENDS
ON SURGERY

SCRUB

VIDEO 1

VIDEO 2*

BACK
TABLE

* Video Position
Change per
physician preference

**REVERSE FOR RIGHT SIDE
PATIENT IN LOW ALLEN STIRRUPS**

Possible equipment needed for the procedure includes a basic laparotomy set and self-retaining retractor.

A brief description of the procedure, doing the surgery through an abdominal incision, includes:

1. Self-retaining retractor is used for visualization after the abdomen is opened.
2. A Doyen intestinal forceps is used for atraumatic bowel clamping.
3. A Carmalt hemostatic forceps is used for hemostasis and blunt dissection.
4. Long Babcock tissue forceps is used for handling the bowel.
5. An Ethicon linear cutter is used for dissection of the bowel.
6. An Ethicon linear stapler is used for reanastomosis of the bowel.

Resection of the sigmoid colon may need a special stapling device (EEA) that also cuts the tissue.

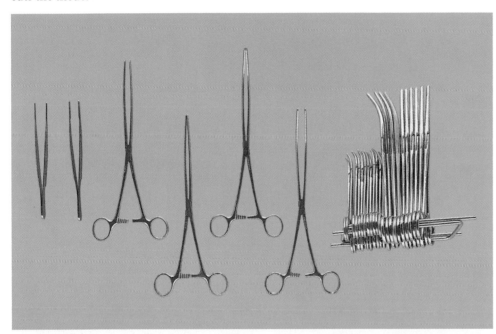

15-1 *Left to right:* 2 DeBakey vascular Autraugrip tissue forceps, short; 2 Doyen intestinal forceps, straight; 2 Doyen intestinal forceps, curved; 12 Halstead mosquito hemostatic forceps, curved; 4 Carmalt hemostatic forceps, long, curved; 6 Carmalt hemostatic forceps, long, straight.

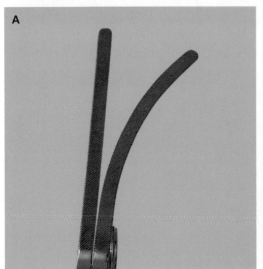

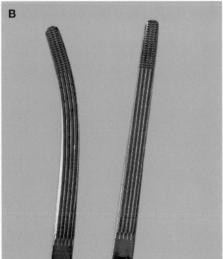

15-2 *Left to right:* Tips: **A**, Doyen intestinal forceps, straight and curved; **B**, Carmalt hemostatic forceps, long, curved and straight.

Sigmoidoscopy

A sigmoidoscopy is the visualization within the sigmoid and descending colon with the aid of a scope and a light source.

A brief description of the procedure follows:

1. The scope is inserted with the obturator in place.
2. The obturator is removed.
3. The air hose and bulb are attached to the scope.
4. The colon is inflated.
5. The light source is attached to the scope.

16-1 *Left to right:* 1 transformer cord; 1 light handle; 1 sigmoidoscope; 1 obturator; 1 colonic insufflator.

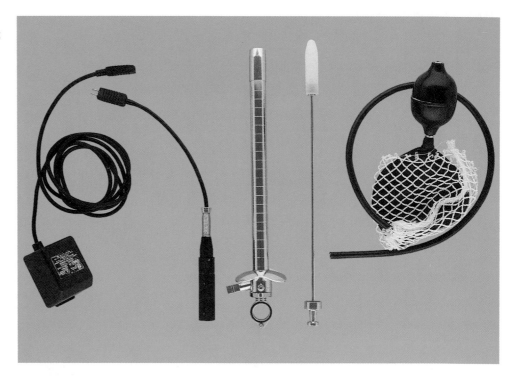

A hemorrhoidectomy is the removal of the hemorrhoidal veins.

A brief description of the procedure follows:

1. A Hirschman anoscope with obturator is inserted to dilate the anus. The obturator is removed to provide visualization.
2. A Hill-Ferguson retractor is used for anterior retraction.
3. A Sullivan rectal retractor with 5 blades is used for visualization.
4. An Allis tissue forceps is used for grasping the hemorrhoidal vein.
5. A Pennington hemostatic forceps is used for hemostasis at the base of the vein.

A pilonidal cyst is a cyst and sinus tract in the intergluteal fold on the sacrum. A pilonidal cystectomy is the procedure performed to remove the sinus tract.

A brief description of the procedure follows:

1. A groove director is used for following the sinus tract.
2. A groove dilator is used to facilitate following the sinus tract.
3. A Rosser crypt hook is used to find all parts of the sinus tract.
4. A Bard-Parker scalpel handle #3 with a #10 blade is used for wide excision of the entire sinus tract.
5. An Allis tissue forceps is used to grasp the specimen during excision.

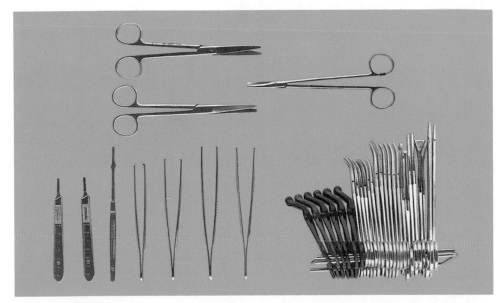

17-1 *Top, left to right:* 2 Mayo dissecting scissors, straight; 1 Metzenbaum scissors, 7 inch. *Bottom, left to right:* 2 Bard-Parker knife handles, #3; 1 Bard-Parker knife handle, #7; 2 thumb tissue forceps with teeth (1 × 2); 2 DeBakey vascular Autraugrip tissue forceps, short; 6 paper drape clips; 6 Crile hemostatic forceps, 5½ inch; 6 Crile hemostatic forceps, 6½ inch; 2 Allis tissue forceps; 2 Ochsner hemostatic forceps, short; 2 Pennington hemostatic forceps; 2 Crile-Wood needle holders, 7 inch.

17-2 *Top:* 1 Poole abdominal suction tube and shield. *Bottom, left to right:* 1 grooved director; 1 probe dilator; 1 Rosser crypt hook; 2 Army Navy retractors, side view and front view; 1 Hirschman anoscope (2 parts); 1 Hill-Ferguson rectal retractor; 1 anoscope, extra large (2 parts).

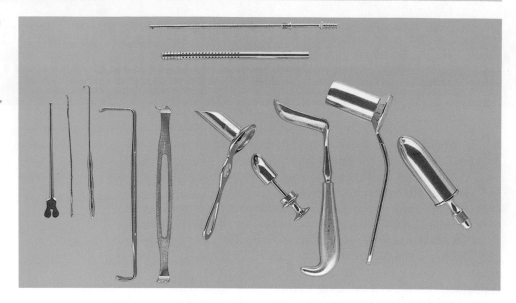

17-3 *Left to right:* Tips: 1 probe dilator; 1 grooved director; 1 Rosser crypt hook; 1 Pennington hemostatic forceps.

17-4 1 Sullivan rectal retractor, self-retaining; 5 blades.

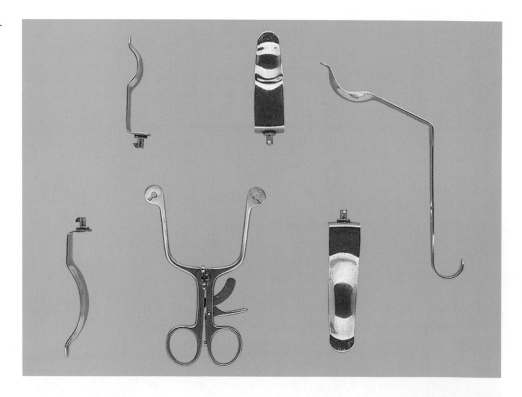

Laparoscopic gastric banding is a type of bariatric surgery. Bariatrics is the field of medicine that deals with obesity and weight-related conditions.

Possible equipment needed for the laparoscopic gastric banding procedure includes a laparoscope, a BioEnteric Lap Band, a camera, a fiberoptic light cord, and special long trocars.

A brief description of the procedure follows:

1. The laparoscope is inserted in the usual manner.
2. The Nathanson retractor is positioned to retract the liver.
3. The Hook scissors are used to make a circular window in the mesenteric layers of the fundus of the stomach.
4. The BioEnteric Lap Band (10 cm long) is introduced through another port and manipulated into the window in the mesenteric layer and around the stomach. The band connects to itself by means of a lasso end and a notched end; it is tightened as much as necessary and secured.
5. The Apple needle holder is used to suture the mesentery if needed. A needlepoint suture passer inserts the suture, and a Ranfac knot pusher is used to tighten the suture.

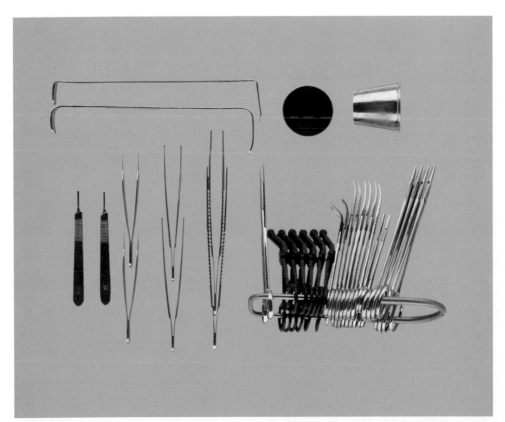

18-1 *Top, left to right:* 2 Army Navy retractors; 2 medicine cups, metal, one upright, one on side. *Bottom, left to right:* 2 Bard-Parker knife handles #3; 2 Adson retractors with teeth (1 × 2); 2 tissue thumb forceps with teeth (1 × 2); 2 DeBakey vascular Autraugrip tissue forceps; 1 Mayo dissecting scissors, straight; 6 paper drape clips; 1 Backhaus towel clip; 1 Halstead mosquito hemostatic forceps, curved; 6 Crile hemostatic forceps, curved; 2 Johnson needle holders, 5 inch; and 4 Crile-Wood needle holders, 6 inch.

18-2 *Left to right:* 2 sets of trocars and obturators, 1 set 5 mm × 100 mm (standard), 1 set 5 mm × 150 mm (bariatric); 2 sets of trocars and obturators, 1 set 11 mm × 150 mm (bariatric), 1 set 12 mm × 150 mm (bariatric); and 1 set Hasson trocar and obturator, 12 mm.

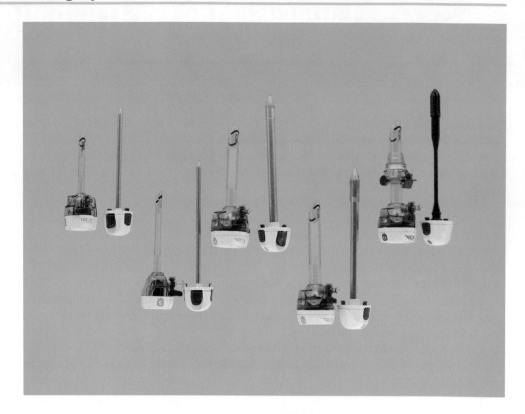

18-3 *Top to bottom:* 1 bariatric telescope, 10 mm, 30 degrees; 3 telescopes, 45, 30, and 0 degrees; bottom telescope, 5 mm, 30 degrees.

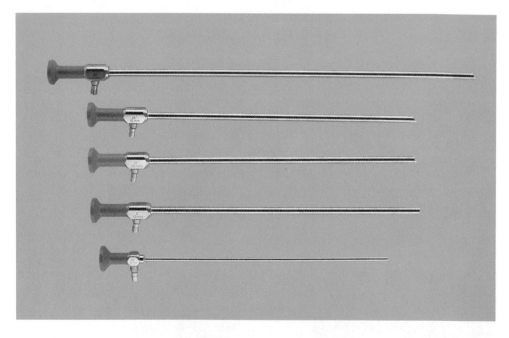

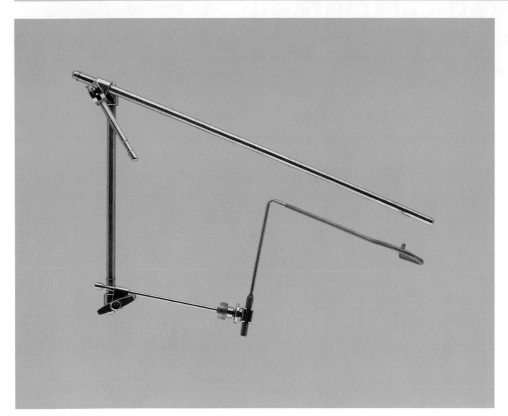

18-4 Nathanson retractor with laparoscopic Thompson retractor holder.

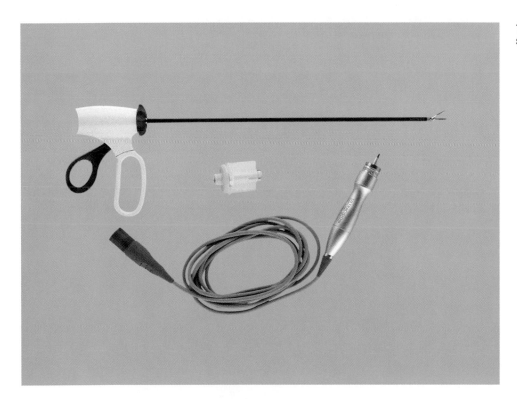

18-5 *Top to bottom:* harmonic scalpel; wrench; and electric cord.

Laparoscopic Gastric Bypass

Possible equipment needed for the procedure includes a laparoscope, a camera, a fiberoptic light cord, and special long trocars and obturators.

19-1 *Left to right:* 1 Bard-Parker knife handle #3; 2 Adson tissue forceps with teeth (1 × 2); 2 thumb tissue forceps without teeth, short; 1 Mayo dissecting scissors, curved; 1 Metzenbaum dissecting scissors, 7 inch; 1 Mayo dissecting scissors, straight; 2 Mayo-Péan hemostatic forceps, curved; 2 Kocher clamps; 1 Crile-Wood needle holder, 7 inch; 1 Crile-Wood needle holder, 5 inch; 6 Crile hemostatic forceps, curved, 6$^1/_2$ inch; 4 Backhaus towel clips; 8 paper drape clips; and 3 non-insulated rotating handles.

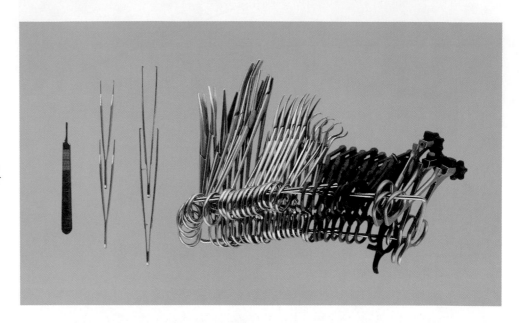

19-2 *Top:* 2 Apple needle holders with locks, 5 mm, right and left curves. *Bottom, left to right:* Inlet fascia closure device; cone, long; 2 medicine cups, metal side view, top view; and Nathanson live retractor.

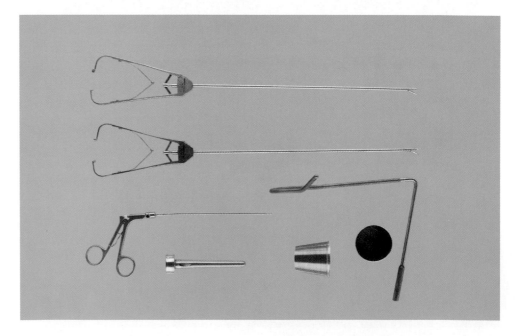

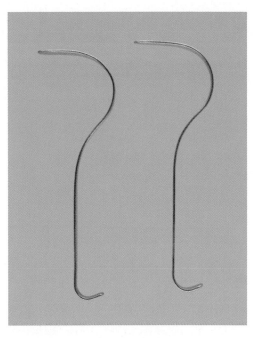

19-3 Two baby Deaver retractors.

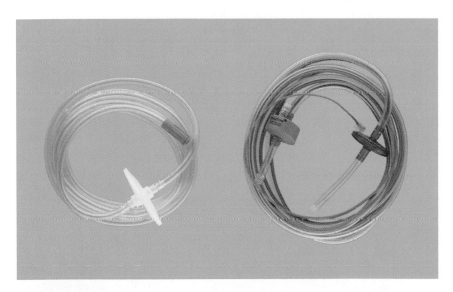

19-4 *Left to right:* Disposable high-flow insufflation tube and InsuFlow heater hydrator insufflation tubing.

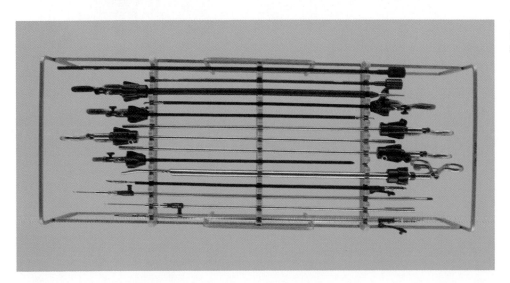

19-5 Rack with laparoscopic instruments that fits inside a sterilization container.

19-6 *Top to bottom:* 1 switchblade scissors, bariatric; 1 switchblade scissors, regular; 1 bariatric spatula; and 1 Nezhat-Dorsey irrigator.

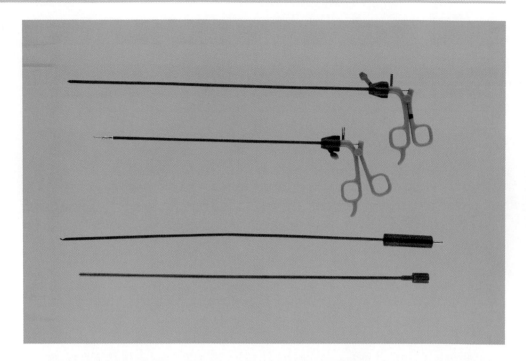

19-7 Top and bottom instruments work together: *bottom:* fenestrated bowel grasper that slides inside the noninsulated sheath at the *top;* both connect to the noninsulated metal handle; *middle:* DeBakey forceps, 10 mm, curved.

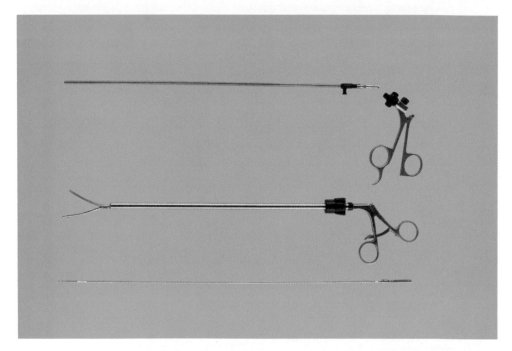

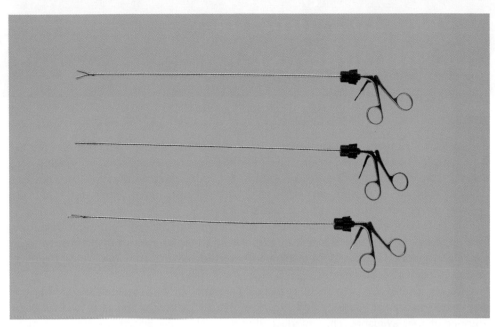

19-8 Three Hunter bowel graspers.

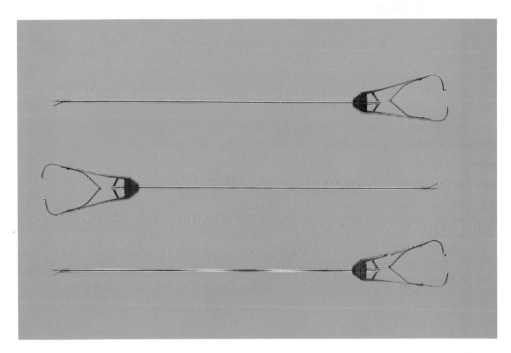

19-9 Three Apple needle holders, 2 left curved, 1 right curved.

The da Vinci® Surgical System and EndoWrist® Instruments (Robotic Instruments)*

EndoWrist instruments are manufactured by Intuitive Surgical, Inc., specifically for use with the *da Vinci* Surgical System. The *EndoWrist* instruments provide surgeons with natural dexterity and a full range of motion for more precise operation through tiny incisions. Similar to the human wrist, an *EndoWrist* instrument allows for rapid and precise suturing, dissection, and tissue manipulation.

The *EndoWrist* instrument line features a variety of specialized tip designs, including forceps, needle drivers and scissors; monopolar and bipolar electrocautery instruments; scalpels and more. The *EndoWrist* instruments are available in 5-mm and 8-mm diameters to meet surgeons' requirements.

After an *EndoWrist* instrument is installed on the *da Vinci* System, the interface is designed to recognize the type and function of the instrument and also to display the number of uses available. This interface allows the *da Vinci* System to detect when an instrument needs replacement.

Because of the delicate nature of these instruments, all handling, cleaning, and sterilization must be performed in strict accordance with the manufacturer's guidelines.

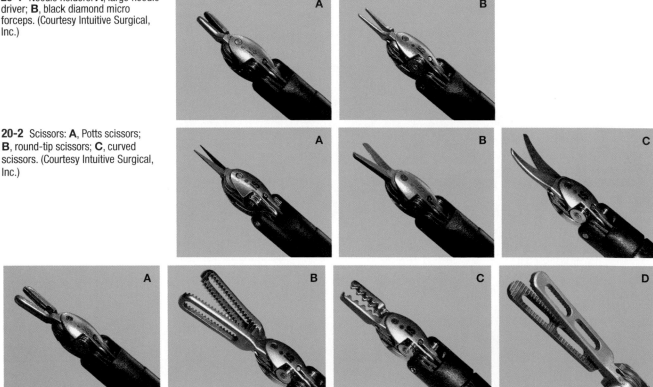

20-1 Needle holders: **A**, large needle driver; **B**, black diamond micro forceps. (Courtesy Intuitive Surgical, Inc.)

20-2 Scissors: **A**, Potts scissors; **B**, round-tip scissors; **C**, curved scissors. (Courtesy Intuitive Surgical, Inc.)

20-3 Graspers: **A**, DeBakey forceps; **B**, Cadiere forceps; **C**, Resano forceps; **D**, double-fenestrated grasper. (Courtesy Intuitive Surgical, Inc.)

*Additional images are available on the Companion CD.

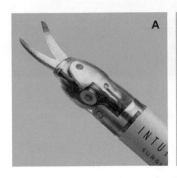
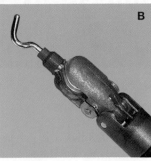
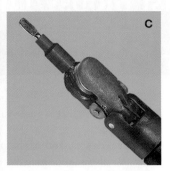

20-4 Monopolar energy instruments: **A**, hot shears, aka monopolar curved scissors; **B**, permanent cautery hook; **C**, permanent cautery spatula. (Courtesy Intuitive Surgical, Inc.)

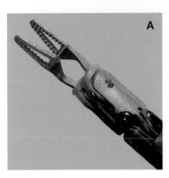
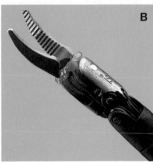

20-5 Bipolar energy instruments: **A**, Precise bipolar forceps; **B**, Maryland bipolar forceps. (Courtesy Intuitive Surgical, Inc.)

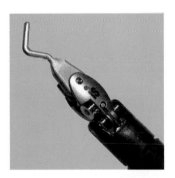

20-6 Specialty instrument: valve hook. (Courtesy Intuitive Surgical, Inc.)

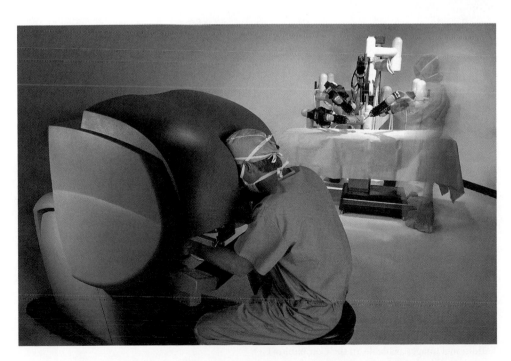

20-7 Surgeon at da Vinci console and nurse at operating table with robotic instrumentation. (Courtesy Intuitive Surgical, Inc.)

Breast Biopsy/Lumpectomy*

A breast biopsy is the removal of suspicious breast tissue for the purpose of microscopic examination.

A brief description of the procedure follows:

1. A Halstead mosquito forceps is used for hemostasis.
2. A DeBakey tissue forceps is used for atraumatic handling of breast tissue.
3. A Lahey thyroid tenaculum is used for grasping the pathology.
4. A Senn retractor is used for deeper retraction.
5. Joseph hooks are used for skin retraction.

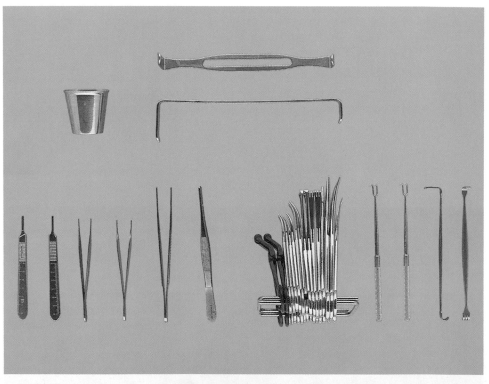

21-1 *Top, left to right:* 1 medicine cup, metal; 2 Army Navy retractors, front view and side view. *Bottom, left to right:* 2 Bard-Parker knife handles #3; 1 Adson tissue forceps (1 × 2); 1 Brown-Adson tissue forceps (9 × 9); 2 DeBakey vascular Autraugrip tissue forceps, short (front view and side view); 2 paper drape clips; 4 Halstead mosquito hemostatic forceps, curved; 2 Crile hemostatic forceps, 5½ inch; 2 Allis tissue forceps; 2 Lahey goiter vusellum forceps; 1 Crile-Wood needle holder, 6 inch; 2 Mayo dissecting scissors, straight and curved; 1 Metzenbaum dissecting scissors, 5 inch; 2 Joseph skin hooks, double; 2 Miller-Senn retractors, side view and front view.

*Additional images available on the Companion CD.

A mastectomy is the removal of a breast (mammary gland).

A brief description of the procedure follows:
1. A Lahey tenaculum is used for grasping skin edges.
2. Prince Metzenbaum scissors are used for dissecting.
3. Hays Martin tissue forceps are used to help with dissection.
4. Volkman (rake) retractors (sharp and dull) are used for visualization.
5. Poole suction tip with tubing is used for visualization.
6. Allis Adair forceps are used for grasping breast tissue.
7. Curved Crile hemostatic forceps are used for hemostasis and blunt dissection.
8. A skin stapler is used for skin closure.

For the axillary node dissection, a brief description of the procedure follows:
1. A Green retractor is used for visualization.
2. A cushing vein retractor is used for retracting small structures.
3. A Yankauer tip is used for visualization.

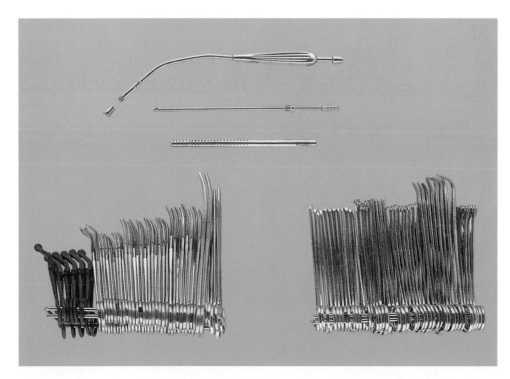

22-1 *Top to bottom:* Yankauer suction tube and tip; Poole abdominal suction tube and shield. *Bottom, left to right:* First instrument stringer: 6 paper drape clips; 2 Backhaus towel forceps, 8 Halsted mosquito hemostatic forceps, curved; 12 Crile hemostatic forceps, 5½ inch; 8 Crile hemostatic forceps, 6½ inch; 2 Mayo-Péan hemostatic forceps, long; 2 Halsey needle holders, serrated, 5 inch; 2 Crile-Wood needle holders, 7 inch; Second instrument stringer: 12 Allis tissue forceps; 4 Babcock tissue forceps; 4 Ochsner hemostatic forceps, straight, short; 8 Adair breast clamps, short; 4 tonsil hemostatic forceps; 4 Westphal hemostatic forceps; 4 Lahey traction forceps.

*Additional images are available on the Companion CD.

22-2 *Top, left to right:* 2 Bard-Parker knife handles #3; 1 Hoen nerve hook; 1 Bard-Parker knife handle #4. *Bottom, left to right:* 2 Metzenbaum dissecting scissors, 5 inch and 6 inch; 1 Prince-Metzenbaum dissecting scissors; Mayo dissecting scissors: 2 straight and 1 curved.

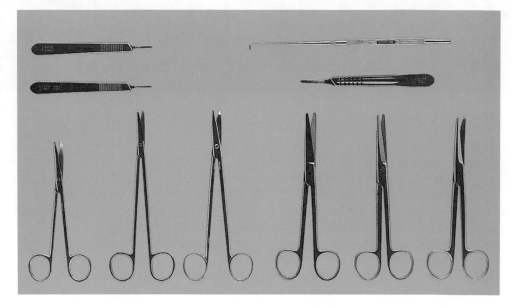

22-3 *Left to right:* 2 Adson tissue forceps with teeth (1 × 2), front view and side view; 2 Brown-Adson tissue forceps (9 × 9), front view and side view; 1 Adson tissue forceps without teeth, front view; 2 DeBakey vascular Autraugrip tissue forceps, short, front view and side view; 2 Hayes Martin tissue forceps, short, front view and side view; 2 DeBakey vascular Autraugrip tissue forceps, medium, front view and side view.

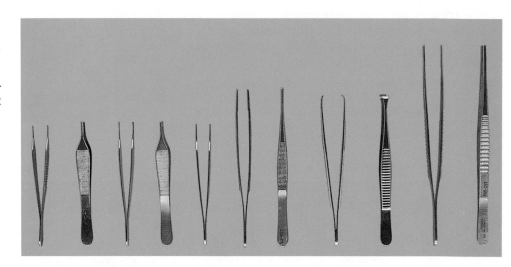

22-4 *Left to right:* 2 Richardson retractors, small and medium; 2 Volkmann retractors, 6 prong, sharp, front view and side view; 2 Volkmann retractors, 6 prong, dull, front view and side view; 2 Volkmann retractors, 4-prong, dull, front view and side view; 2 Volkmann retractors, 4 prong, sharp, front view and side view.

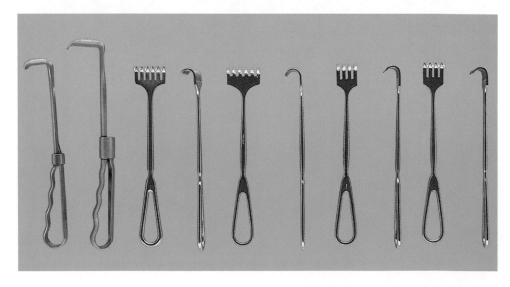

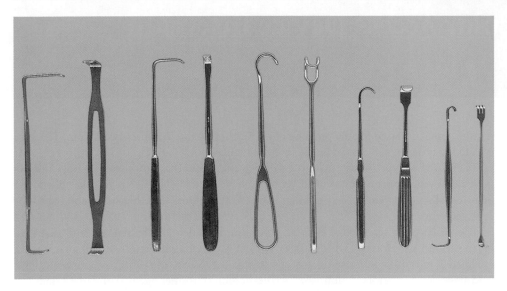

22-5 *Left to right:* 2 Army Navy retractors, side view and front view; 2 Langenbeck retractors, side view and front view; 2 Green goiter retractors, side view and front view; 2 Cushing vein retractors, side view and front view; 2 Miller-Senn retractors, side view and front view.

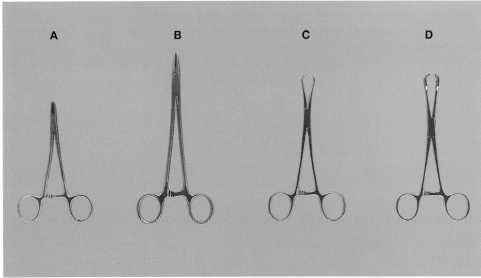

22-6 *Left to right:* **A**, Halsey needle holder, serrated, 5 inch, and tip; **B**, Crile-Wood needle holder, 7 inch, and tip; **C**, Adair breast clamp and tip; **D**, Lahey goiter vusellam forceps and tip.

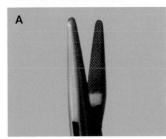
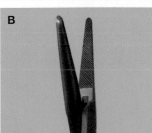
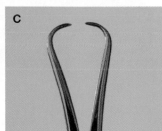
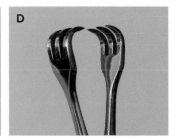

Vascular Access Device Insertion

A large vein is accessed for the purpose of administering medication or nutrition. The vein selected may be the subclavian or the internal jugular.

There are two types of vascular access device insertions, the central venous port and the peripheral venous port. The central venous ports and catheters are placed in subclavian or internal jugular veins. The peripheral venous ports (PAS) are placed in the basilic or cephalic veins.

The instrument set needed for the procedure includes 2 Bard-Parker knife handles, #3; 1 Adson tissue forceps with teeth (1 × 2); 1 Metzenbaum dissecting scissors, 5 inch; 3 Halsted mosquito hemostatic forceps, curved; 1 Mayo dissecting scissors, straight; 2 Miller-Senn retractors; 1 Johnson needle holder; 1 tunneling instrument (Takahashi nasal forceps, straight, or Pratt dilators, #13-15, 17-19). If using the central venous port or catheter, add the central venous port or catheter kit. If using the peripheral venous port, add the peripheral venous port kit and catheter finder and delete the tunneling instrument.

To place the catheter, Takahashi nasal forceps (straight) or a Pratt dilator are used for tunneling. The catheters that may be used are Groshong or Hickman.

23-1 *Top, left to right:* Groshong catheter for central venous access; peripheral venous port with catheter attached. *Bottom, left to right:* Central venous port with catheter attached; Hickman catheter for central venous access.

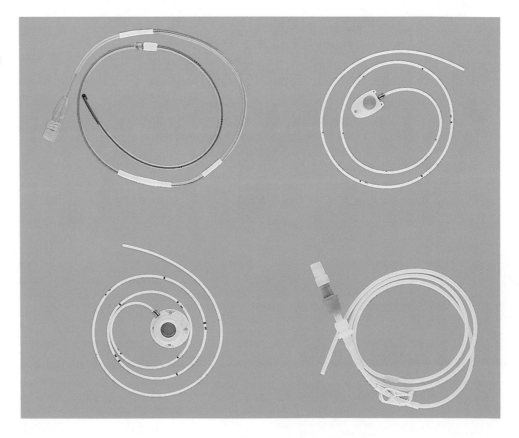

Dilation and Curettage of the Uterus (D and C)

Chapter

24

A dilation and curettage of the uterus (D and C) is performed to treat illness or to obtain a specimen for microscopic evaluation.

A description of the procedure follows:

1. An Auvard speculum is placed to open the posterior wall of the vagina.
2. A Heaney right-angle retractor is placed to elevate the anterior wall of the vagina.
3. A Schroeder tenaculum is placed on the cervix to stabilize the uterus.
4. A Sims uterine sound is inserted to determine the depth of the uterus.
5. Hegar dilators are inserted to dilate the cervix (from the smallest to the largest).
6. A Sims uterine curette is inserted to scrape tissue from the uterus.
7. A Thomas dull curette is used to remove any remaining tissue.

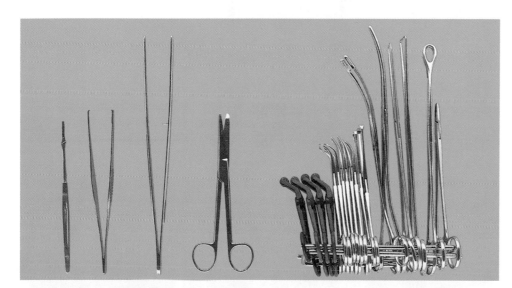

24-1 *Left to right:* 1 Bard-Parker knife handle, #7; 1 Ferris Smith tissue forceps; 1 dressing forceps, long; 1 Mayo dissecting scissors, curved; 4 paper drape clips; 2 Backhaus towel forceps; 4 Crile hemostatic forceps, 5½ inch; 2 Allis tissue forceps; 1 Randall stone forceps, ¼ curve; 1 Bozeman uterine forceps, S-shaped; 2 Schroeder uterine tenaculum forceps, single tooth; 1 Foerster sponge forceps; 1 Crile-Wood needle holder, 7 inch.

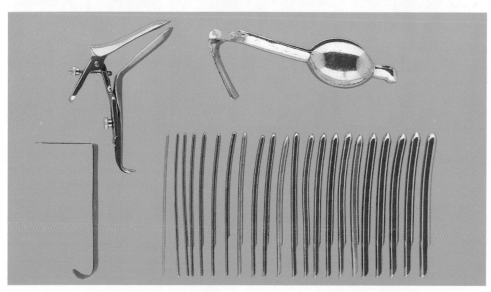

24-2 *Top, left to right:* 1 Graves vaginal speculum; 1 Auvard weighted vaginal speculum, medium lip. *Bottom, left to right:* 1 Heaney retractor; 1 set of Hegar dilators, sizes 3 to 13½ (including half sizes).

24-3 *Left to right:* 1 Sims uterine sound; 1 Heaney uterine biopsy curette, sharp, serrated, 5 mm wide; 1 Thomas uterine curette, semirigid, dull, small, 0.6-mm wide loop; 1 Sims uterine curette, semirigid, sharp, medium, 2.8 mm loop; 1 Kevorkian-Younge endocervical biopsy curette, 2-mm loop.

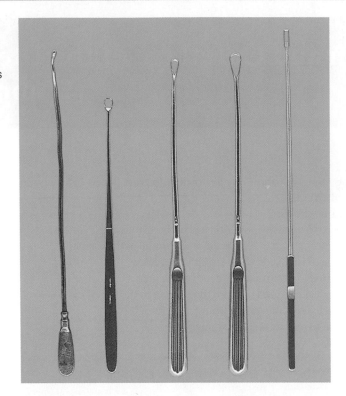

24-4 *Left to right:* Tips: **A**, Sims uterine sound; **B**, Heaney uterine biopsy curette, sharp, serrated, 5 mm wide; **C**, Thomas uterine curette, semirigid, dull, small, 0.6-mm wide loop; **D**, Sims uterine curette, semirigid, sharp, medium, 2.8-mm loop; **E**, Kevorkian-Younge endocervical biopsy curette, 2-mm loop; **F**, Bozeman uterine forceps, S-shaped.

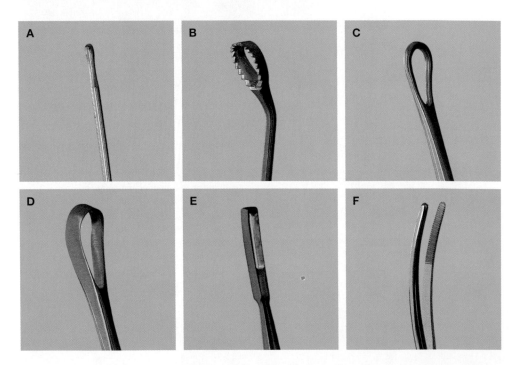

Hysteroscopy

Hysteroscopy is an endoscopic visualization of the uterine cavity and is usually performed to aid in the diagnosis and treatment of intrauterine diseases.

Possible equipment needed for the procedure includes a hysteroscope, D and C instruments, and possibly, if surgeon wishes to examine inside the abdomen, a laparoscope, a fiberoptic light source, polyethylene tubing, a hysteroscopic insufflator, a video camera, and a monitor.

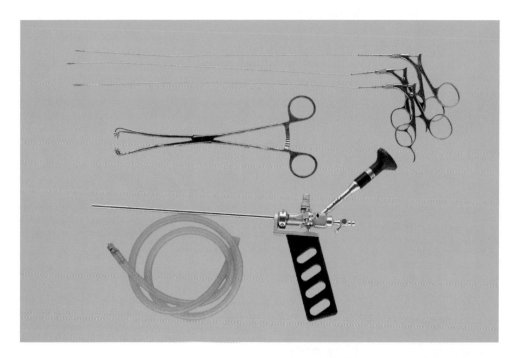

25-1 *Top to bottom:* Multitoothed semirigid grasping forceps, 5 Fr; semirigid Metzenbaum scissors, 5 Fr; semirigid cup biopsy forceps, 5 Fr; Gimpelson tenaculum; 20 degrees angled hysteroscope (adapter, on scope); and cable with adapter.

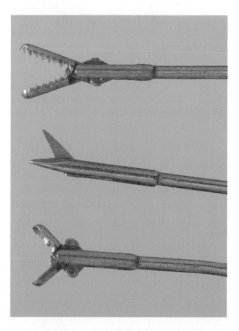

25-2 *Top to bottom:* Enlarged tips of multitoothed semirigid grasping forceps, 5 Fr; semirigid Metzenbaum scissors; and semirigid cup biopsy forceps.

Abdominal Hysterectomy

Abdominal hysterectomy is the removal of the uterus through an abdominal incision. Additional structures that may be removed through the same incision and at the same time are the ovaries (oophorectomy) and fallopian tubes (salpingectomy).

Instruments needed for the procedure include a basic laparotomy set and an O'Sullivan-O'Connor retractor.

A brief description of the procedure follows:

1. Schroeder uterine tenaculum forceps or Skene uterine vulsellum forceps are used for grasping the uterus.
2. Heaney or Heaney-Ballantine hysterectomy forceps are used for clamping uterine ligaments.
3. A Jorgenson dissecting scissors is used for dissection.
4. A Heaney needle holder is used for suture ligation.

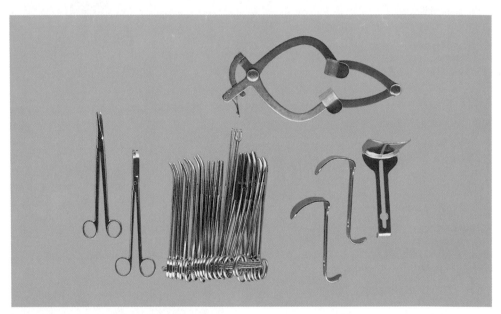

26-1 *Top, right:* 1 O'Sullivan-O'Connor retractor body. *Bottom, left to right:* 1 Mayo dissecting scissors, curved, 9 inch; 1 Jorgenson dissecting scissors, curved, 9 inch; 4 Ochsner hemostatic forceps, 8 inch; 2 Heaney hysterectomy forceps, single tooth; 2 Heaney-Ballantine hysterectomy forceps, single tooth; 4 Ochsner hemostatic forceps, 8 inch; 1 Schroeder uterine tenaculum forceps, single tooth; 1 Schroeder uterine vulsellum forceps, double tooth; 2 Jarit hysterectomy forceps, straight, 8½ inch; 2 Jarit hysterectomy forceps, curved, 8½ inch; 2 Heaney needle holders; 2 medium blades for O'Sullivan-O'Connor retractor, side view; 1 large blade, front view.

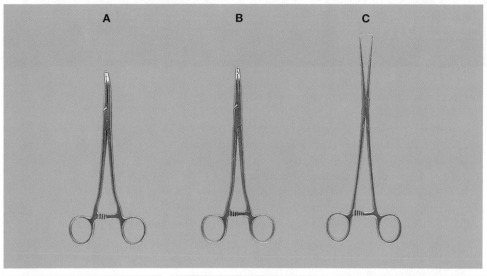

26-2 *Left to right:* **A**, Heaney hysterectomy forceps, single tooth, and tip; **B**, Heaney-Ballantine hysterectomy forceps, single tooth, and tip; **C**, Schroeder uterine tenaculum forceps, straight, single tooth, and tip; **D**, Tip of Schroeder uterine vulsellum forceps, double tooth.

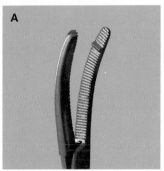
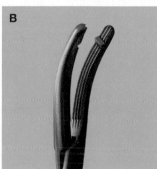
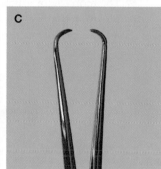
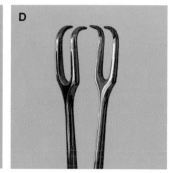

26-3 *Left to right:* **A**, Jarit hysterectomy forceps, straight, 8½ inch, and tip; **B**, Jarit hysterectomy forceps, curved, 8½ inch, and tip; **C**, Heaney needle holder, curved, 8½ inch, and tip. Tip of Jorgenson dissecting scissors: **D**, front view; **E**, side view.

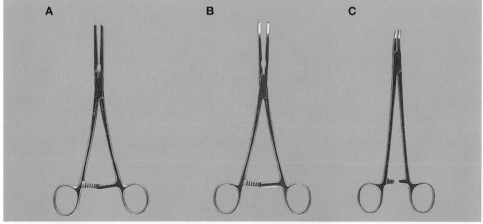

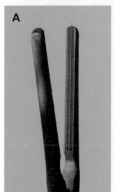
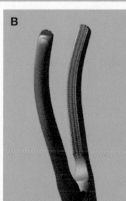
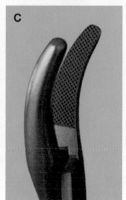
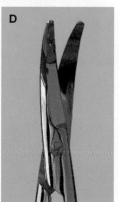
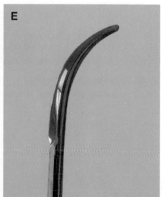

Supracervical Laparoscopic Hysterectomy

Supracervical laparoscopic hysterectomy is the removal of the uterus without the cervix through a laparoscope.

Possible equipment needed for the procedure includes a laparoscope, a Harmonic scalpel, an electrosurgical unit, a morcellator, a generator and foot pedal, and minor laparoscopic instruments.

A brief description of the procedure follows:

1. The laparoscope is inserted in the usual manner.
2. The Gimpelson tenaculum is used to grasp the uterus.
3. The Harmonic scalpel is used to dissect and cauterize the uterine ligaments and vessels.
4. The Harmonic scalpel is used to transect and cauterize the uterus above the cervix.
5. The morcellator is inserted through another port.
6. The morcellator is used to shave the uterus into pieces so it may be removed.
7. A heavy grasper is inserted through the morcellator to remove the uterine tissue fragments.

27-1 *Top to bottom:* UltraCision 5-mm Harmonic scalpel with curved shears; wrench; and then connecting cable.

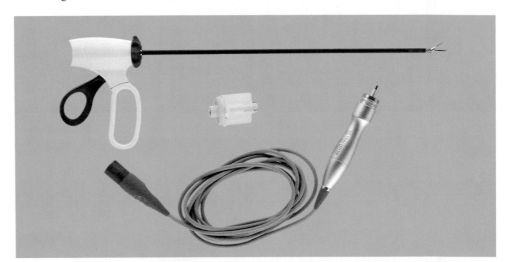

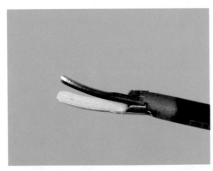

27-2 Tip of UltraCision 5-mm Harmonic scalpel with curved shears.

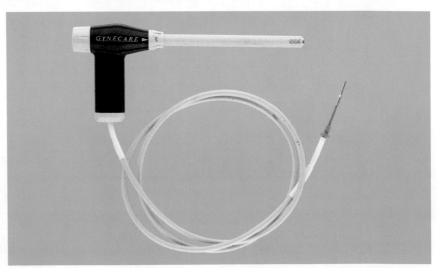

27-3 Morcellator.

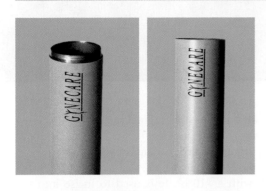

27-4 Tip of morcellator; left blade is out, right blade is inside.

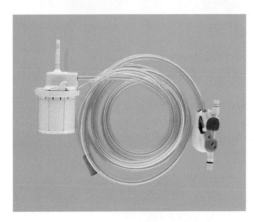

27-5 Suction/irrigator with pump.

27-6 Position for hysteroscopic procedures.

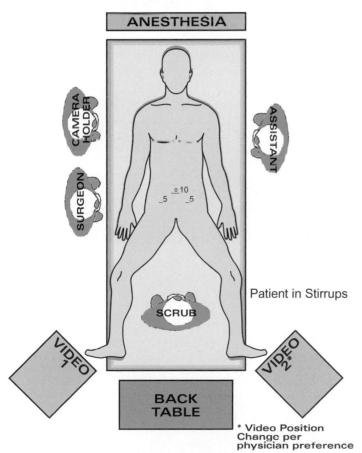

ANESTHESIA

CAMERA HOLDER

ASSISTANT

SURGEON

°10
_5   _5

Patient in Stirrups

SCRUB

VIDEO 1

VIDEO 2*

BACK TABLE

* Video Position Change per physician preference

REVERSE FOR RIGHT SIDE
PATIENT IN LOW ALLEN STIRRUPS

Chapter 28

Vaginal Hysterectomy

A vaginal hysterectomy is the removal of the uterus through a vaginal incision.

A brief description of the procedure follows:

1. An Auvard speculum and Heaney retractor are placed to visualize the cervix.
2. A Schroeder vulsellum is used to grasp the cervix.
3. A Bard-Parker long scalpel handle #3 with a #10 blade is used to incise into the peritoneum.
4. Heaney forceps or Heaney-Ballantine forceps are used to clamp the uterine ligaments and vessels.
5. A long curved Mayo scissors is used to bisect the ligaments and vessels.
6. A curved Heaney needle holder is used to ligate the ligaments and vessels with the use of Russian tissue forceps.
7. Foerster forceps with 4 × 4 sponges are used for hemostasis and visualization.
8. Allis-Adair forceps are used to approximate the peritoneum edges.
9. A long Crile-Wood needle holder is used to suture the peritoneum edges.

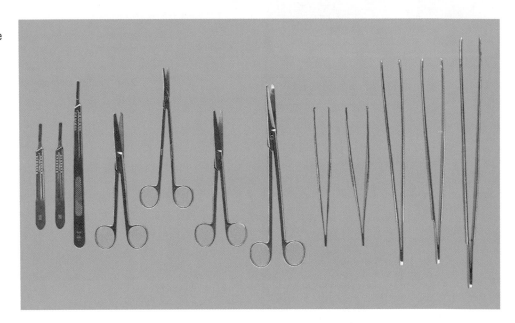

28-1 *Left to right:* 2 Bard-Parker knife handles, #4; 1 Bard-Parker knife handle, #4, long; 1 Mayo dissecting scissors, straight; 1 Metzenbaum scissors, 7 inch; 1 Mayo dissecting scissors, curved; 1 Mayo dissecting scissors, long, curved; 2 Ferris Smith tissue forceps; 2 Russian tissue forceps; 1 tissue forceps without teeth, long.

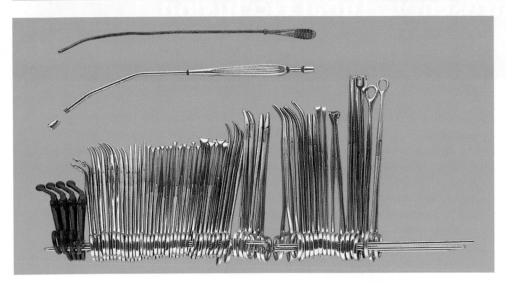

28-2 *Top to bottom:* 1 uterine sound; 1 Yankauer suction tube with tip. *Bottom, left to right:* 4 paper drape clips; 2 Backhaus towel clips; 8 Crile hemostatic forceps, 6½ inch; 4 Halsted hemostatic forceps; 12 Allis tissue forceps; 6 Allis-Adair tissue forceps; 4 tonsil hemostatic forceps; 2 Heaney needle holders; 2 Crile-Wood needle holders, 8 inch; 2 Heaney hysterectomy forceps, single tooth, curved; 2 Heaney-Ballantine hysterectomy forceps, single tooth, curved; 2 Ochsner hemostatic forceps, 8 inch; 2 Allis tissue forceps, long; 2 Babcock tissue forceps, medium; 2 Schroeder uterine tenaculum forceps, single tooth; 1 Schroeder uterine vulsellum forceps, double tooth, straight; 2 Foerster sponge forceps.

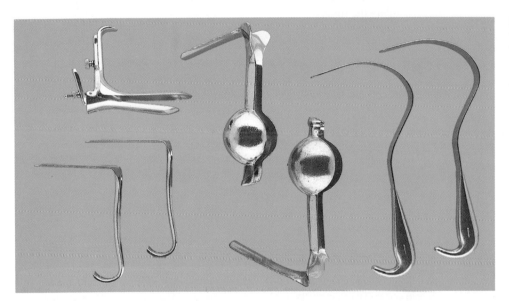

28-3 *Top, left to right:* 1 Graves vaginal speculum; 1 Auvard weighted vaginal speculum, medium lip. *Bottom, left to right:* 2 Heaney retractors; 1 Auvard weighted vaginal speculum, long lip; 2 Deaver retractors, narrow.

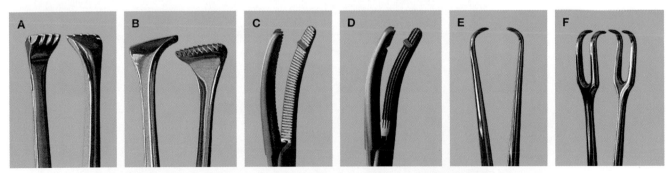

28-4 *Left to right:* Tips: **A**, Allis tissue forceps; **B**, Allis-Adair tissue forceps; **C**, Heaney hysterectomy forceps, single tooth, curved; **D**, Heaney-Ballantine hysterectomy forceps, single tooth, curved; **E**, Schroeder uterine tenaculum forceps, single tooth; **F**, Schroeder uterine vulsellum forceps, double tooth, straight.

Chapter 29

Laparoscopic Tubal Occlusion

Tubal occlusion is the interruption of the fallopian tubes for the purpose of permanent sterilization.

Possible equipment needed for the procedure includes a laparoscope, an electrosurgical unit, Falope rings, and D and C retractors.

A brief description of the procedure follows:

1. A Cohen cannula is inserted into the cervix vaginally to elevate the uterus.
2. The laparoscope is inserted in the usual manner.
3. A manipulation probe is used to expose the fallopian tube.
4. The Endoflex retractor is used to retract the structures away from the tube.
5. Babcock forceps are used to stabilize the tube.
6. A Falope ring applier with Silastic band is introduced.
7. The ring is placed over a loop of the fallopian tube or the Jarit bipolar forceps are used to coagulate the tube.

29-1 *Left to right, bottom:* I Verres needle stylet with adapter. *Top to bottom:* bipolar forceps; bipolar cord; telescope; Cohen cannula; and two black tips.

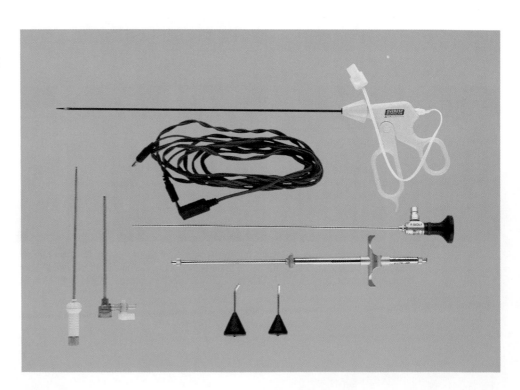

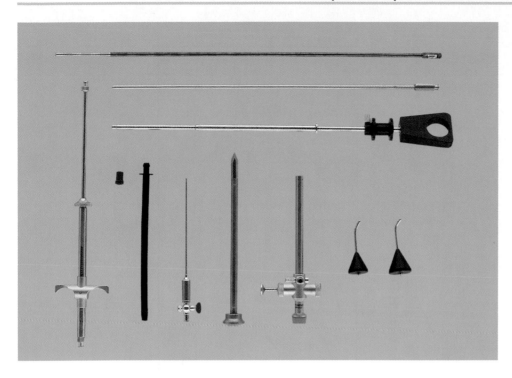

29-2 *Top to bottom:* 1 manipulation probe; 1 suction/irrigation cannula; 1 fallopian ring applicator. *Bottom, left to right:* 1 Cohen cannula, black nipple; 1 reducer cannula, 5 mm; 1 Verres needle stylet, medium; 1 trocar; trumpet-valve cannula; and 2 black Cohen nipples.

29-3 Position for tubal occlusion.

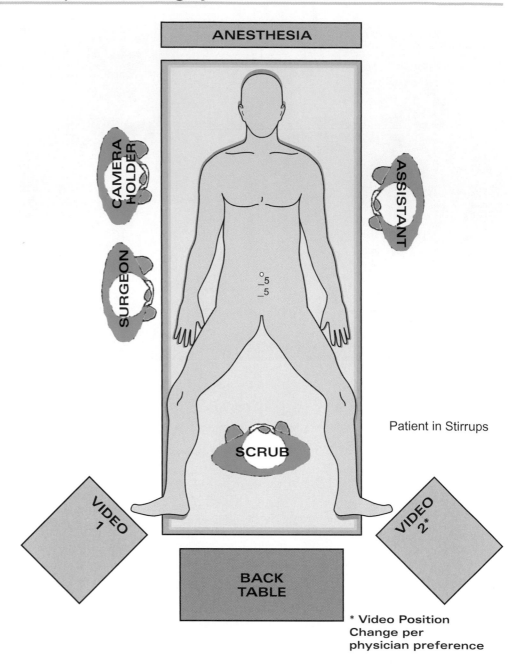

ANESTHESIA

CAMERA HOLDER

ASSISTANT

SURGEON

Patient in Stirrups

SCRUB

VIDEO 1

VIDEO 2*

BACK TABLE

* Video Position Change per physician preference

REVERSE FOR RIGHT SIDE
PATIENT IN LOW ALLEN STIRRUPS

Microtuboplasty

Microtuboplasty is the surgical repair of an occluded fallopian tube with the assistance of the operating microscope.

Equipment needed for the procedure includes a basic laparotomy set and self-retaining retractor.

For the procedure, very fine atraumatic instruments are used. A brief description of the procedure after the abdomen is opened and a self-retaining retractor placed is as follows:

1. A Frazier suction tip is used with a stylet.
2. A Gomel irrigator is used to lubricate delicate tissue.
3. Halstead mosquito forceps are used for stabilizing the tube.
4. Cottle hooks are used to hold the tube.
5. A Swolin Teflon angled rod, 1 mm, is used for probing the tube.
6. A Swolin Teflon angled rod, 3.5 mm, is used for dilating the tube.
7. Westcott scissors are used for dissection.
8. Storz microforceps are used for handling the tube during suturing.
9. A Barraquer needle holder is used for suturing.
10. Kelman-McPherson suture tying forceps are used for atraumatic knot tying of the suture.

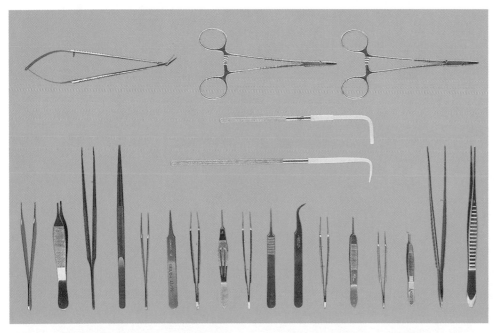

30-1 *Top, left to right:* 1 Castroviejo needle holder, curved, without lock; 2 Crile-Wood needle holders, 6 inch; 2 Swolin Teflon angled rods on handles, 1 mm and 3.5 mm. *Bottom, left to right:* 2 Brown-Adson tissue forceps (9 × 9), front view and side view; 2 titanium tying forceps, front view and side view; 3 jeweler's forceps #3, straight, front view, side view, and front view; 2 Castroviejo suturing forceps, 0.12 mm, with tying platforms, side view and front view; 1 Castroviejo suturing forceps, 0.5 mm, with tying platforms, side view; 1 jeweler's forceps, curved, side view; 2 Harms tying forceps without teeth, front view and side view; 1 McPherson tying forceps, straight, front view; 1 Kelman-McPherson tying forceps, curved, side view; 2 Cushing thumb forceps, front view and side view.

30-2 *Left to right:* **A**, Brown-Adson tissue forceps (9 × 9) and tip; **B**, Castroviejo suturing forceps, 0.12 mm, and tip; **C**, McPherson tying forceps, straight, 4.5 mm, tying platform, and tip; **D**, jeweler's forceps, curved, very fine, and tip; **E**, tip of jeweler's forceps, straight, very fine; **F**, tip of Kelman-McPherson suture tying forceps, angled, 7 mm, tying platform.

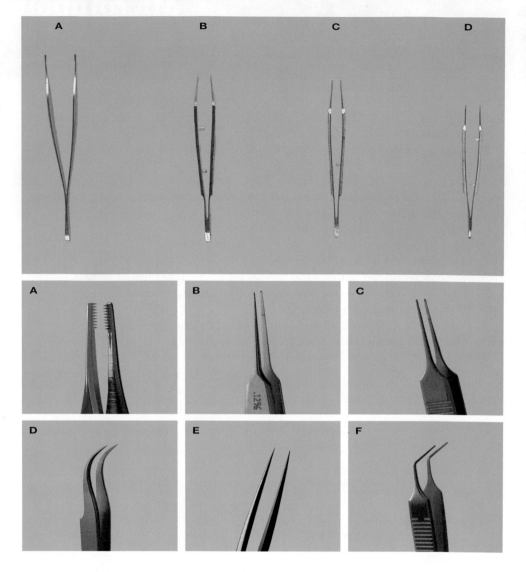

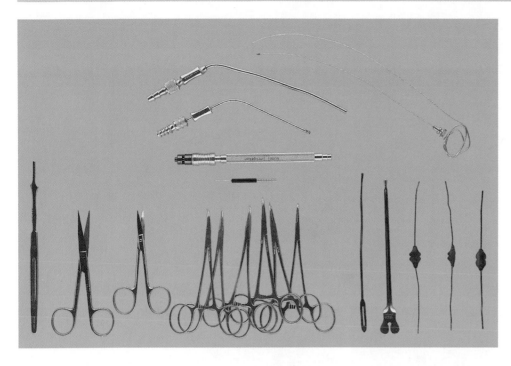

30-3 *Middle, top to bottom:* 1 Frazier suction tube, 11 Fr; 1 Frazier suction tube, 8 Fr; 1 Gomel irrigator; 1 nondisposable needle electrode, $^7/_8$ inch. *Top, right:* 2 suction tube stylets, 11 Fr, 8 Fr. *Bottom, left to right:* 1 Bard-Parker knife handle, #7; 2 plastic scissors, straight and curved; 6 Halsted mosquito hemostatic forceps, curved, delicate; 1 probe dilator; 1 grooved director; 3 Bowman (lacrymal) probes, 00-0, 1-2, 3-4.

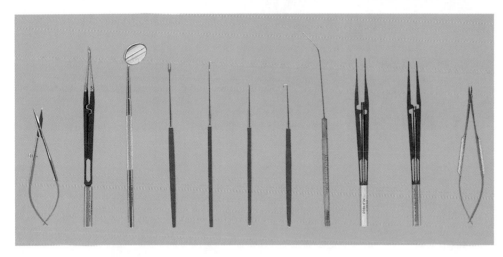

30-4 *Left to right,* 1 Westcott tenotomy scissors; 1 Vannas microscissors, curved; 1 front surface dental mirror (DMS-5 rhodium only); 2 Guthrie hooks, double, sharp, front view and side view; 2 Cottle skin hooks, single, front view and side view; 1 microprobe; 1 Storz microforceps with teeth; 1 Storz microforceps without teeth; 1 Barraquer needle holder, curved, without lock.

30-5 *Left to right.* **A**, Guthrie fixation hook, double, sharp, and tip; **B**, Cottle skin hook, single, and tip; **C**, Storz microforceps, without teeth, and tip; **D**, titanium tying forceps and tip.

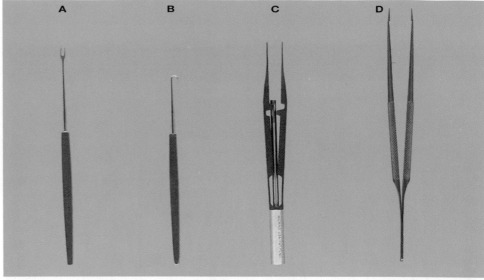

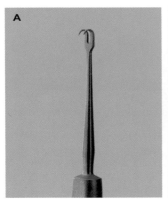
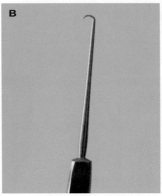
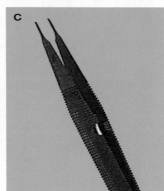
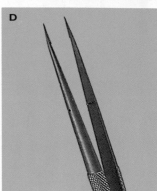

30-6 *Left to right:* Tips: Westcott tenotomy scissors; Barraquer needle holder, curved, without lock; Vannas microscissors, curved; microprobe.

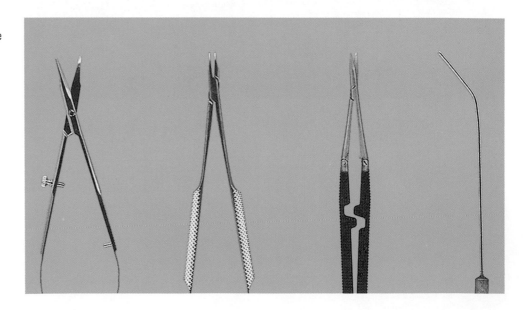

Cystoscopy*

Cystoscopy is the visualization of the urinary bladder via a cystoscope.

If a biopsy is done, possible equipment needed for the procedure includes biopsy forceps, which are used for taking tissue specimens, and a Bugbee electrode, which is used to cauterize bleeders.

If the urethra is constricted for any reason, possible equipment needed for the procedure includes an Otis urethrotome, with blade to incise the stricture, and van Buren dilators used for dilating.

A brief description of the procedure follows:

1. A sheath and obturator are lubricated and inserted into the urethra.
2. An obturator is removed and the cystoscope is inserted.
3. Irrigation tubing is attached, and the bladder is filled with solution for visualization.
4. A light cord is attached to the fiberoptic unit.

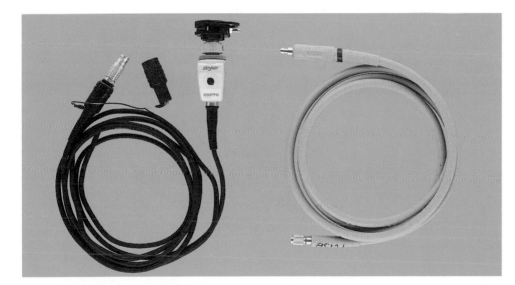

31-1 Standard cystoscopy set: camera, light cable.

*Additional images are available on the Companion CD.

31-2 *Left to right:* paper drape clip; Halstead hemostatic forceps, straight; Mayo dissecting scissors, straight; Crile hemostatic forceps, straight; and paper drape clip.

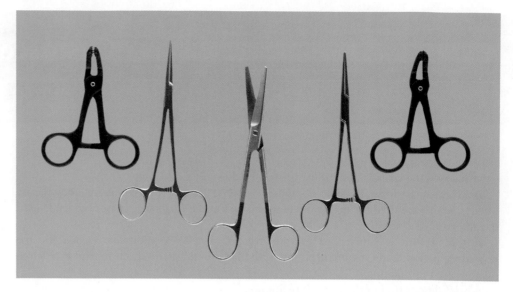

31-3 *Left to right:* 30-degree telescope; 70-degree telescope; Albarrán deflecting mechanism with double ports; obturator, 22 Fr; cystoscope sheath, 22 Fr. *Top to bottom:* 1 stopcock; 1 red port cap; 2 gray nipples; 2 bridges; and light cord.

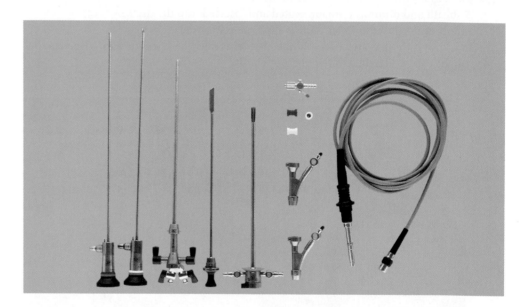

31-4 *Left to right:* double-action stent grasper; biopsy forceps, straight; and biopsy forceps, angled.

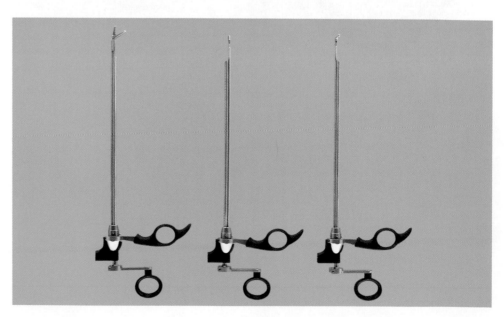

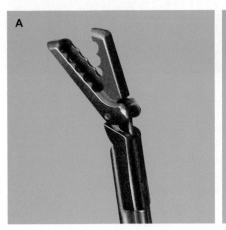
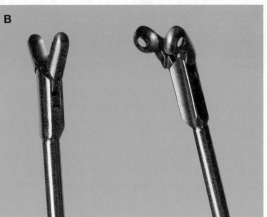

31-5 *Left to right.* Tip: **A** double-action stent grasper; **B**, biopsy forceps, angled and straight.

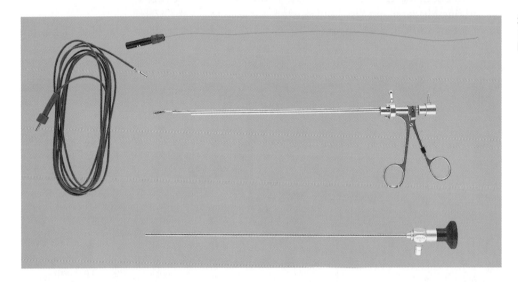

31-6 *Left:* 1 cautery cord. *Right, top to bottom:* 1 Bugbee electrode; 1 biopsy forceps; 1 telescope, 0 degree.

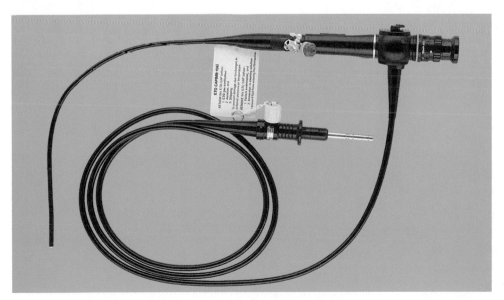

31-7 Olympus flexible cystoscope with cord.

Nephrectomy and Ureteroplasty

A nephrectomy is the removal of a kidney.

Equipment needed for the procedure includes a basic laparotomy set and self-retaining retractor.

A brief description of the nephrectomy procedure follows:

1. A Thompson retractor is used to expose the kidney area.
2. Metzenbaum dissecting scissors are used to incise Gerota's capsule.
3. Adson tissue forceps are used for blunt dissection and hemostasis.
4. Curved Mayo dissecting scissors are used for sharp dissection.
5. Mixter hemostatic forceps are used to double-clamp the ureter.
6. Long Metzenbaum dissecting scissors are used to cut the ureter.
7. A Guyon-Péan vessel clamp or Herrick kidney clamps are used to double-clamp the kidney pedicle.

32-1 *Left to right:* 1 Lincoln-Metzenbaum scissors, narrow dissecting tip; 1 Potts-Smith cardiovascular scissors, 45-degree angle; 1 probe dilator; 1 grooved director; 2 Hoen nerve hooks; 2 Love nerve retractors, straight, front view, 90-degree angle, side view; 2 Little retractors, medium; 4 Gil-Vernet retractors, assorted sizes.

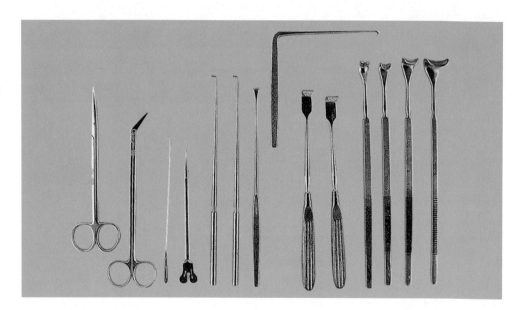

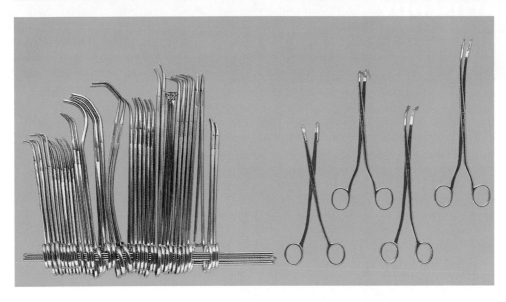

32-2 *Left to right:* 4 Westphal hemostatic forceps; 6 tonsil hemostatic forceps; 2 Adson hemostatic forceps, fine, curved; 1 Guyon-Péan vessel kidney clamp; 2 Herrick kidney clamps; 2 Satinsky (vena cava) clamps; 6 tonsil hemostatic forceps, 9½ inch; 2 tonsil hemostatic forceps, 10½ inch; 2 Babcock tissue forceps, extra long; 4 Mixter hemostatic forceps, 10½ inch, fine tip; 2 Ayers needle holders, extra long; 2 Heaney needle holders, long; 4 Randall stone forceps: full curve, ¾ curve, ½ curve, and ¼ curve.

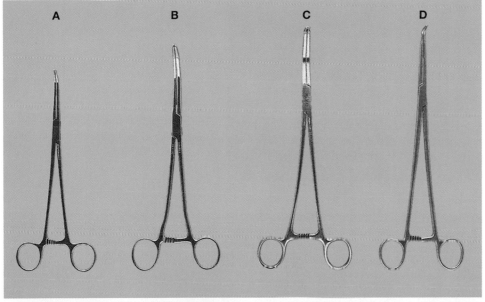

32-3 *Left to right:* **A**, Adson hemostatic forceps, fine curve, and tip; **B**, Herrick kidney clamp and tip; **C**, Satinsky (vena cava) clamp, medium, 4 cm, 9½ inch, and tip; **D**, Mixter hemostatic forceps, fine tip, 10½ inch, and tip; **E**, tip of Guyon-Péan vessel clamp, 9½ inch.

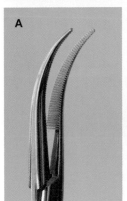
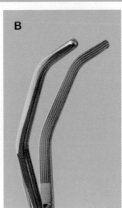
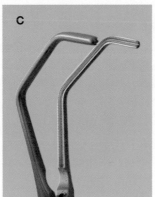
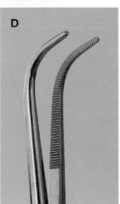
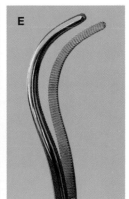

Urethroscopy

33-1 *Left to right:* 1 obturator; 1 urethroscope sheath; 1 telescope adapting bridge; 1 telescope, 0 degree; 1 urethrotome blade.

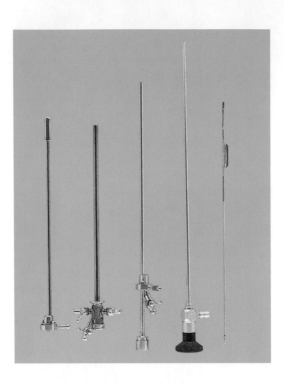

33-2 *Top to bottom:* Otis urethrotome: blade, urethrotome.

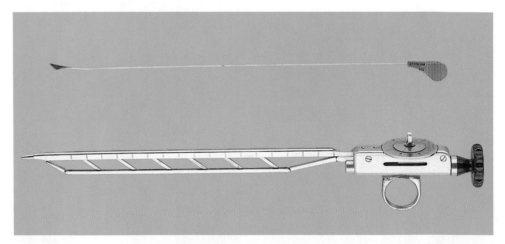

Prostatectomy

A prostatectomy is the removal of the prostate gland. The prostate may be removed in three ways: abdominally by a suprapubic or a retropubic approach; by a perineal approach; or transurethrally.

Instruments needed for a suprapubic approach include an electrosurgical unit, additional retractors, and a disposable skin stapler.

A brief description of the procedure follows:

1. After the abdomen is opened, a Balfour retractor with blades may be placed for visualization.
2. A Harrington retractor may be needed to retract the abdominal structures superiorly.
3. Long Allis forceps may be used to stabilize the bladder.
4. A Bard-Parker long scalpel handle #3 with a #10 blade may be used to incise into the bladder.
5. Long curved Metzenbaum dissecting scissors may be used to extend the incision.
6. A small Richardson retractor may be used to hold the bladder walls open.
7. The prostate gland is enucleated manually.
8. Horizon clip appliers and clips may be used for hemostasis.
9. A long, fine needle holder and long Autraugrip may be used to close the bladder.
10. After closing the abdominal layers, the skin may be closed with staples with the aid of Adson tissue forceps.

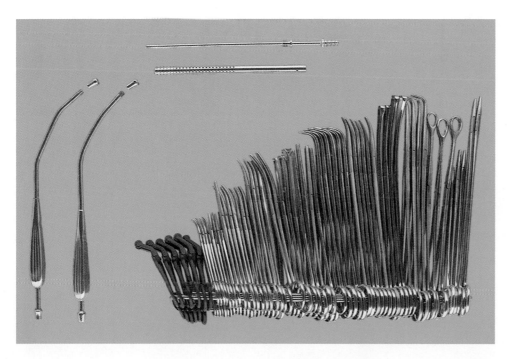

34-1 *Top:* 1 Poole abdominal suction tube and shield. *Left to right:* 2 Yankauer suction tubes and lips; 6 paper drape clips; 4 Halsted mosquito hemostatic forceps, curved; 4 Halsted mosquito hemostatic forceps, straight; 1 Halsted hemostatic forceps; 6 Crile hemostatic forceps, 6½ inch; 4 tonsil hemostatic forceps; 2 Mayo-Péan hemostatic forceps, curved; 2 Allis tissue forceps, medium; 1 Babcock tissue forceps, medium; 4 Ochsner hemostatic forceps, straight, long jaw; 6 Mixter hemostatic forceps, 9 inch; 6 tonsil hemostatic forceps, long; 4 Allis tissue forceps, extra long, curved; 4 Mixter hemostatic forceps, extra long; 3 Foerster sponge forceps; 2 Crile-Wood needle holders, 7 inch; 2 Crile-Wood needle holders, 8 inch; 2 Mayo-Hegar needle holders, 12 inch.

34-2 *Left to right:* 2 Bard-Parker knife handles #4; 1 Bard-Parker knife handle #3, long; 2 Mayo dissecting scissors, curved and straight; 2 Metzenbaum dissecting scissors, 7 inch and extra long; 2 Snowden-Pencer scissors, straight and curved; 1 Jorgenson dissecting scissors; 1 Mayo dissecting scissors, long, curved.

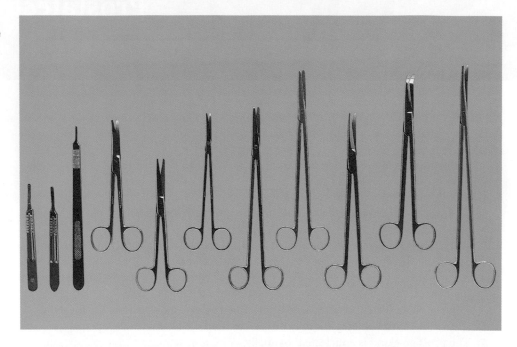

34-3 *Left to right:* 2 Adson tissue forceps (1 × 2), front, side view; 2 Ferris Smith tissue forceps (1 × 2), front, side view; 2 Russian tissue forceps, front, side view; 2 thumb tissue forceps with teeth (1 × 2), long, front, side view; 2 DeBakey vascular Autraugrip tissue forceps, long, front, side view; 2 DeBakey vascular Autraugrip tissue forceps, extra long, front, side view.

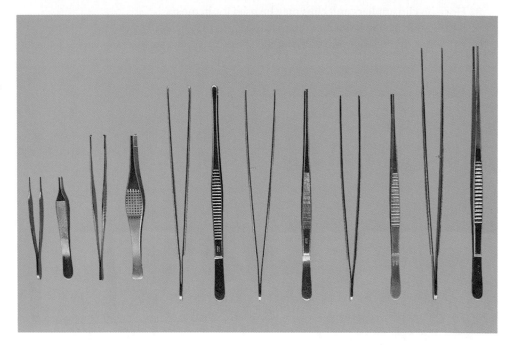

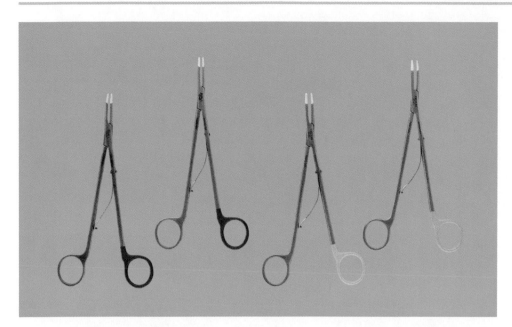

34-4 *Left to right:* Hemoclip-applying forceps, 2 medium, 2 large.

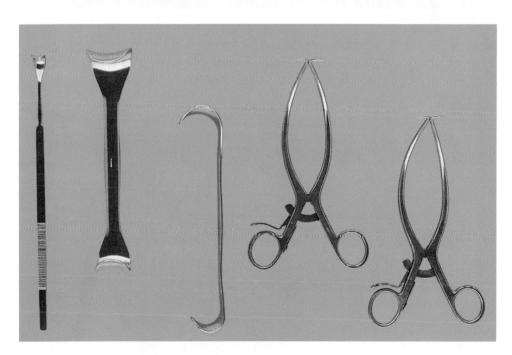

34-5 *Left to right:* 1 Gil-Vernet retractor; 2 Goelet retractors, front view and side view; 2 Gelpi retractors.

34-6 *Left to right:* 2 Greenwald suture guides, 24 Fr and 28 Fr; 3 Deaver retractors: narrow, side view; medium, front view; and wide, side view; 2 Harrington splanchnic retractors, small and large, side view.

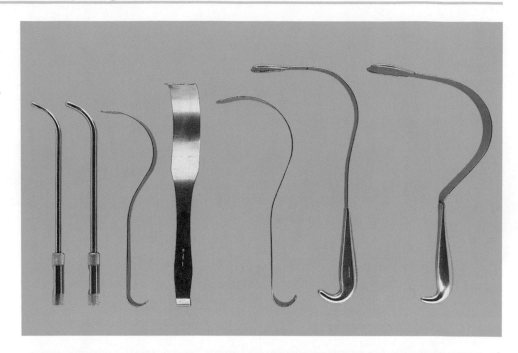

34-7 *Top:* 2 Balfour abdominal retractor fenestrated blades, large. *Left to right:* 1 Balfour abdominal retractor frame; 2 Balfour abdominal retractor fenestrated blades, small; 2 Balfour abdominal retractor center blades, large and small; 2 Richardson retractors, medium and large; 3 Ochsner malleable retractors, narrow (side view), medium, and large.

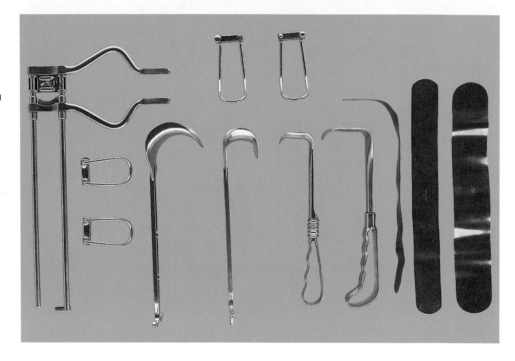

Transurethral Resection of the Prostate (TURP)*

Chapter 35

TURP is the removal of the enlarged portion of the prostate gland with a resectoscope.

Possible equipment needed for the procedure includes an electrosurgical unit, volumes of irrigating solution, a light source, and Ellik evacuator.

A brief description of the procedure follows:

1. A van Buren dilator is inserted to enlarge the urethra.
2. The resectoscope sheath with obturator is passed into the bladder.
3. Irrigating tubing is attached, and the bladder is filled with solution.
4. A fiberoptic cord and electrosurgery cord are connected.
5. An obturator is removed and the Iglesias working element is inserted.
6. A cutting electrode is inserted to remove prostate tissue.
7. A ball electrode is used to cauterize bleeders.
8. An Ellik evacuator is used to retrieve the specimen that has floated into the bladder.
9. A spoon is used for prostate tissue that is drained from the bladder and collects on the screen of the drape.

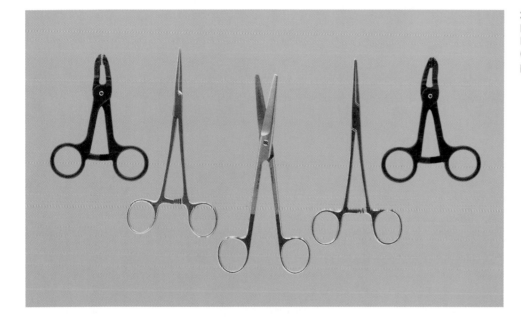

35-1 *Left to right:* paper drape clip; Halsted hemostatic forceps, straight; Mayo dissecting scissors, straight; Crile hemostatic forceps, straight; paper drape clip.

---

*Additional images are available on the Companion CD.

35-2 Resectoscopes: 30-degree telescope; obturator; inner sheath; outer sheath; working element. *Top to bottom:* 1 red port cap; 1 gray nipple; stopcock; 2 metal tubing connectors; bridge; and 2 peg clamps.

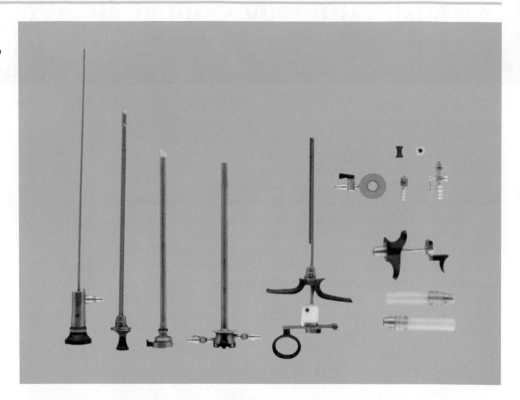

35-3 *Top, left to right:* plastic tubing; spoon. *Bottom, left to right:* inner sheath; obturator; outer sheath; light cord; van Buren urethral male sounds, 30 Fr to 22 Fr.

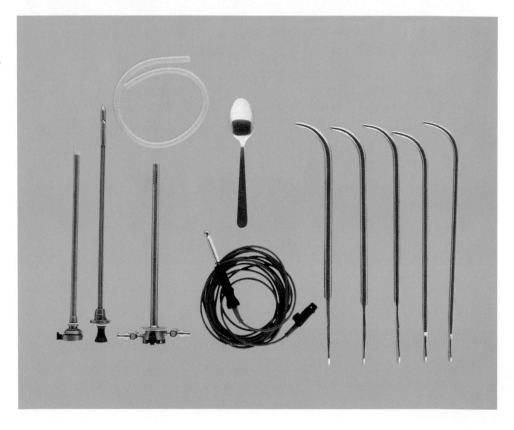

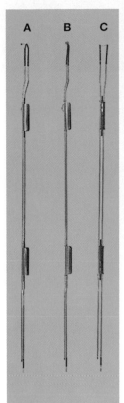

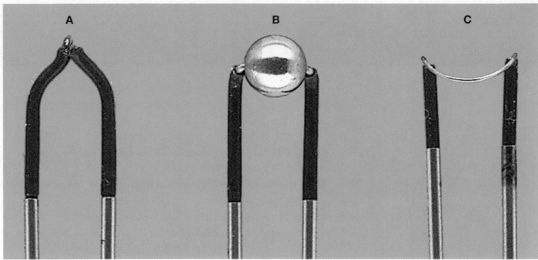

35-4   A, *Left to right:* **A**, cutting electrode with pointed end and tip; **B**, coagulating electrode with ball end and tip; **C**, cutting electrode with round wire and tip.

Vasectomy

A vasectomy is the transection of both vas deferens in the scrotum for the purpose of permanent sterilization.

A brief description of an open procedure follows:

1. A Beaver knife is used to make an incision over the vas.
2. Providence Hospital hemostatic forceps are used for clamping bleeders.
3. Westcott tenotomy scissors are used for blunt dissection of the vas.
4. Jeweler's forceps are used to grasp the vas.
5. Providence Hospital hemostatic forceps are used for clamping the vas.
6. A Beaver knife is used to bisect the vas.
7. DeBakey tissue forceps are used to assist in closing the incision.
8. A Barraquer needle holder is used to suture the incision.

36-1 *Top to bottom, left to right:* 1 Beaver knife handle, knurled, with tip; 1 jeweler's forceps; 2 DeBakey vascular Autraugrip tissue forceps, short. *Bottom, left to right:* 1 iris scissors, straight, sharp; 1 Stevens tenotomy scissors; 4 Providence Hospital hemostatic forceps; 2 Backhaus towel forceps.

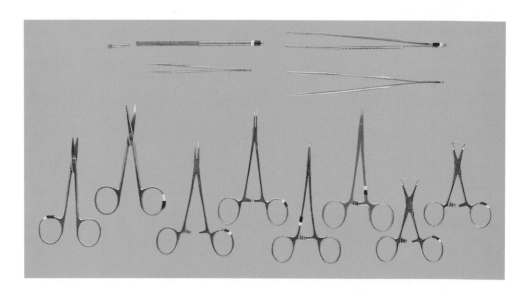

36-2 *Left to right:* 1 Vannas capsulotomy scissors; 1 Westcott tenotomy scissors; 3 Henle probes, assorted sizes; 1 lacrimal probe, 0-00; 1 titanium microneedle holder, nonlocking; 1 Barraquer needle holder, extra delicate, tapered, curved, with lock; 1 Troutman tier needle holder with lock.

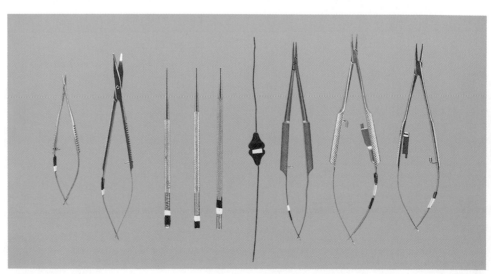

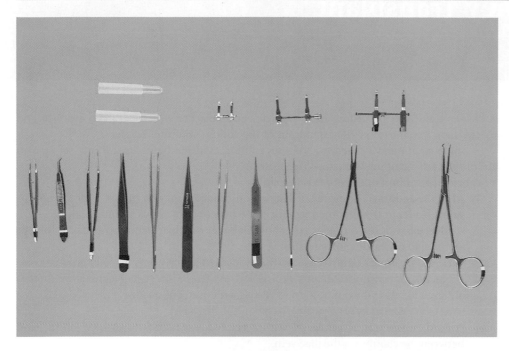

36-3 *Top, left to right:* 2 chamber maintainers; 1 Silber vasovasostomy clamp; 1 Strauch vasovasostomy approximator, hinged, small; 1 vasovasostomy approximator, hinged, large. *Bottom, left to right:* 2 McPherson tying forceps, angled, front view and side view; 1 Castroviejo suturing forceps, 0.12 mm, front view; 3 jeweler's forceps #3, side view, front view, and side view; 2 jeweler's forceps #4, front view and side view; 1 jeweler's forceps #5, front view; 1 Snowden-Pencer dissecting forceps; 1 Snowden-Pencer fixation forceps.

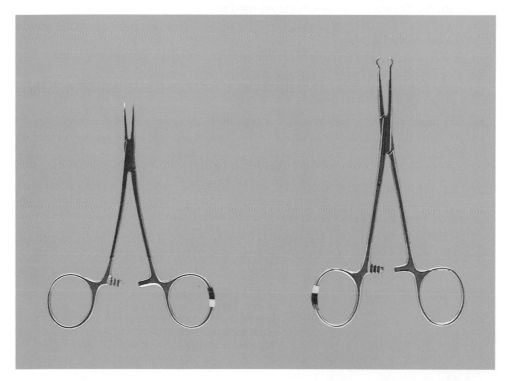

36-4 *Left to right:* 1 Snowden-Pencer dissecting forceps; 1 Snowden-Pencer fixation forceps.

Kidney Transplant

A kidney transplant procedure takes a kidney and adjacent structures from a donor and places them into the lower right quadrant of the abdomen of the recipient.

Possible equipment needed for the procedure includes a basic laparotomy set and an abdominal self-retaining retractor (Thompson).

A brief description of the procedure follows:

1. After the abdomen is opened, a Thompson retractor may be placed with the appropriate blades in the abdomen to deflect the peritoneum above and medially.
2. A Metzenbaum dissecting scissors and DeBakey vascular Autraugrip tissue forceps are used to dissect the internal iliac vessels.
3. A DeBakey vascular clamp is used to hold the internal iliac artery for later anastomosis.
4. A Hartmann mosquito forceps, an iris scissors, and a short DeBakey tissue forceps are used to revise the donor kidney, vessels, and ureter as needed.
5. Two Geary-DeBakey forceps are placed on the iliac vein.
6. A Bard-Parker scalpel handle #7 with a #11 blade is used to make a small incision between the clamps on the iliac vein.
7. Potts-Smith cardiovascular scissors are used to extend the incision, if needed.
8. A Fell needle holder and jeweler's forceps are used to anastomose the renal vein to the side of the iliac vein.
9. The renal artery and iliac artery are anastomosed using the same instruments.
10. Two long Babcock tissue forceps are used to grasp the bladder.
11. A Bard-Parker long scalpel handle #3 with a #10 blade is used to make an incision into the bladder.
12. The ureter is inserted between the layers of the bladder for a short distance.
13. An Ayers needle holder and a Gerald tissue forceps are used to suture the ureter into the bladder.

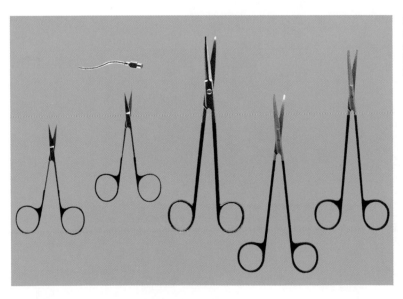

37-1 *Top:* Webster infusion cannula. *Bottom, left to right:* 2 iris scissors, straight, sharp, 4 inch; 1 facelift scissors, curved, 7¾ inch; 2 Metzenbaum scissors, curved, 7 inch.

37-2 Webster infusion cannula.

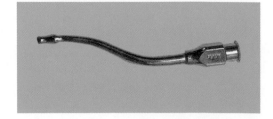

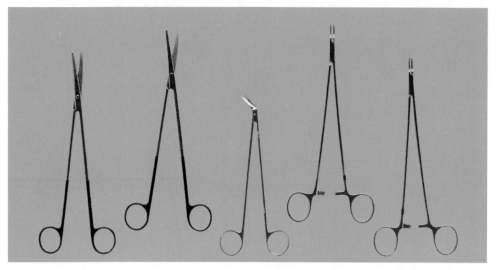

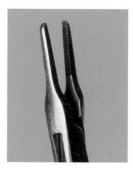

37-3 *Left to right:* 2 Metzenbaum scissors, curved, 9 inch; 1 Potts-Smith cardiovascular scissors; and 2 Ryder needle holders, 9 inch.

37-4 Tip of Ryder needle holder.

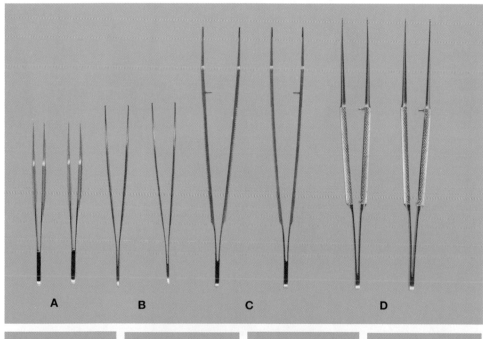

37-5 *Left to right:* **A**, 2 jeweler's forceps; and tip; **B**, 2 Adson tissue forceps with teeth (1 × 2), and tip; **C**, 2 Gerald-DeBakey tissue forceps, 7 inch, and tip; **D**, and 2 micro diamond dust ring forceps, 7 inch, and tip.

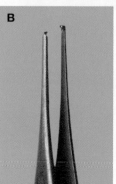

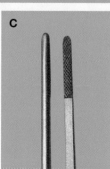

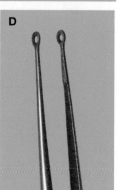

37-6 *Left to right:* **A**, 2 Autraugrip tissue forceps, titanium, and tips; **B**, 1 Kay aortic clamp, and tip; **C**, 2 Cushing vein retractors, and tips; **D**, 1 nerve hook, dull, and tip; **E**, 1 bulldog clamp applier, and tip; and **F**, 1 Lahey gall duct forceps, and tip.

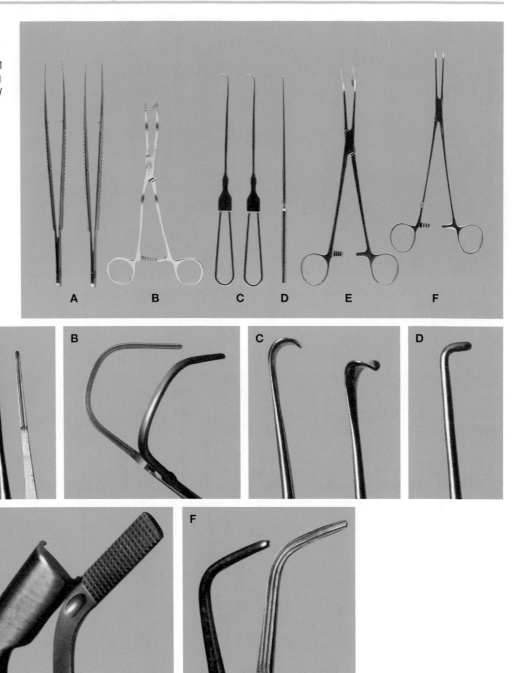

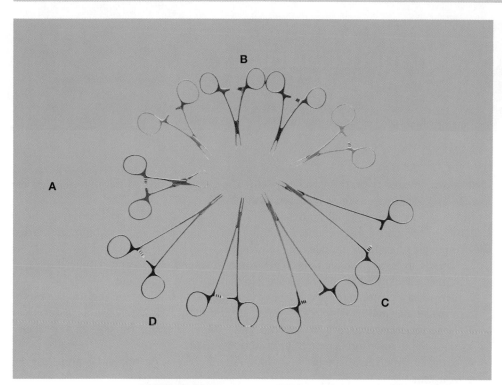

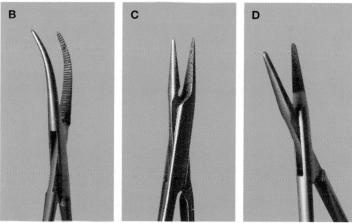

37-7 *Left center and clockwise:*
A, 1 Backhaus towel clip; **B**, 4 Hartmann mosquito forceps, curved, and tip; **C**, 2 micro diamond dust needle holders, 6¼ inch, and tip; and **D**, 2 Fell carbon inlay needle holders, 6 inch, and tip.

Chapter

38

Basic Orthopedic Surgery

Orthopedics is surgery on the skeletal system. The variety of procedures that may be performed are too numerous to be included in this book.

In most surgeries, a small soft-tissue dissection set is needed to expose the bony structures. The general instrumentation and a description of possible equipment needed for orthopedic procedures include the following:

1. Chisels are used to shape bone. They come in several widths and require the use of a mallet. Hoke and Hibbs chisels are two that are used commonly.
2. Periosteal elevators are used for removing periosteum. They too require the use of a mallet. Key and Langenbeck elevators are commonly used.
3. Bone curettes are used to scrape and shape bone. They are available in several cup sizes. Spratt and Cobb curettes are commonly used.
4. Rongeurs, used to shape bone, include Luer, Kerrison, Adson, and Smith-Petersen rongeurs.
5. Bone cutters are used to cut bone for removal. They include Ruskin-Liston and Horsley bone cutters.
6. Bone clamps are used to stabilize the long bones during fixation. They include Lowman and Kern clamps.
7. Retractors are used for visualization and sometimes for supporting structures during surgery. There are, among others, Hibbs, Taylor, Doane, and Bennett retractors.
8. Rasps are used to smooth the bone or to ream the shaft of a long bone for implantation. They include Putti, Aufricht, Wiener, and Lewis rasps.
9. Gouges are used for removing large pieces of bone. They are used with a mallet and include such names as Smith-Petersen, Hibbs, and Cobb.

38-1 *Top, left to right:* 1 metal medicine cup, 2 oz; 1 Mayo dissecting scissors, straight; 1 Metzenbaum scissors, 5 inch. *Bottom, left to right:* 2 Bard-Parker knife handles, #3; 1 plastic scissors, straight, sharp; 1 plastic scissors, curved, sharp; 2 thumb tissue forceps with teeth (1 × 2), front view and side view; 2 Adson tissue forceps with teeth (1 × 2), front view and side view; 2 Brown-Adson tissue forceps with teeth (9 × 9), front view and side view; 2 paper drape clips; 2 Backhaus towel forceps; 6 Halsted mosquito hemostatic forceps, curved; 2 Crile hemostatic forceps, curved, 5½ inch; 2 Allis tissue forceps; 2 Ochsner hemostatic forceps; 2 Crile-Wood needle holders, 6 inch; 1 Crile-Wood needle holder, 7 inch.

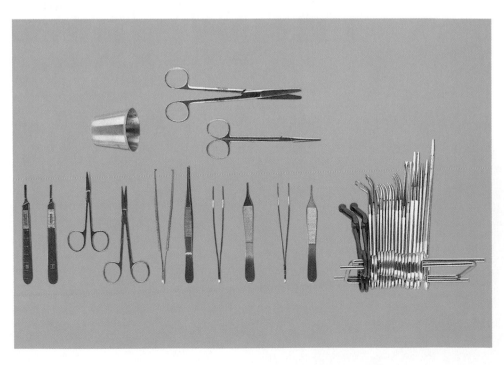

10. Bone hooks are used to stabilize bone.
11. Bone forceps such as the Joplin forceps are used to hold bone.
12. Mallets are used with chisels, periosteal elevators, gouges, impactors, and osteotomes. Some mallets are the Lucae, Mead, Heath, and Kirk mallets.
13. Osteotomes are used to shape bone and are used with a mallet. Cottle and Converse are the names of two osteotomes.

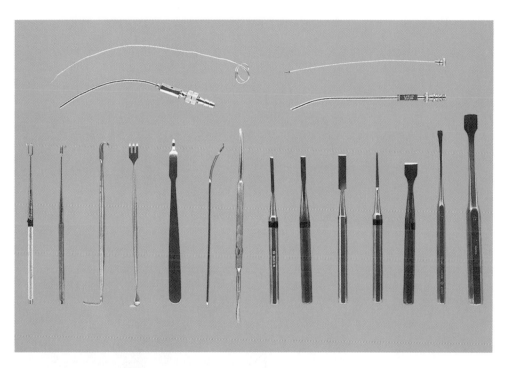

38-2 *Top:* 2 Adson suction tubes with finger valve controls and stylets: 9 Fr and 11 Fr. *Bottom, left to right:* 2 Joseph skin hooks, double prong, front view and side view; 2 Miller-Senn retractors, side view and front view; 2 Hohmann retractors, mini, front view and side view; 1 Freer elevator; 5 Hoke chisels, assorted sizes; 3 front view, 4th side view, and 5th front view; 1 Key periosteal elevator, ¼ inch; 1 Key periosteal elevator, ½ inch.

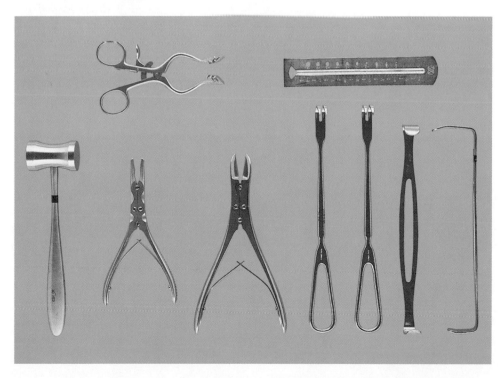

38-3 *Top, left to right:* 1 Weitlaner retractor, baby, curved; 1 metal ruler, 6 inch. *Bottom, left to right:* 1 Lucae mallet; 1 Ruskin rongeur, double-action; 1 Ruskin-Liston bone-cutting forceps; 2 Volkmann retractors, 2 prong, sharp; 2 Army Navy retractors, front view and side view.

39-1 *Left, top to bottom:* 1 Mayo dissecting scissors, straight; 1 Bard-Parker knife handle #7; 2 Bard-Parker knife handles #3. *Top right:* 2 Adson suction tubes, curved, with finger valve controls, and stylets. *Bottom, left to right:* 1 Mayo dissecting scissors, curved; 1 Metzenbaum dissecting scissors, 7 inch; 2 Adson tissue forceps with teeth (1 × 2), front view and side view; 2 thumb tissue forceps with teeth (1 × 2), front view and side view; 2 thumb tissue forceps with multiteeth (4 × 5), front view and side view; 2 Ferris Smith tissue forceps, front view and side view; 6 paper drape clips; 4 Halsted mosquito hemostatic forceps, curved; 2 Backhaus towel forceps; 4 Crile hemostatic forceps, 5½ inch; 4 Crile hemostatic forceps, 6½ inch; 2 Allis tissue forceps; 4 Ochsner hemostatic forceps, short; 2 tonsil hemostatic forceps; 2 Crile-Wood needle holders, 6 inch; 2 Crile-Wood needle holders, 7 inch.

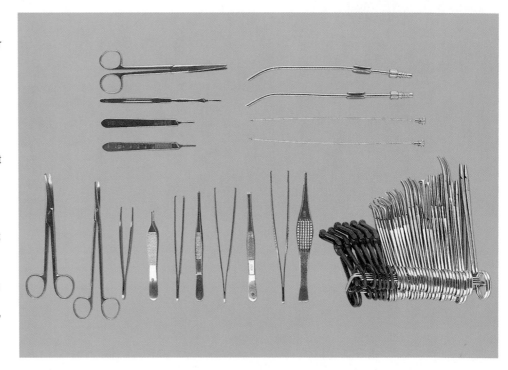

39-2 *Left to right:* 1 pliers; 1 Luer bone rongeur; 1 Adson rongeur, double-action; 1 Ruskin-Liston bone-cutting forceps, double-action; 1 Smith-Petersen laminectomy rongeur, double-action.

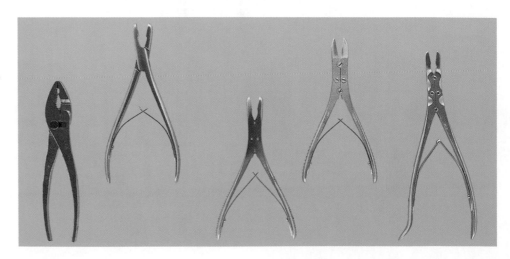

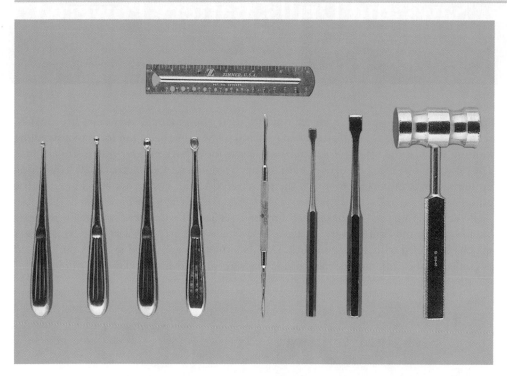

39-3 *Top:* 1 metal ruler, 6 inch. *Bottom, left to right:* 4 Spratt curettes, #2 through #5; 1 Freer elevator; 1 Key periosteal elevator, ¼ inch; 1 Key periosteal elevator, ½ inch; 1 metal mallet.

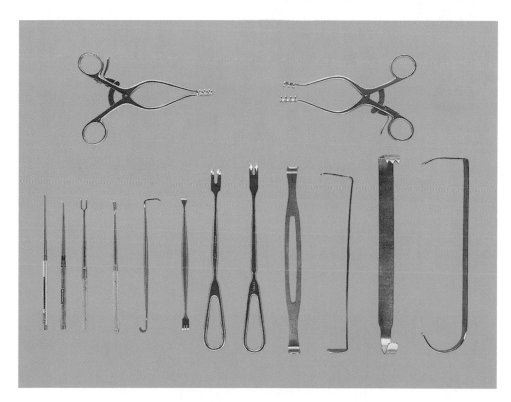

39-4 *Top:* 2 Weitlaner retractors, sharp prong, medium. *Bottom, left to right:* 2 Joseph skin hooks, single prong, side view; 2 Joseph skin hooks, double prong, front view and side view; 2 Miller-Senn retractors, side view and front view; 2 Volkmann retractors, 2 prong, sharp; 2 Army Navy retractors, front view and side view; 2 Hibbs laminectomy retractors, narrow, front view and side view.

Power saws and power drills are commonly used equipment. Power saws are used to remove or shape bone. The blades of an oscillating saw move back and forth in a swinging motion, whereas the blades of a reciprocating saw move back and forth in a straight line. The power source may be a battery pack, compressed nitrogen, or electricity. When setting up the saw, it is important to attach the power cord to the saw before attaching it to the power source.

Power drills are used to make holes for the insertion of wires or screws or for reaming long bones. Some drill bits are attached by a chuck that requires a key, whereas others may be tightened with a keyless chuck. Drill bits may be cannulated so wires can be used as guides for the drill. Power drills include the Maxi driver, Mini Stryker, and MicroAire.

40-1 Stryker System 5 in case: drills, batteries, and most of the attachments are shown in the top right of the case. *For right, top:* pin collet.

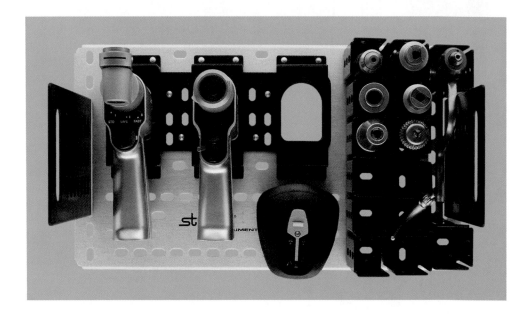

---

*Additional images available on the Companion CD.

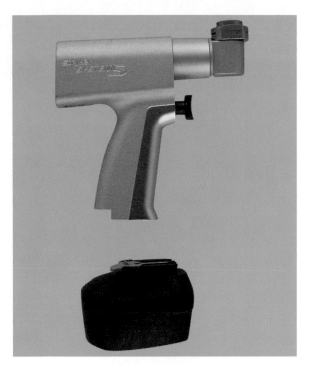

40-2 *Top to bottom:* Oscillating saw and battery.

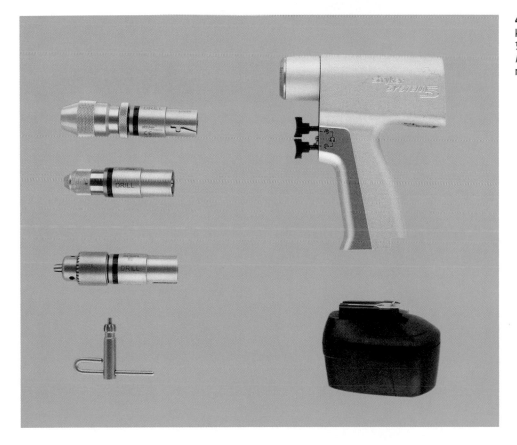

40-3 *Left, top to bottom:* ¼ inch keyless drill attachment; drill; ¼ inch drill; and chuck key. *Right, top to bottom:* dual trigger rotary handpiece; and battery.

40-4 Stryker Mini 4200 Driver in case.

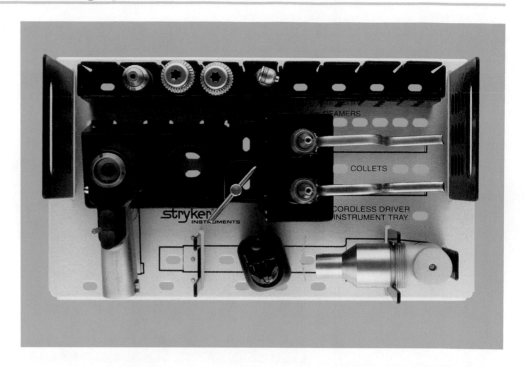

40-5 *Left, top to bottom:* Dual-trigger rotary handpiece; battery. *Middle:* pin collet. *Right, top to bottom:* Jacobs chuck attachment; chuck key; oscillating saw attachment; and Synthes chuck.

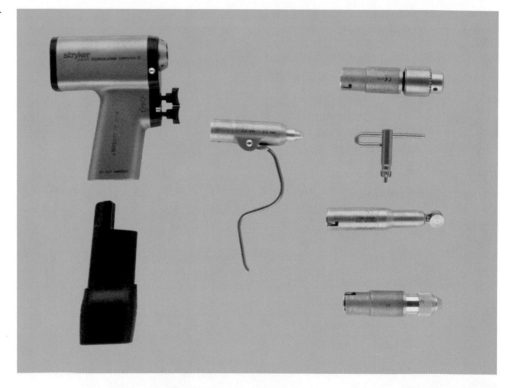

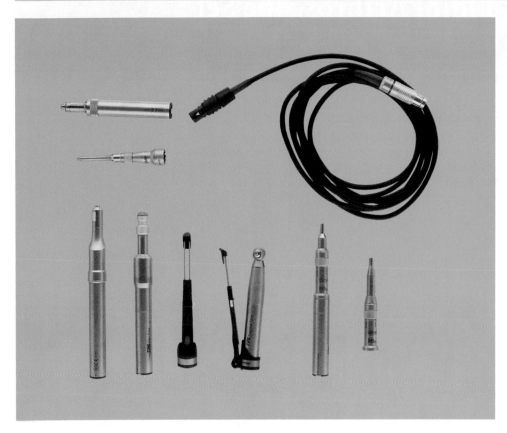

40-6 Stryker TPS Ortho Power System, electricity powered (micro driver). *Left to right, top to bottom:* Drill attachment; drill and burr attachment; and power cord. *Bottom, left to right:* Straight saw; right-angle saw; TPS elite medium attachment; saw handpiece; reciprocating saw; and drill and burr.

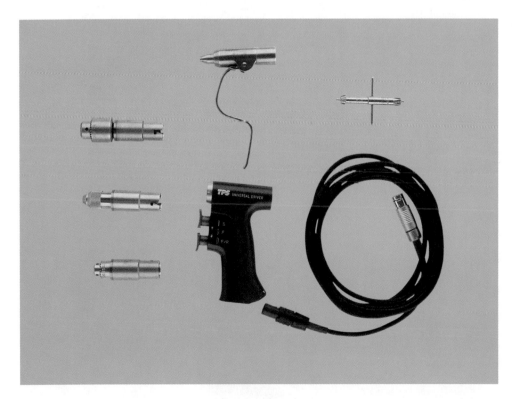

40-7 *Left to right, top to bottom:* ¼ inch drill; Synthes drill; and ⁵/₃₂ inch Jacobs drill; wire collet; and dual trigger handpiece. *Right, top to bottom:* chuck key; and power cord.

Small Joint Arthroscope Set

Arthroscopy is the visualization of a joint via a scope. The diameter and length of the scope vary according to the size of the joint.

Possible equipment needed for the procedure includes 1 Bard-Parker knife handle #3; 1 Adson tissue forceps with teeth (1 × 2); 1 Mayo dissecting scissors, straight; 1 Halsted mosquito hemostatic forceps, curved; and 1 Webster needle holder.

41-1 *Left to right:* 1 trocar sleeve, 2.7 mm; 1 pyramidal trocar; 1 blunt obturator; 1 probe; 1 telescope lens, 25-degree.

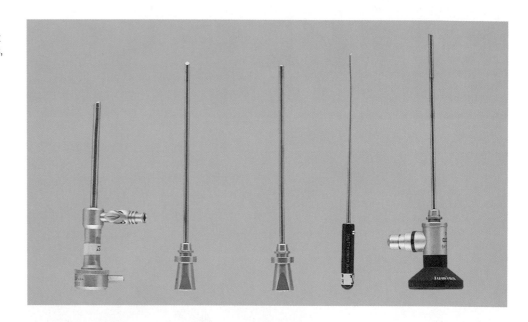

41-2 *In case, left:* 1 blunt probe; 1 hook probe; 1 straight rasp; 1 angled-down rasp; 1 angled-up rasp; 1 lateral-release knife; 1 retrograde knife; 1 serrated banana knife; 1 meniscectomy knife, right; 1 meniscectomy knife, left; 1 handle. *In case, right top:* 1 blunt obturator; 1 pyramidal trocar; *Right bottom:* 2 trocar sleeves; telescope lens, 30 degree. *Right, top to bottom, not in case:* 1 cup forceps; 1 scissors; 1 grasper.

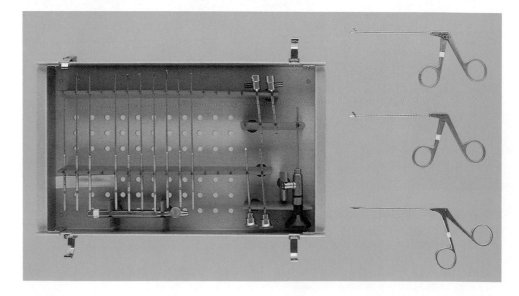

Arthroscopic Carpel Tunnel Instruments

Carpal tunnel syndrome is the narrowing of the space where the median nerve enters the hand from the wrist. An arthroscope is used for the arthroscopic carpal tunnel release procedure. Lactated Ringer's solution or saline is often used to distend the joint for visualization.

Possible carpal tunnel instruments needed for the procedure include a small joint arthroscope set, 1 Bard-Parker knife handle #3; 1 Mayo dissecting scissors, straight; 1 Adson tissue forceps with teeth (1 × 2); and 1 Crile-Wood needle holder.

A brief description of the arthroscopic carpal tunnel release procedure follows:
1. A small arthroscope is inserted with the usual attachments into the carpal tunnel.
2. A retrograde knife incises the flexor reticulum with the aid of the arthroscope.

A brief description of the open carpal tunnel release procedure follows:
1. A Bard-Parker scalpel handle #3 with a #10 blade is used to make a small incision in the palm of the hand.
2. A probe is inserted along the carpal tunnel narrowing.
3. A #3 Hegar dilator may be inserted to open the space.
4. A blunt dissector may be used to release the stricture.

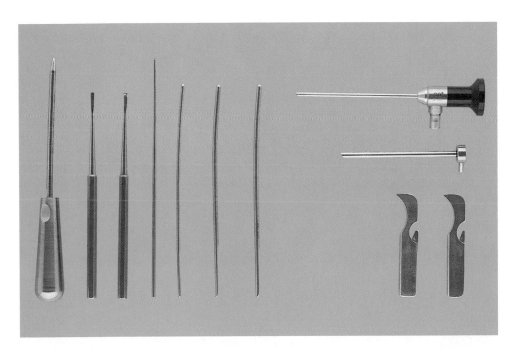

42-1 *Left to right:* 1 ridged obturator; 1 straight blunt dissector; 1 curved blunt dissector; 1 right-angle probe; 3 Hegar dilators (3, 4, and 5). *Right, top to bottom:* 1 carpal tunnel video endoscope, 30 degree; 1 slotted cannula; 2 gold handles for disposable carpal tunnel blades.

Small/Minor Joint Replacement

Small joints are replaced with Silastic prosthetics to relieve pain and improve function.

Possible equipment needed for the procedure includes a small bone set; a prosthesis; and a mini drill with bits and burrs.

A brief description of the procedure follows:

1. A Bard-Parker scalpel handle #3 with #15 blade is used to make an incision on the dorsal side of the joint.
2. A Weitlaner retractor is placed to expose the joint.
3. A Ruskin-Liston bone cutter is used to cut the distal and proximal ends of the bones of the joint.
4. An Adson rongeur is used to round the bone ends.
5. The mini drill is used to ream both bone canals.
6. The caliper is used to measure the length of the bone for sizing the prosthesis.
7. The Silastic prosthesis is inserted.
8. The ligaments and tendons are reattached as needed.
9. The incision is closed.

43-1 *Top to bottom, left to right:* 1 Metzenbaum dissecting scissors, 7 inch; 1 Mayo dissecting scissors, straight; 1 bandage scissors, 8 inch; 1 Mayo dissecting scissors, curved. *Bottom, left to right:* 2 Bard-Parker knife handles #3; 1 Bard-Parker knife handle #4; 2 Adson tissue forceps with teeth (1 × 2), front view and side view; 2 Ferris Smith tissue forceps, front view and side view; 2 Cushing tissue forceps with teeth (1 × 2), 8 inch, front view and side view; 6 paper drape clips; 2 Backhaus towel forceps; 6 Crile hemostatic forceps, 5½ inch; 2 tonsil hemostatic forceps; 2 Ochsner hemostatic forceps, long; 2 Allis tissue forceps, long; 2 Crile-Wood needle holders, 7 inch.

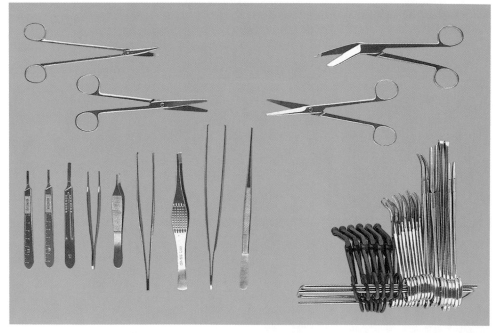

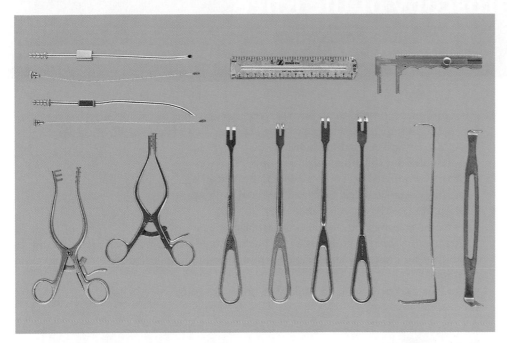

43-2 *Top, left to right:* 2 Adson suction tubes with finger valve controls: 1 straight, 1 curved, with stylets; 1 metal ruler, 6 inch; 1 caliper, inside/outside. *Bottom, left to right:* 2 Weitlaner retractors, sharp, medium; 2 Volkmann retractors, 2 prong, sharp; 2 Volkmann retractors, 2 prong, dull; 2 Army Navy retractors, side view and front view.

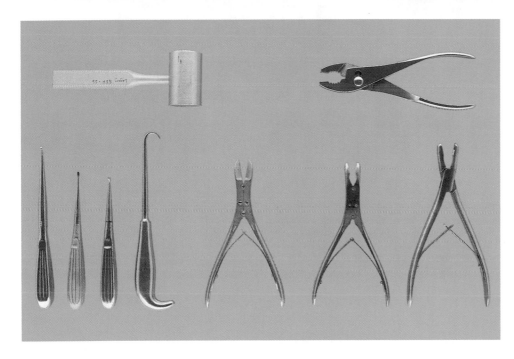

43-3 *Top, left to right:* 1 Heath mallet; 1 pliers. *Bottom, left to right:* 3 Spratt curettes: long curved, 2-0, and 3-0; 1 Ruskin-Liston bone-cutting forceps, double-action; 1 Adson rongeur, double action; 1 Luer bone rongeur.

Arthroscopy of the Knee

Possible equipment needed to perform surgery through an arthroscope includes:

1. An Acufex punch, used to grasp "tough" tissue, such as periosteum or cartilage.
2. An Acufex basket, used to remove tissue.
3. An Acufex duckbill biter, used to remove cartilage.
4. Acorn cannulated drill bits, used for femoral drilling.
5. Acufex cannulated drill bits, used for tibial drilling.
6. Rasp tips used to smooth bone.
7. A meniscectomy knife, used to cut cartilage.
8. Arthrex tips, used as graft pushers to push the tendon into position; a femoral tunnel notcher for graft attachment; and a femoral positioning drill guide for placing guide wires.
9. An Isotac screwdriver used with suture to secure graft.

44-1 *Top, right:* Large bandage scissors. *Bottom, left to right:* 1 Bard-Parker knife handle, #3; 1 self-locking trocar sleeve, 4 mm; 1 blunt obturator, 4 mm; 1 LUMINA telescope, 25 degree, 4 mm; 1 egress cannula, 4.5 mm; 1 pyramidal trocar, 3.7 mm; 1 conical obturator, 3.7 mm; 2 probes; 1 Adson tissue forceps with teeth (1 × 2); 1 Crile-Wood needle holder, 6 inch; 1 Mayo dissecting scissors, straight.

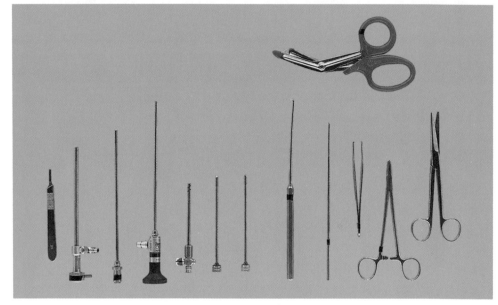

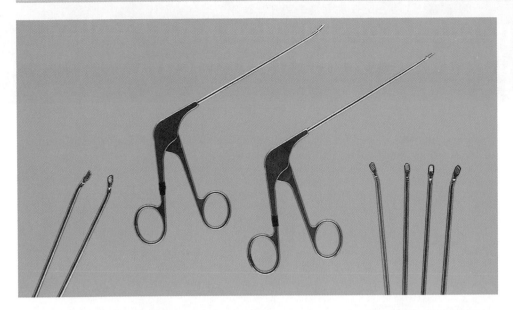

44-2 *Left to right:* Tips: 1 Acufex duckbill biter, right; 1 Acufex duckbill biter, left. 1 Acufex duckbill biter, upbite; 1 Acufex duckbill biter, straight bite. Tips: 4 Acufex ducklings bill biters: right; upbite; straight; left.

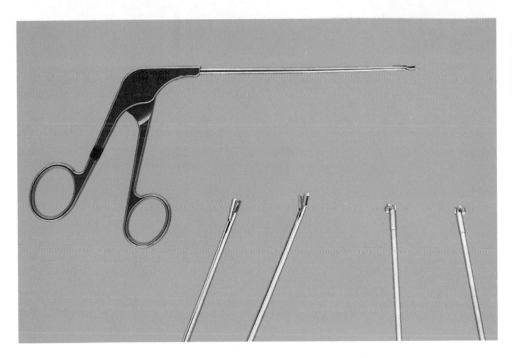

44-3 *Left to right:* 1 grasper. Tips: I Acufex upbiting linear punch, 1.3 mm; 1 Acufex upbiting linear punch, 1.5 mm; 1 Acufex basket, 90 degree, 2.2 mm, left; 1 Acufex basket, 90 degree, 2.2 mm, right.

Chapter 45

Arthroscopic Anterior Cruciate Ligament Reconstruction with Patellar Tendon Bone Graft Instruments

Possible equipment needed for the procedure includes a knee arthroscopic instrument set, an arthroscopic wand, and an arthroscopic shaver.

45-1 *Top, left to right:* 1 tonsil hemostatic forceps, straight; 1 Webster needle holder, 5 inch; 1 small sharp scissors. *Middle:* 1 Jacobs chuck. *Bottom, left to right:* 7 Acufex graft sizers, 6 mm to 12 mm; 3 Acufex isometric centering guides, 7 to 8 mm, 9 to 10 mm, 11 mm; 1 parallel drill guide, 5 mm; 1 isometric positioner; 6 acorn cannulated drill bits for femoral drilling; 6 Acufex cannulated drill bits for tibial drilling.

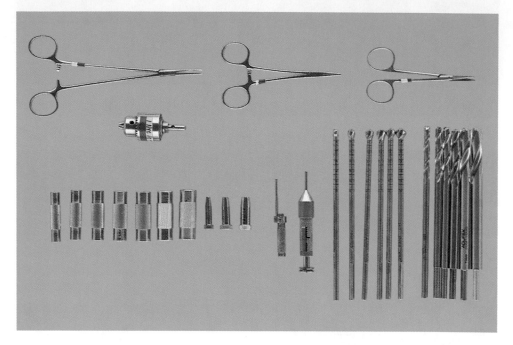

130

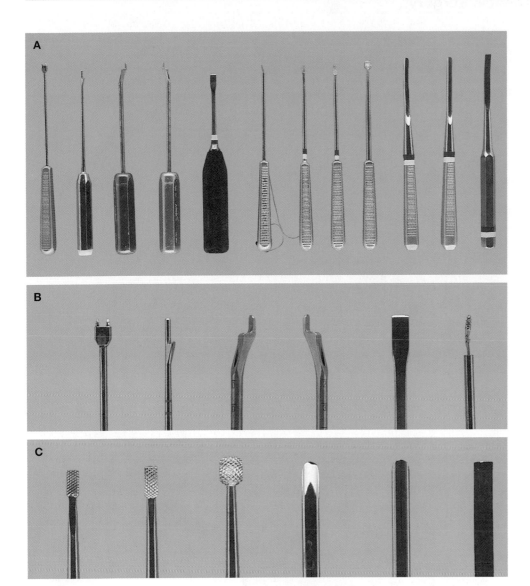

45-2 A, *Left to right:* 1 Arthrex graft pusher; 1 Arthrex femoral tunnel notcher; 1 Arthrex over-the-top femoral positioning drill guide, 6 mm; 1 Arthrex over-the-top femoral positioning drill guide, 7 mm; 1 osteotome, thin, ¼ inch; 1 Isotac screwdriver with suture and Isotac in place; 3 chamfering rasps, convex, concave, half-round; 2 gouges, ¼ inch, straight and curved; 1 osteotome, ¼ inch, curved. **B,** *Left to right:* 5 Arthrex tips: graft pusher; femoral tunnel notcher; over-the-top femoral positioning drill guide, 6 mm; over-the-top femoral positioning drill guide, 7 mm; osteotome ¼ inch, thin; Isotac screwdriver with suture and Isotac in place. **C,** *Left to right:* 3 rasp tips: convex, concave, and half-round; 2 gouges ¼ inch, tips: straight and curved; 1 osteotome ¼ inch, curved.

45-3 *Top to bottom:* 2 Hyperflex guide wires; 2 Beath passing pins; 1 K-wire; 1 drill bit, ¹/₁₆ inch. *Bottom, left to right:* 3 templates: 8 and 9, side view; 10, front view; 1 Beyer rongeur curved; 1 Ferris Smith rongeur, cup jaw (Martin); 1 pituitary rongeur.

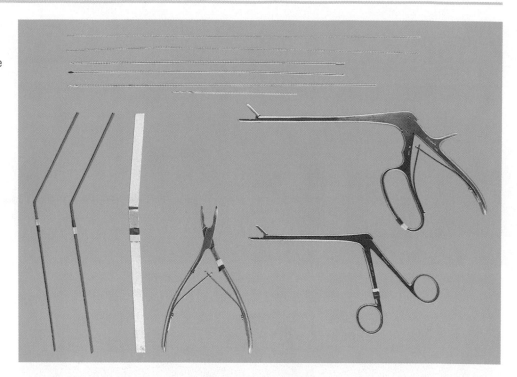

45-4 *Left to right:* 2 tibial aiming hooks, right and left, for Arthrex tibial guide; 1 K-wire sleeve for Concept precise tibial aiming guide; 1 K-wire sleeve for Arthrex tibial aiming guide; 1 notchplasty gouge. *Right, top to bottom:* 1 Concept precise tibial aiming guide; 1 Arthrex tibial aiming guide.

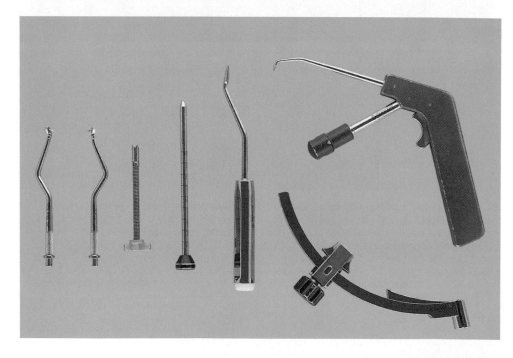

A total knee replacement is the removal of the distal end of the femur and the proximal end of the tibia. A prosthesis is used to reestablish the joint.

Possible equipment needed for the procedure includes a small/minor joint replacement set and Stryker battery powered drills.

A brief description of the procedure follows:

1. A Doane retractor is used to protect the medial collateral ligament.
2. An alignment guide is placed lateral to the tibial tubercle.
3. A power saw is used to resect the proximal end of the tibia.
4. Spacer/alignment blocks are used to check for valgus alignment.
5. The AP cutting guide is used to determine where to cut the femur.
6. The saw is used to resect the distal end of the femur.
7. Tibial and femoral ends are checked for size.
8. The trial components are placed and secured.
9. The joint is evaluated and the trials are removed.
10. A prosthesis is chosen and placed. Both a femoral impactor and a tibial impactor are needed. A mallet is used to seat each component.

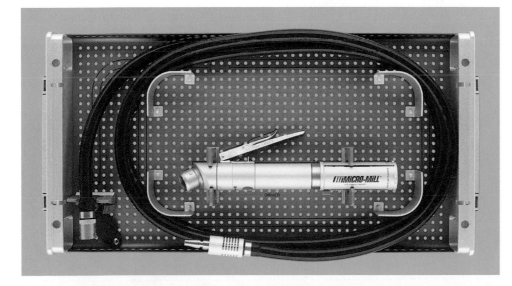

46-1 Micro-mill driver and attachments.

*Instrumentation in Figures 46-1 through 46-13 was provided by Zimmer-Pasion, Inc., Beaverton, OR.

46-2 Intramedullar (IM) instruments.

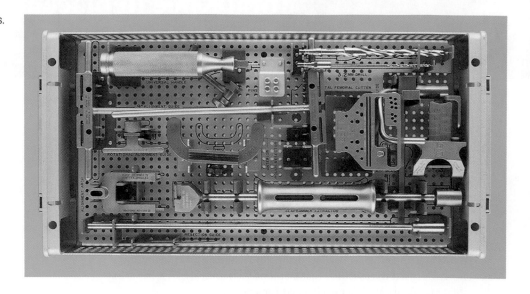

46-3 Femoral resection/finishing (5 in 1) instruments.

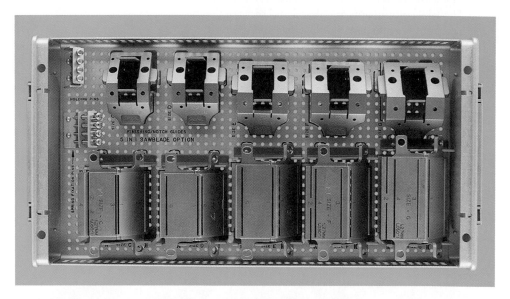

46-4 IM femoral finishing instruments.

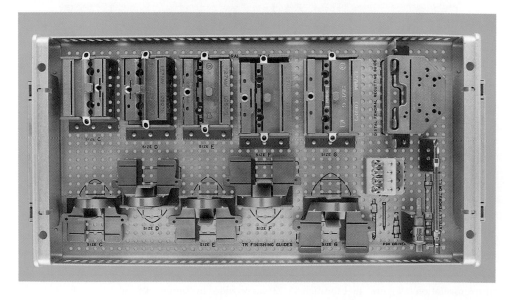

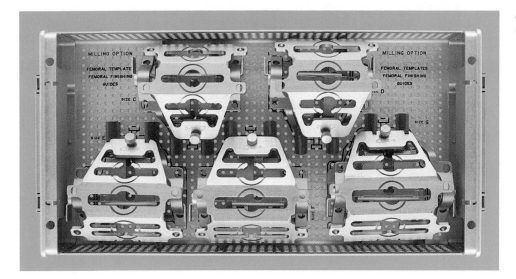

46-5 Femoral resection/finishing milling instruments.

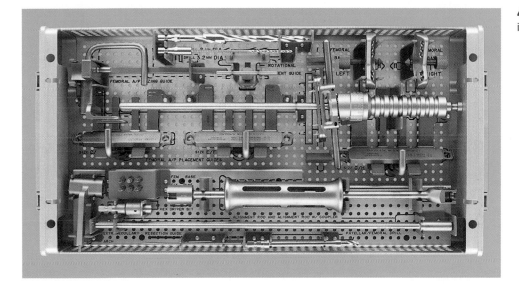

46-6 Femoral sizing/alignment instruments.

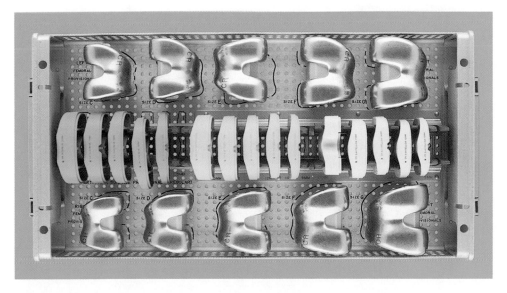

46-7 Cruciate retaining (CR) provisionals.

46-8 IM tibial alignment/finishing instruments.

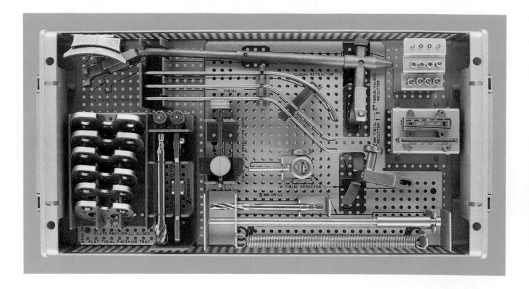

46-9 Tibial alignment/resection instruments.

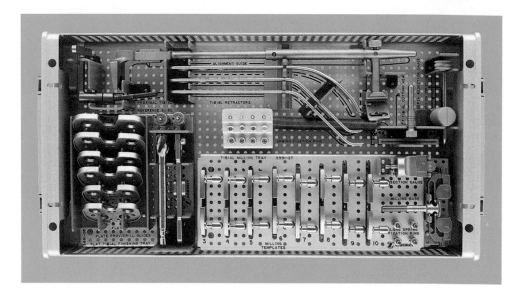

46-10 Patellar/spacer guide instruments (first tray): spacer/alignment guides, recutting blocks.

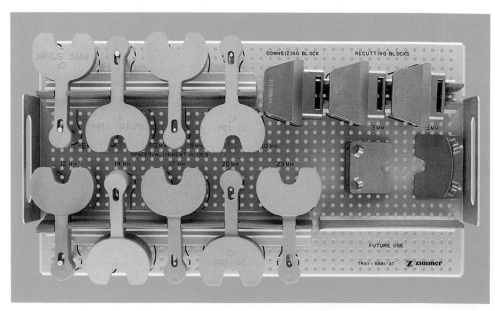

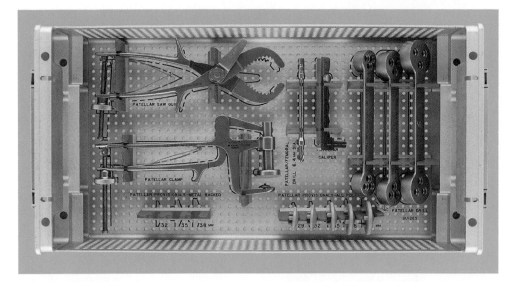

46-11 Patellar/spacer guide instruments (second tray).

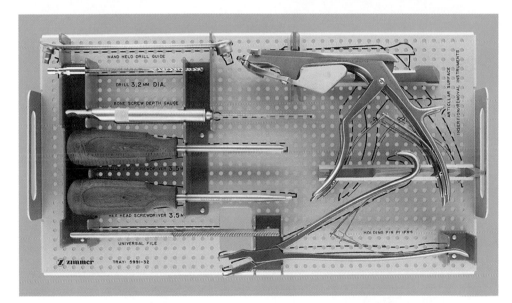

46-12 Tibial/femoral implant instruments (first tray).

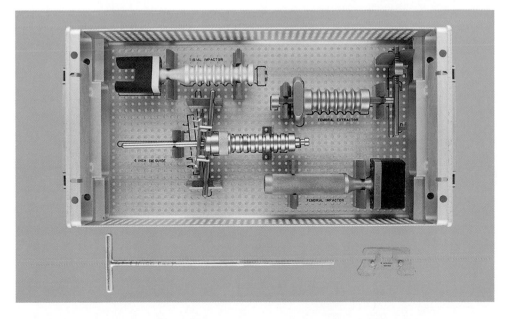

46-13 Tibial/femoral implant instruments (second tray).

46-14 Alvarado knee support.

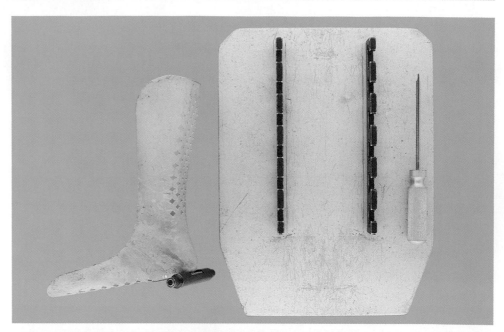

46-15 Stryker cement gun.

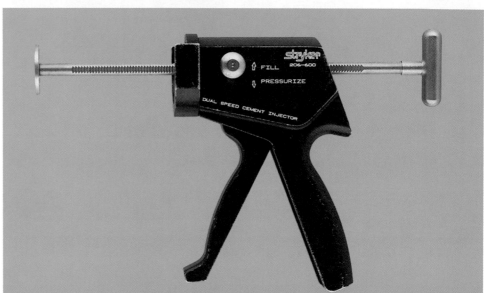

46-16 *Left to right:* 1 impactor; 2 Doane retractors, side view and front view.

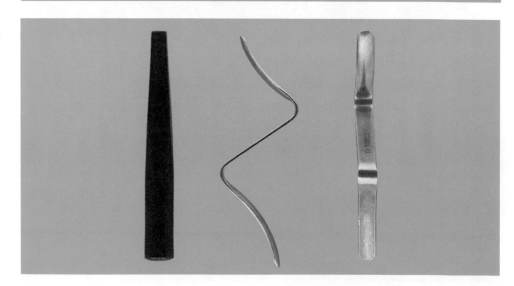

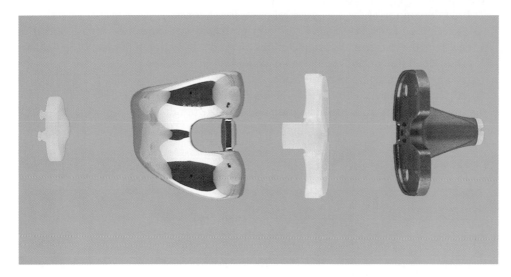

47-1 NexGen system. *Left to right:* 1 patella button; 1 femoral component; 1 articulating surface; 1 stem–tibial base plate.

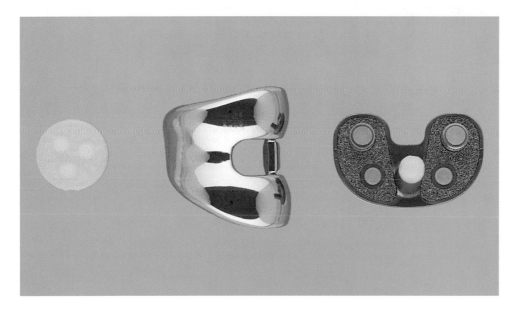

47-2 NexGen system. *Left to right:* 1 patella button; 1 femoral component; 1 porous stem–tibial base plate.

Shoulder Surgery Instruments

Possible equipment needed for the arthroscopic procedure in the shoulder includes an arthroscope; arthroscopic knee instruments; a bipolar wand coagulator, used for hemostasis; and a bipolar cord, used to connect to the power source.

A brief description of the open surgical procedure follows:

1. Retractors that help visualize the joint and hold structures out of the operative field are the humeral head retractor, the glenoid self-retaining retractor, the Bankart shoulder retractor, and the Bateman glenoid retractor.
2. A bone file is used to shape the bone.
3. A glenoid punch is used to grasp the cartilage.
4. Joplin bone forceps are used to grasp and stabilize bone.

48-1 *Left to right:* 2 humeral head retractors, side view and front view; 2 Richardson retractors, small, side view and front view; 2 Richardson retractors, medium, side view and front view; 2 Hibbs laminectomy retractors, side view and front view.

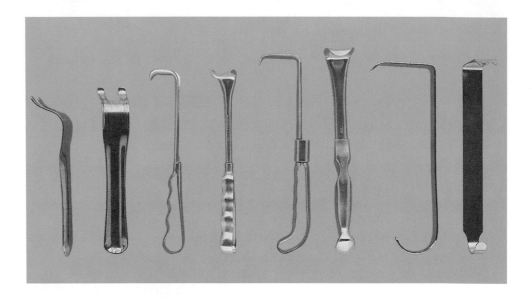

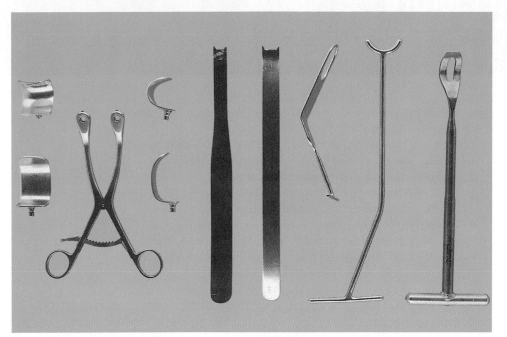

48-2 *Left to right:* 1 glenoid self-retaining retractor with 4 blades: 2 short, 2 long, front view and side view; 1 glenoid (Bateman) retractor, narrow; 1 glenoid (Bateman) retractor, medium; 1 shoulder retractor, angled, short; 1 Bankart shoulder retractor; 1 shoulder retractor, angled, long.

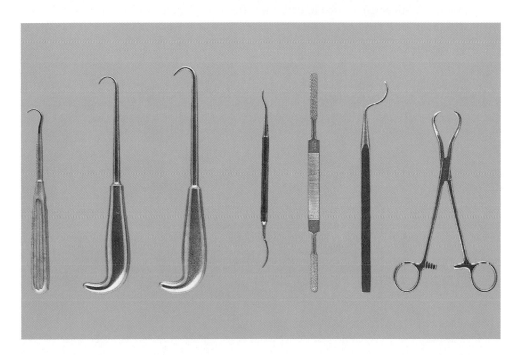

48-3 *Left to right:* 1 shoulder ligature carrier; 2 bone hooks; 1 double ended blunt elevator; 1 Foman rasp, double-ended; 1 glenoid punch; 1 Joplin bone forceps.

Hip Fracture

A hip fracture is usually a break in the neck of the femur. The fracture may be pinned with a nail, a screw, or a screw and plate.

Possible equipment needed for the procedure includes hip retractors.

A brief description of the hip-pinning procedure follows:

1. An Israel retractor is used for muscle retraction.
2. A Hibbs retractor is used for visualization of the hip joint.
3. A Bennett elevator is used to raise the femur into position.
4. A Scott-McCracken elevator is used to remove periosteum.
5. A Hohmann retractor is used to hold soft tissue back from operative site.
6. An Adson suction tip with tubing is used for visualization.
7. A drill guide is used to show the angle of drilling.
8. A drill is used to make a hole for the nail or the screw.
9. A depth gauge is used to determine the length of the dynamic hip screw (DHS).
10. A nail is inserted.
11. If a plate is needed, it is chosen to fit the femur. A drill is used to start the screw holes; a depth gauge is used to determine the screw length; and a screwdriver is used to tighten the screws.

49-1 *Top, left to right:* 2 Mayo dissecting scissors, straight; 1 Metzenbaum dissecting scissors, 7 inch; 1 Mayo dissecting scissors, curved. *Bottom, left to right:* 2 Bard-Parker knife handles #4; 2 Adson tissue forceps with teeth (1 × 2), front view and side view; 2 thumb tissue forceps with teeth (1 × 2), front view and side view; 2 thumb tissue forceps with multiteeth (4 × 5), front view and side view; 2 Ferris-Smith tissue forceps, front view and side view.

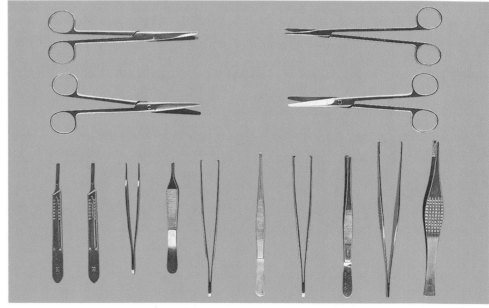

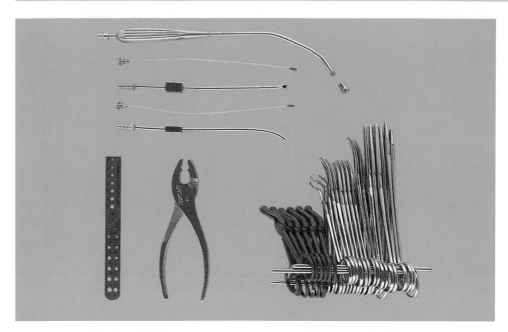

49-2 *Top to bottom:* 1 Yankauer suction tube with tip; 2 Adson suction tubes with finger valve controls and stylets, large. *Bottom, left to right:* 1 metal ruler, 6 inch; 1 pliers; 6 paper drape clips; 2 Backhaus towel forceps; 6 Crile hemostatic forceps, 6½ inch; 2 tonsil hemostatic forceps; 4 Ochsner hemostatic forceps, 8 inch; 2 Crile-Wood needle holders, 8 inch.

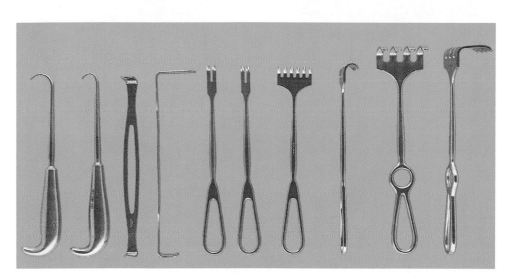

49-3 *Left to right:* 2 bone hooks; 2 Army Navy retractors, front view and side view; 2 Volkmann retractors, 2 prong, sharp; 2 Volkmann retractors, 6 prong, sharp, front view and side view; 2 Israel retractors, front view and side view.

49-4 *Left to right:* 2 Weitlaner retractors, medium, sharp; 2 Bennett bone elevators and retractors, side view and front view; 2 Hibbs laminectomy retractors, medium, side view and front view.

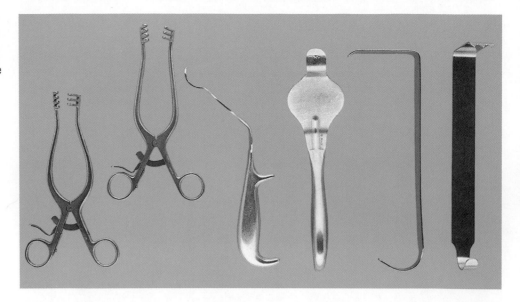

49-5 *Left to right:* 1 Scott-McCracken elevator; 1 Key periosteal elevator, ¾ inch; 1 Heath mallet; 1 Luer bone rongeur; 2 Lowman bone-holding clamps, front view.

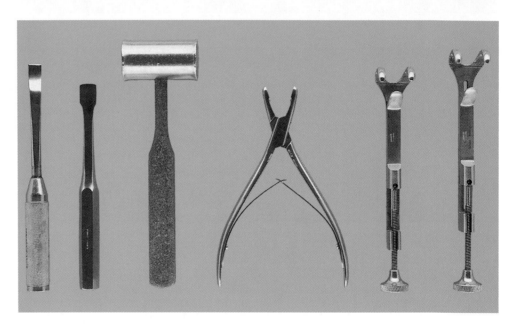

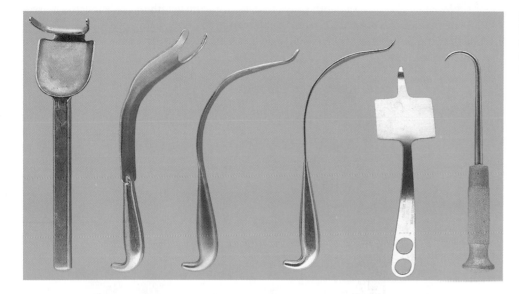

50-1 *Left to right:* 1 Antler retractor, front view; 1 double Cobra retractor, side view; 2 blunt Cobra retractors, side view; 1 Hohmann retractor, front view; 1 bone hook.

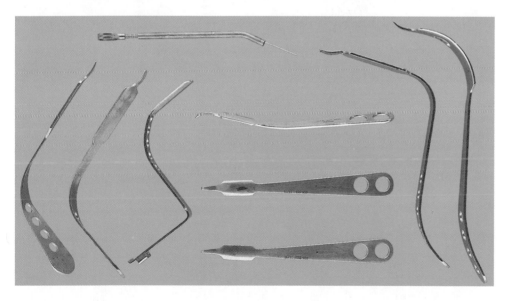

50-2 *Top:* 1 flexible depth gauge. *Bottom, left to right:* 2 anterior retractors, left and right; 1 superior retractor; 3 Hohmann retractors, narrow, 1 side view and 2 front views; 1 posterior/inferior retractor; 1 femoral retractor.

Internal Fixation with Screws and Plates*

A brief description of the procedure follows:

1. Drill holes are made so as to pass wires that stabilize bone fragments, to prepare the site for screw fixation, and to prepare the site for screw and plate fixation. That is followed by the use of a depth gauge to determine the length of the screw to be used.
2. Plate benders are needed to shape the plate to fit the bone being plated.
3. Following screw insertion by using a drill, a manual screwdriver is needed to tighten the screw safely.

51-1 Association for the Study of Internal Fixation (ASIF) basic low-contact–dynamic compression plate (LC-DCP) and dynamic compression plate (DCP) instrument set.

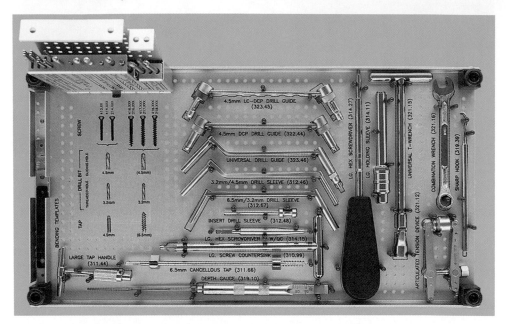

51-2 *Top, left to right:* 2 Bard-Parker knife handles #3; 1 Adson suction tube with stylet, 14 Fr. *Bottom, left to right:* 1 Metzenbaum dissecting scissors, 7 inch; 1 Mayo dissecting scissors, curved; 1 Mayo dissecting scissors, straight; 2 Adson tissue forceps with teeth (1 × 2), front view and side view; 2 thumb tissue forceps with teeth (1 × 2), front view and side view; 6 paper drape clips; 2 Halsted mosquito hemostatic forceps; 2 Backhaus towel forceps; 4 Crile hemostatic forceps, 5½ inch; 2 tonsil hemostatic forceps; 2 Ochsner hemostatic forceps; 2 Crile-Wood needle holders, 7 inch.

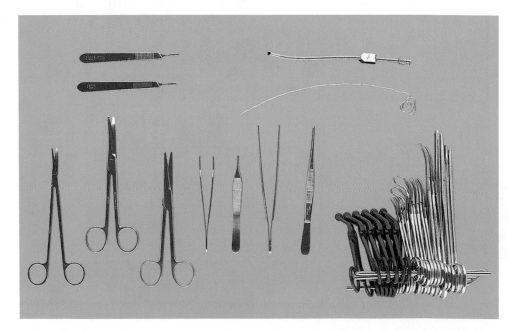

*Additional images are available on the Companion CD.

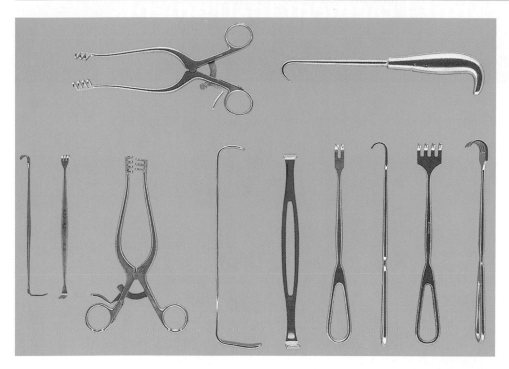

51-3 *Top, left to right:* 1 Weitlaner retractor, sharp, medium; 1 bone hook. *Bottom, left to right:* 2 Miller-Senn retractors, side view and front view; 1 Weitlaner retractor, sharp, medium; 2 Army Navy retractors, side view and front view; 2 Volkmann retractors, 2 prong, sharp, front view and side view; 2 Volkmann retractors, 4 prong, sharp, front view and side view.

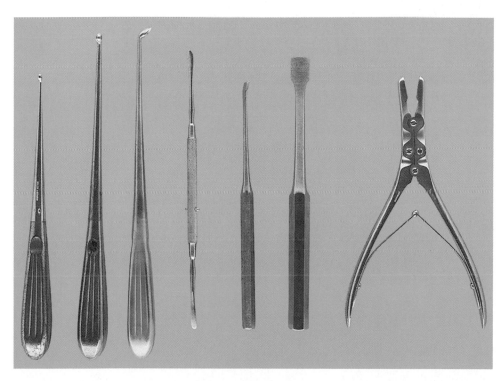

51-4 *Left to right:* 1 Spratt (Brun) curette, long, #00; 1 Spratt (Brun) curette, long, #2; 1 Spratt (Brun) curette, long, #3, angled; 1 Freer double-ended elevator; 1 Key periosteal elevator, ¼ inch, side view; 1 Key periosteal elevator, ½ inch, front view; 1 Ruskin rongeur, double-action.

ASIF Mini-Fragment Instruments

Possible equipment needed for the procedure includes an ASIF basic set.

52-1 ASIF mini-fragment set (labeled).

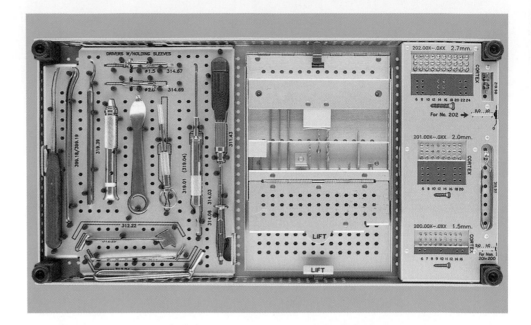

52-2 *Left to right:* bottom compartment of tray in Figure 52-1 (under drills); some instrumentation from tray.

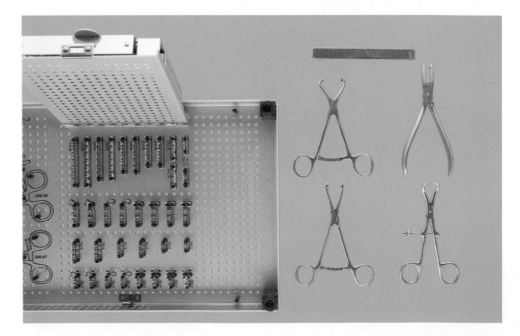

ASIF Small-Fragment Instruments

Possible equipment needed for the procedure includes an ASIF basic set.

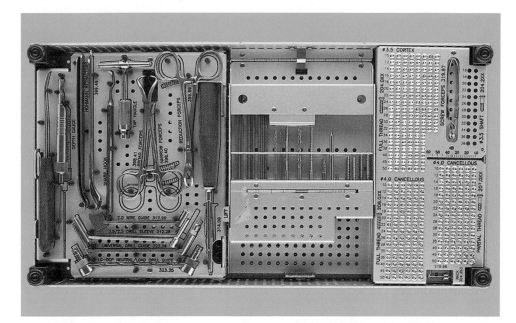

53-1 ASIF small-fragment set (labeled).

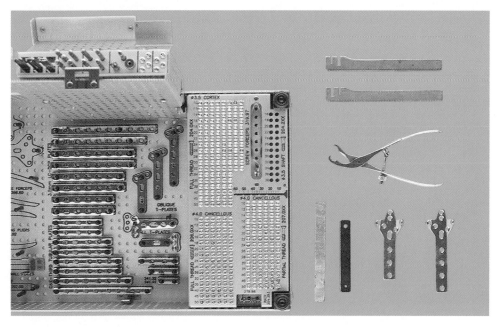

53-2 *Left to right:* bottom compartment of tray in Figure 53-1 (under drills); some instrumentation from tray.

ASIF Basic LC-DCP and DCP Instrument Set

Possible equipment needed for the procedure includes an ASIF basic set.

54-1 ASIF basic LC–DCP and DCP instruments.

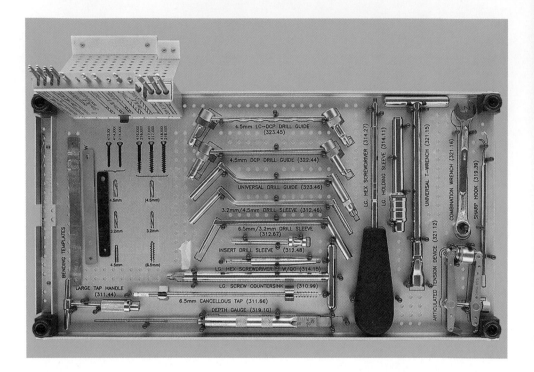

Possible equipment needed for the procedure includes an ASIF basic set and ASIF instruments.

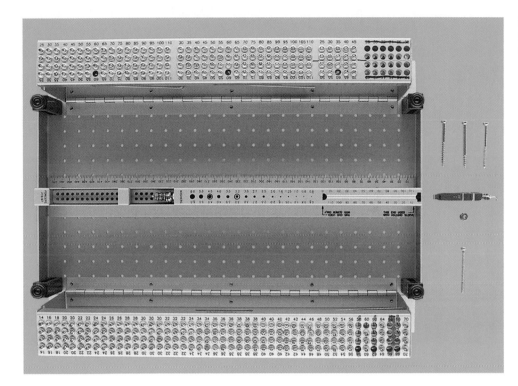

55-1 ASIF standard screw set in tray (labeled); some screws from tray *(right)*.

ASIF Standard Plates

Possible equipment needed for the procedure includes an ASIF basic set, ASIF standard instruments, and ASIF standard screws.

56-1 ASIF standard plate set in tray (labeled).

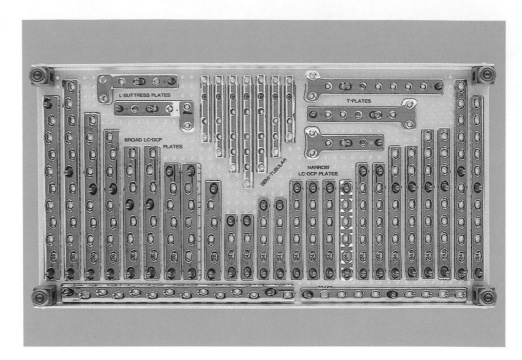

Dynamic Hip Screw (DHS) Instruments and Screws

Possible equipment needed for the procedure includes an open reduction set.

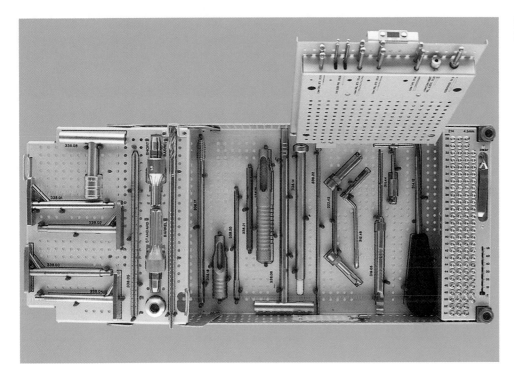

57-1 DHS instrument and screw set (labeled).

DHS Implants

Possible equipment needed for the procedure includes an open reduction set and DHS instruments and screws.

58-1 DHS implants in tray (labeled).

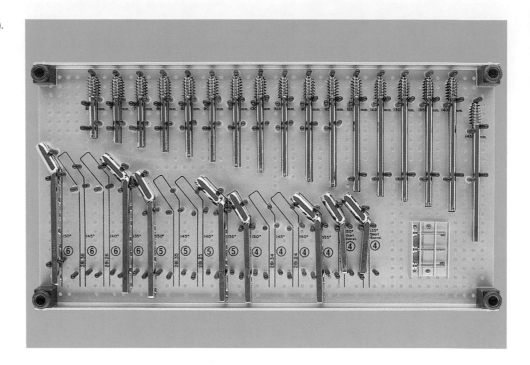

Total Hip Replacement

A total hip replacement is the removal of the acetabulum and the head of the femur, which are replaced with prosthetic implants.

Possible equipment needed for the procedure includes power saws and blades; power drill, bits, and reamers; a hip prosthesis; and hip retractors.

A brief description of the procedure follows:

1. Bennett and Hibbs retractors are used for visualization and stabilization of the hip joint.
2. A power saw is used to remove the head of the femur.
3. A power drill is used to ream the shaft of the femur.
4. An acetabular reamer set is used to prepare the acetabulum.
5. The sizer sets are used to determine the size of the acetabular component.
6. A trochanter reamer set is used to prepare the proximal femur.
7. A reamer tray with drill is used to prepare the femoral shaft.
8. A rasp tray with a mallet is used to prepare the femur for the femoral component.
9. The complete set of hip prostheses is used to select the correct size of the prosthetic to be used.

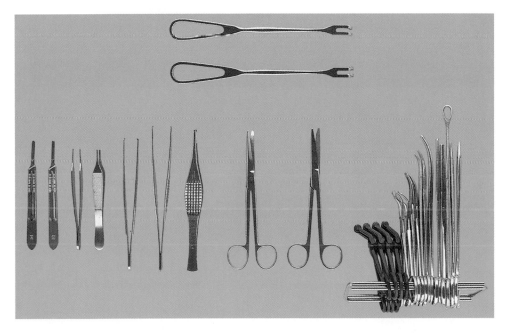

59-1 *Top:* 2 Volkmann retractors, 2 prong, sharp. *Bottom, left to right:* 2 Bard-Parker knife handles #4; 2 Adson tissue forceps with teeth (1 × 2), front view and side view; 1 thumb tissue forceps with teeth (1 × 2); 2 Ferris Smith tissue forceps, front view and side view; 1 Mayo dissecting scissors, curved; 1 Mayo dissecting scissors, straight; 4 paper drape clips; 2 Backhaus towel forceps; 2 Crile hemostatic forceps, 6½ inch; 2 tonsil hemostatic forceps; 1 Mayo-Péan hemostatic forceps; 2 Ochsner hemostatic forceps; 1 Foerster sponge forceps; 2 Crile-Wood needle holders, 8 inch.

59-2 *Top, left to right:* 2 Yankauer suction tubes with tips; 2 Volkmann retractors, 6 prong, sharp. *Bottom, left to right:* 1 Bard-Parker knife handle #4, long; 1 Russian tissue forceps, long; 1 Mayo dissecting scissors, curved, long; 1 bandage scissors, large; 1 Spratt curette, straight, short; 1 Spratt curette, angled, long; 2 Weitlaner retractors, medium.

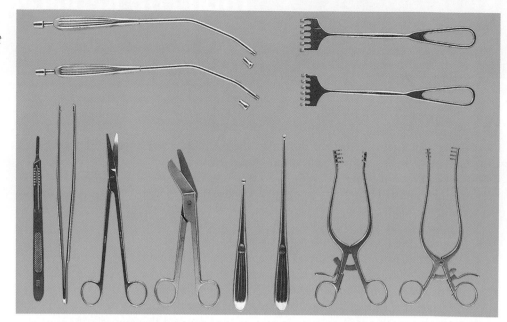

59-3 *Top left:* 1 metal mallet. *Right, top to bottom:* 1 metal ruler, 12 inch; 1 Townley femur caliper; 2 Steinmann pins, $9/64$. *Bottom, left to right:* 3 Cobb spinal elevators: small, medium, and large; 1 Key periosteal elevator, 1 inch; 1 bone hook; 1 pliers; 1 Smith-Petersen laminectomy rongeur, double-action; 1 Luer bone rongeur.

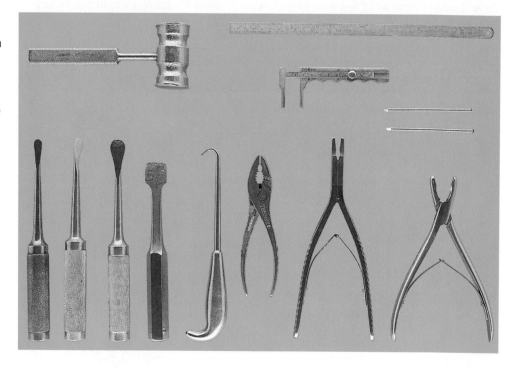

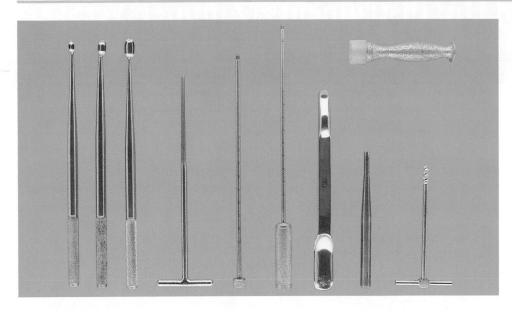

59-4 *Top right:* 1 prosthesis driver. *Bottom, left to right:* 3 Richards bone curettes, long, assorted sizes; 1 tapered T-handle femoral shaft reamer; 1 Buck cement restrictor inserter; 1 Stryker cement restrictor inserter; 1 Murphy bone lever or skid; 1 impactor; 1 corkscrew femoral head remover.

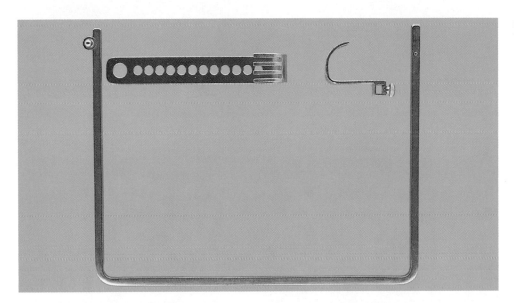

59-5 Initial incision retractor with two blades: long and short.

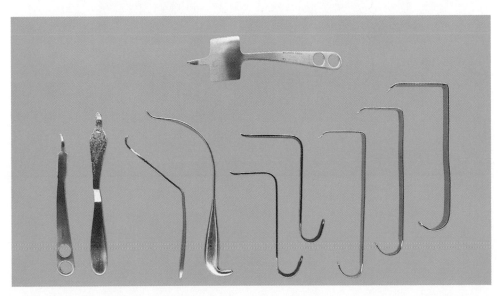

59-6 *Top:* 1 Hohmann retractor, large. *Bottom, left to right:* 1 Hohmann retractor, small; 1 cobra retractor, straight, front view; 1 cobra retractor, angled, side view; 1 cobra retractor, slightly angled, side view; 1 Taylor spinal retractor, black finish, short; 1 Taylor spinal retractor, black finish, long; 3 Hibbs laminectomy retractors: small, medium, and large.

Total Hip Instruments (Zimmer-VerSys)

Possible equipment needed for the procedure includes a basic total hip set and hip retractors.

60-1 Instruments (Trilogy acetabular).

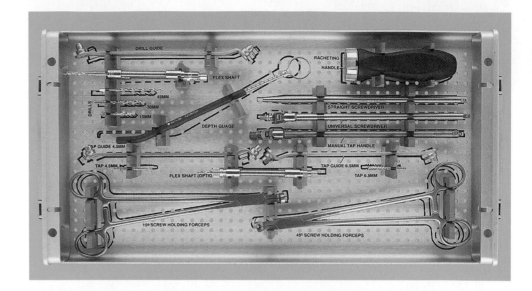

60-2 Hall surgical acetabular reamer set.

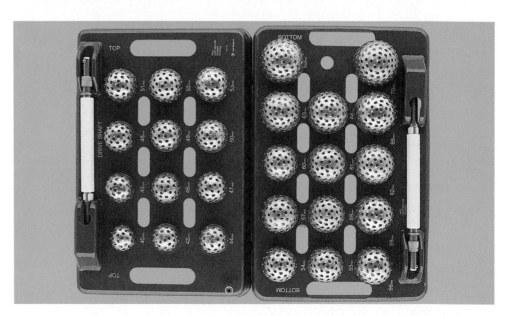

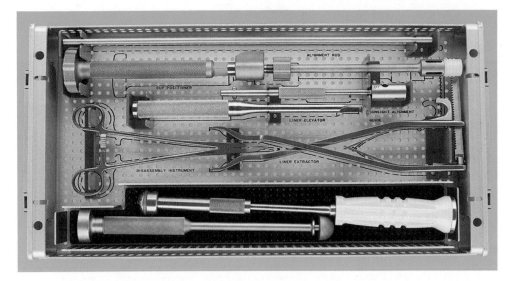

60-3 Shell provisionals and acetabular instruments.

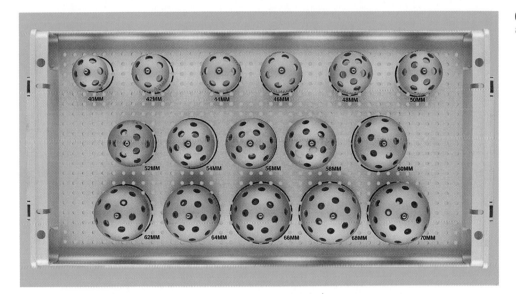

60-4 Shell provisionals and acetabulars.

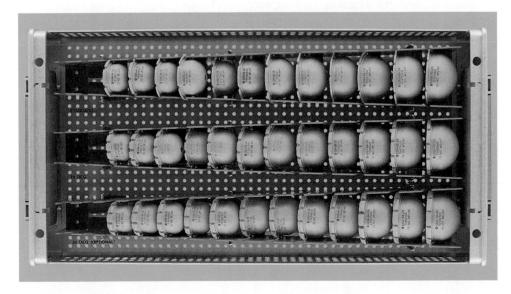

60-5 Linear provisionals.

60-6 General instruments: stem.

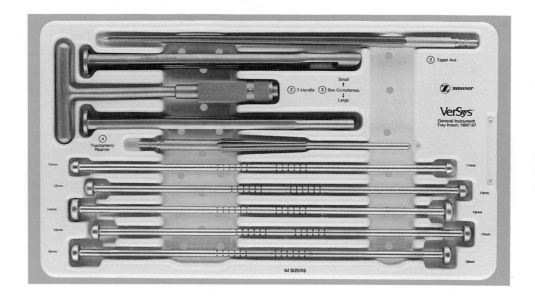

60-7 General instruments: femoral.

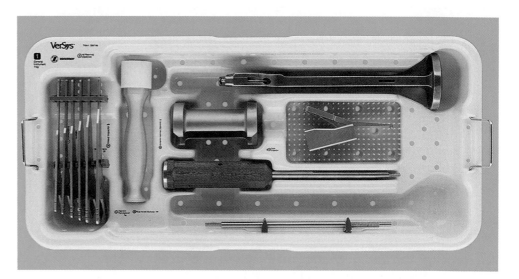

60-8 Rasp tray.

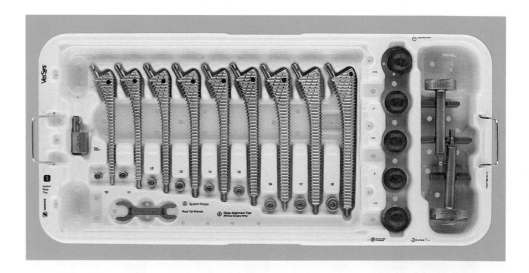

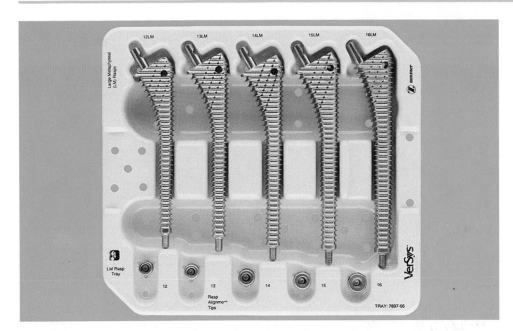

60-9 Large metaphyseal tray.

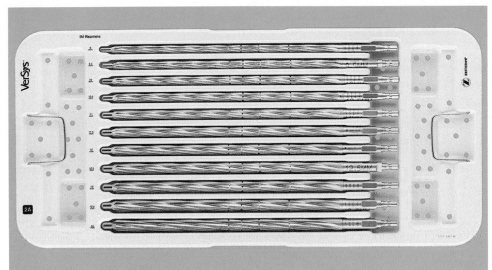

60-10 Reamer tray 2A.

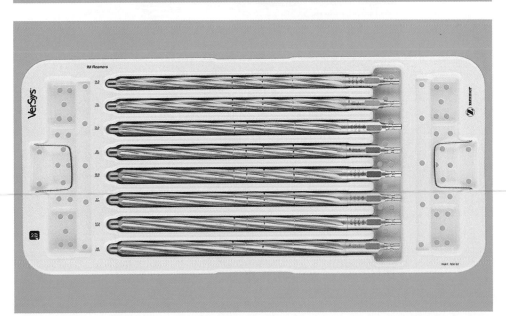

60-11 Reamer tray 2B.

60-12 *Left to right:* V-Lign instrument tray; intramedullary taper reamers. *Bottom, left to right:* stabilizer; 1 Crile template.

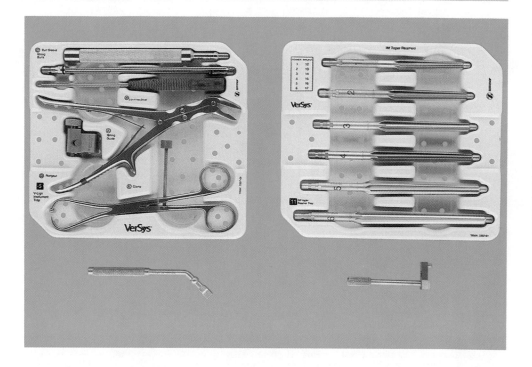

60-13 Cone provisionals. **A,** Size options: **B,** Porous and enhanced taper. **C,** *Left,* cemented. *Right,* cemented extended offset.

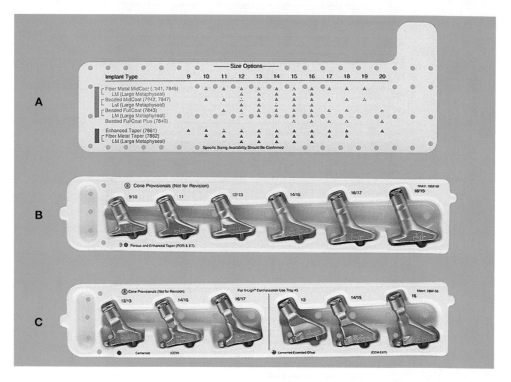

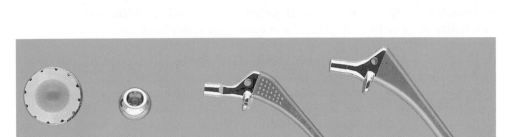

61-1 *Left to right:* 1 acetabular prothesis; 1 femoral head prothesis; 1 femoral stem prosthesis, plain; 1 femoral stem prosthesis, cemented.

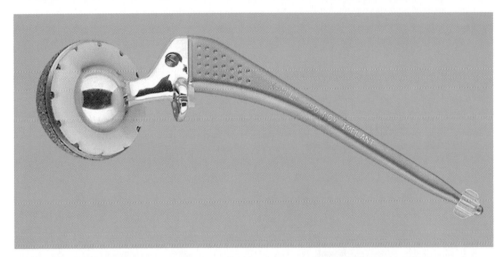

61-2 Acetabular prothesis; femoral head prosthesis; femoral stem prosthesis together.

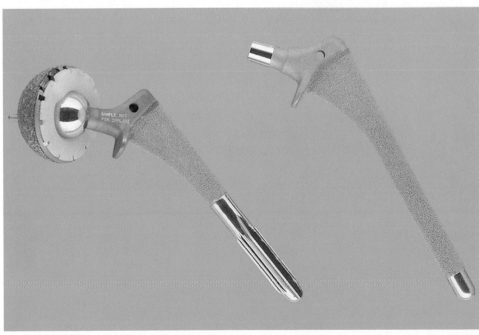

61-3 *Left to right:* prosthesis: midcoat porous stem; prosthesis: fully porous stem.

Spinal Fusion with Rodding

A spinal fusion with rod attachment is performed to correct curvature of the spine. The fusion may use bone from the iliac crest or bone from a bone bank. The soft tissue around the vertebra is removed and the bone graft is placed for the fusion.

Possible equipment needed for the procedure includes an open reduction set.

A brief description of rods and systems used for the procedure follows:

1. A Harrington rod insertion uses distraction rods and compression rods to straighten the spine as much as possible.
2. Luque rods are placed and fixed at multiple points so corrective forces are spread throughout the length of the deformity.
3. The Texas Scottish Rite Hospital (TSRH) system uses a cross-link to stabilize the rods, thus preventing rod migration.
4. The Cotrel-Dubousset system can be used for the correction of scoliosis, kyphosis, and lordosis. The rod can be derotated, compressed, and distracted.

62-1 Texas Scottish Rite Hospital (TSRH) implant tray (labeled).

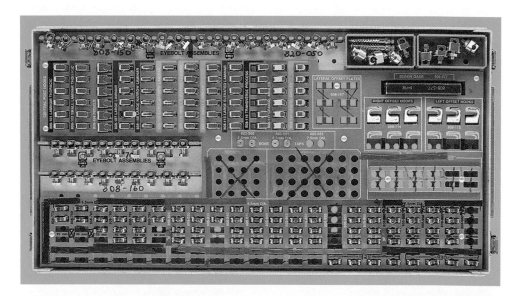

62-2 TSRH top tightening implant tray (labeled).

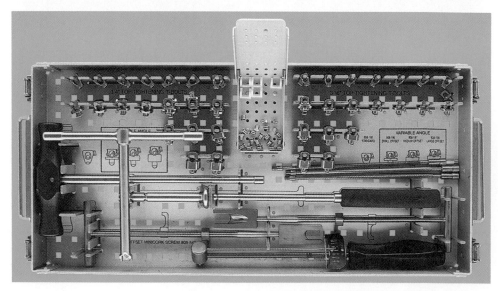

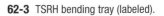

62-3 TSRH bending tray (labeled).

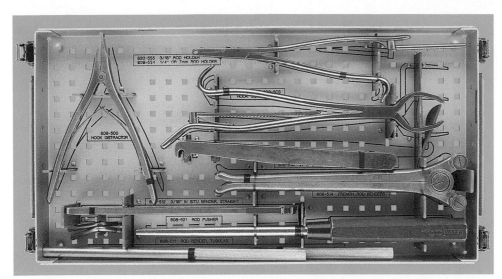

62-4 TSRH rod tray (labeled).

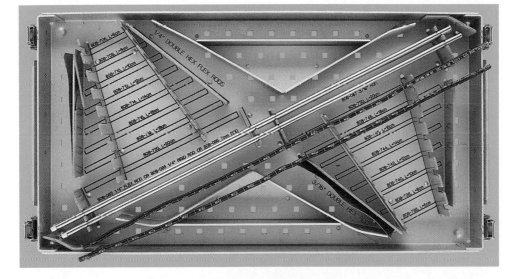

62-5 TSRH pediatric instrument, bottom tray (labeled).

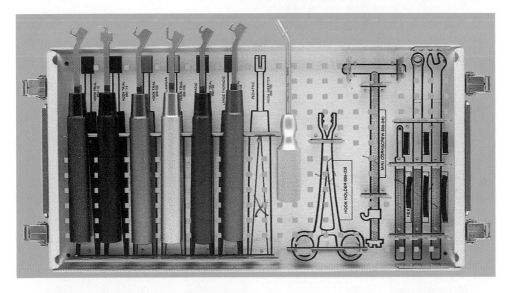

62-6 TSRH pediatric instrument, top tray (labeled).

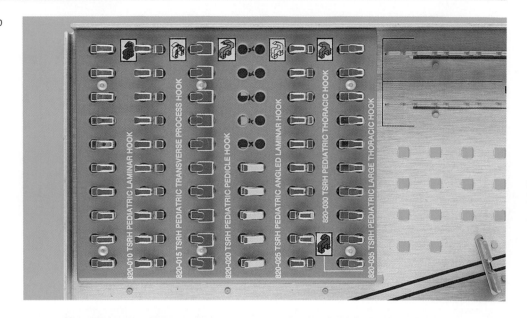

62-7 TSRH hook trials (labeled).

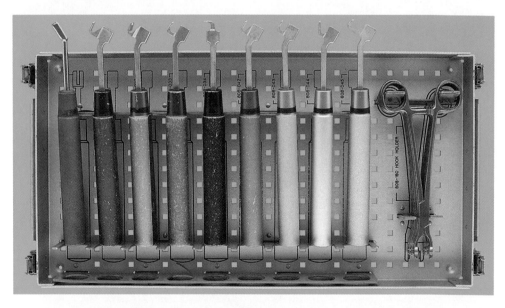

62-8 TSRH cross-link tray (labeled).

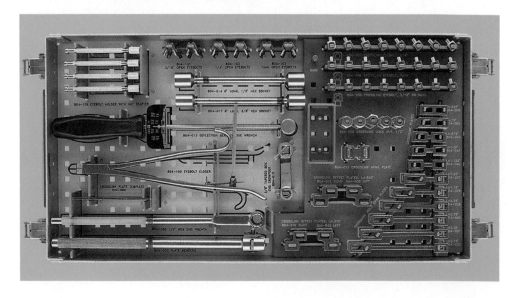

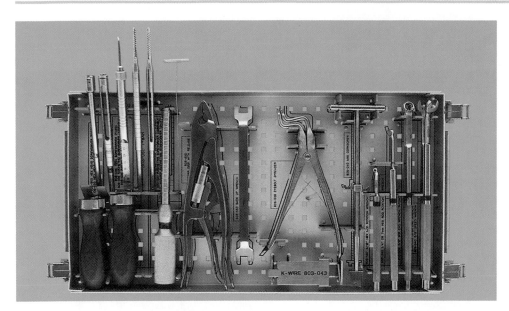

62-9 TSRH wrench tray (labeled).

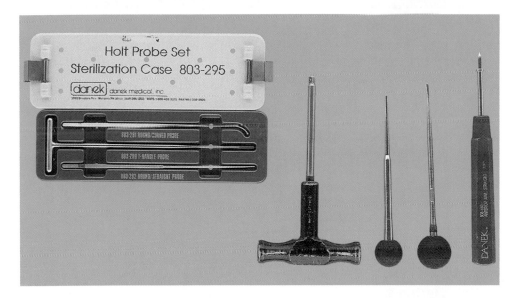

62-10 *Left, top to bottom:* Holt probe set: curved probe, T-handle probe, round/straight probe. *Bottom, left to right:* 1 T handle wrench; 2 probes (DePuy AcroMed); 1 anterlor awl, straight.

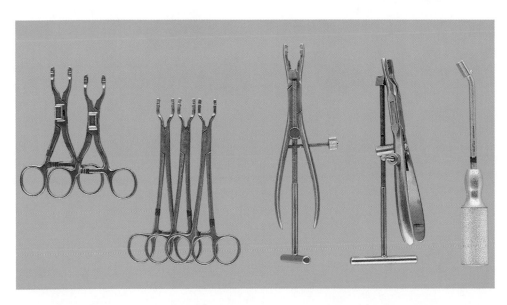

62-11 *Left to right:* 2 mini–hook holders with attachments; 3 hook holders, 4 pegs; 2 hook holders with rod movers, front view and side view; 1 hook inserter.

62-12 *Left to right:* 1 Harrington outrigger (3 pieces), assembled; 1 Harrington outrigger nut, pin, wrench; 1 large compressor; 1 curved spreader (Sofamor); 1 large distractor.

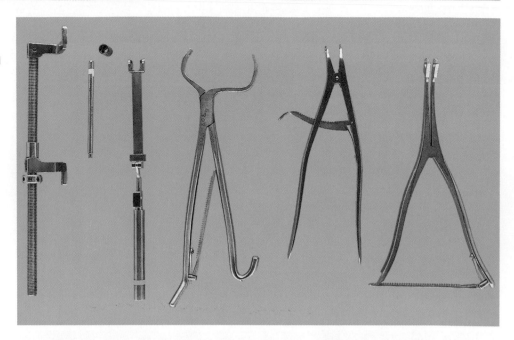

62-13 Rod cutter.

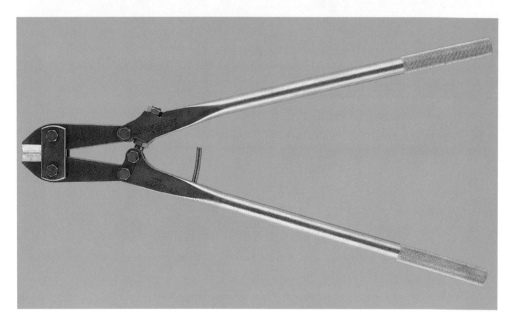

Possible equipment needed for the procedure includes an ASIF basic set.

A brief outline of the procedure follows:

1. A small dissection set is needed to make a small incision on the proximal end of the bone to be reduced.
2. A cannulated drill bit with the aid of fluoroscopy is placed through a drill sleeve.
3. A calibrated guide wire is placed down the shaft across the fracture site.
4. The size and length of the rod (nail) is determined.
5. A slide hammer is attached to the rod.
6. A mallet drives the rod down the shaft.
7. Screws may be placed on either end of the rod for stabilization.

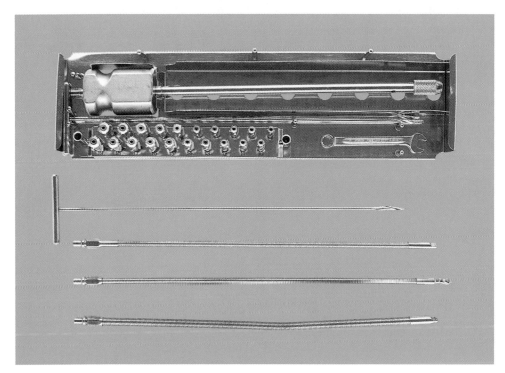

63-1 *Top:* tray that includes reamer heads, flexible shafts and reamer, ram, cannulated guide rod. *Middle:* wrench. *Bottom:* 3 hand reamers.

63-2 *Top:* 2 plastic medullary tubes. *Bottom, left to right:* 1 diameter gauge; 1 awl; 1 socket wrench for conical bolts. *Middle, top to bottom:* 3 threaded conical bolts; 1 guide handle for nails; 1 quick-coupling adapter; 4 reamer heads, assorted sizes; 1 holder for reaming rod and guide shaft; 1 curved driver (2 pieces); 1 tissue protector.

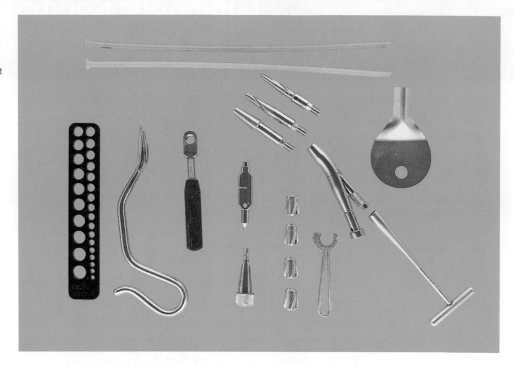

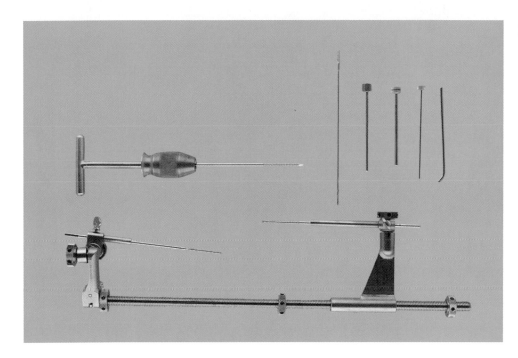

64-1 *Top, left to right:* Universal T-handle and shank pin; 1 drill bit; 3 drill guides; and 1 pin wrench. *Bottom, left:* stationary pin bar on distractor bar; traveling pin bar on right.

Titanium Unreamed Femoral Nail Instruments

65-1 Titanium unreamed femoral nail instrument set: bottom tray (labeled).

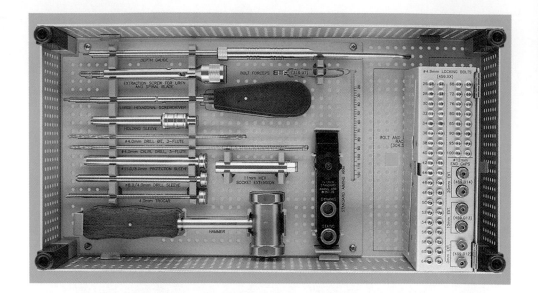

65-2 *Top:* 1 radiographic ruler. *Bottom:* Titanium unreamed femoral nail instrument set: top tray (labeled).

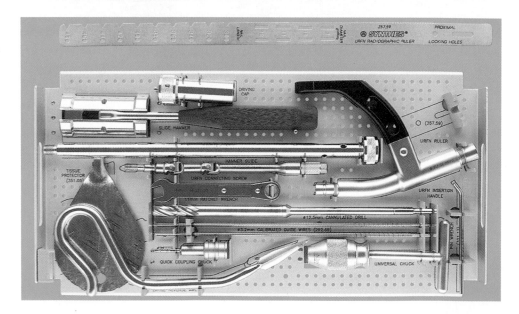

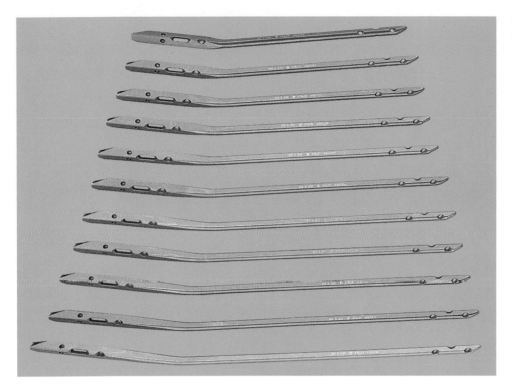

66-1 Synthes unreamed tibial nail set, assorted sizes.

*Additional images are available on the Companion CD.

67-1 Synthes unreamed tibial nail insertion and locking set (labeled). 5 sizes of locking bolts.

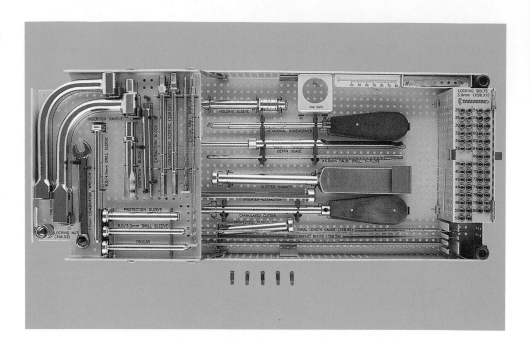

Condyle*

A condyle is the rounded portion at the end of a bone. Fractures of the distal femur (condyles) may be nailed, screwed, or plated. The accurate calculation of the angles of the condyles before internal fixation is very important to help prevent future degenerative changes.

Possible equipment needed for the procedure includes a soft tissue set.

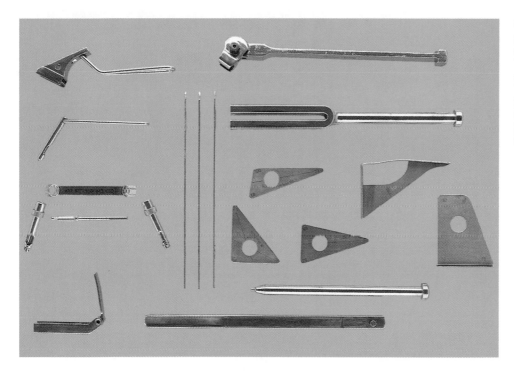

68-1 *Left, top to bottom:* 1 triple drill guide; 1 drill sleeve for plates; DCP drill guide (4 pieces); 1 chisel guide, 16 mm. *Middle:* 3 guide pins. *Right, top to bottom:* 1 inserter/extractor; 1 slotted hammer; 3 triangular positioning plates, assorted sizes; 1 condylar plate guide; 1 quadrangular positioning plate; 1 impactor; 1 seating chisel.

---

*Additional images are available on the Companion CD.

ASIF Angular Blade Plate Set

Possible equipment needed for the procedure includes a soft tissue set.

69-1 *Left, top to bottom:* 1 chisel guide/adjuster, angular; 1 triple drill guide. *Right, top to bottom:* 1 seating chisel, adolescent; 1 seating chisel; 4 quick-coupling drill bits, 4.5 mm; 4 guide pins. *Bottom, left to right:* 2 routers; 3 triangular positioning plates, assorted sizes; 1 quadrangular positioning plate; 1 condylar plate guide.

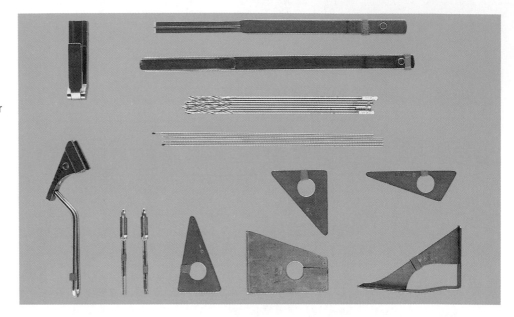

69-2 *Left to right:* 1 slotted hammer; 1 impact adolescent plate; 1 inserter/ extractor; 1 wrench, 11 mm; 1 insert-bifurcated plate; 1 impactor; 1 seating chisel, infant.

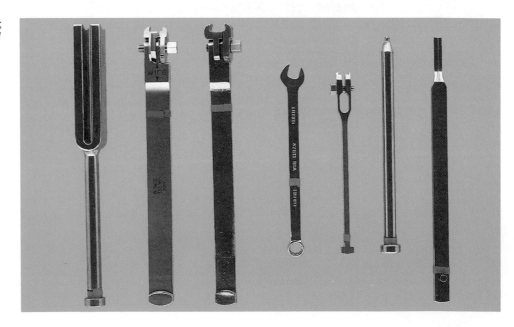

ASIF Cannulated Screw Set

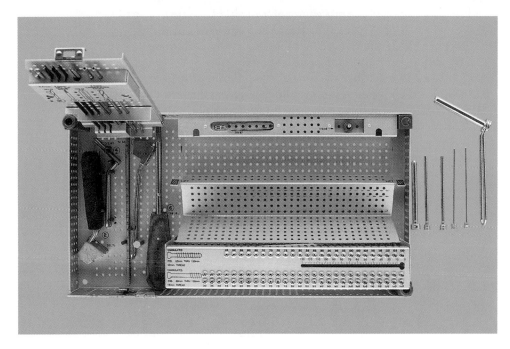

70-1 Synthes cannulated screw set (labeled).

External Fixation of Fractures*

External fixation is the attachment of a framework outside the body to stabilize complex fractures.

Possible equipment needed for the procedure includes an ASIF basic set.

A brief description of the procedure follows:

1. A small incision is made at each insertion and each exit of the pins.
2. A periosteal elevator is used for blunt dissection to the bone.
3. The drill sleeve is placed to protect the soft tissue.
4. Pins are drilled through the bone above and below the fracture or fractures.
5. This process is repeated for every bone fragment that must be stabilized.
6. Universal joints are placed over the ends of each pin.
7. The frame is placed.
8. A wrench is used to tighten the frame.
9. A pin cutter is used to cut the pins as needed.

71-1 The Evolution Tray has the instruments to put together the Taylor Spatial framework. (The Evolution Tray was prepared by Dr. Douglas N. Beaman.)

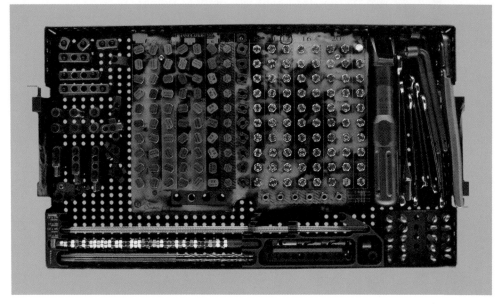

---

*Additional images are available on the Companion CD.

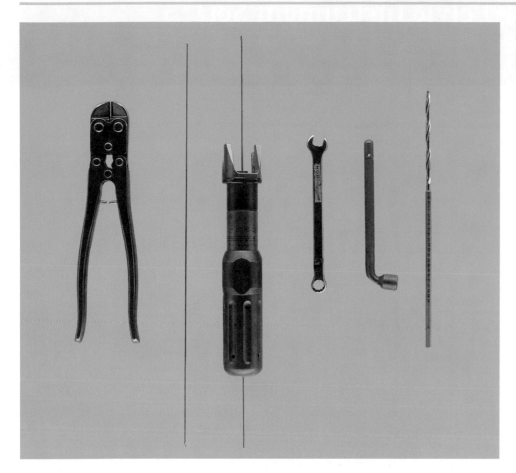

71-2 *Left to right:* pin cutter; wire; tensioner; wrench; box wrench; and drill. (The Evolution Tray was prepared by Dr. Douglas N. Beaman.)

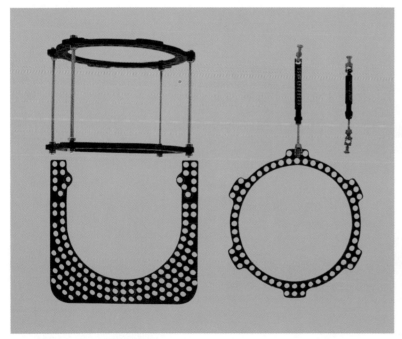

71-3 *Left, top to bottom:* Taylor Spatial rings with struts in place; and Taylor Spatial foot plate. *Right, top to bottom:* 2 struts and 1 Taylor Spatial ring.

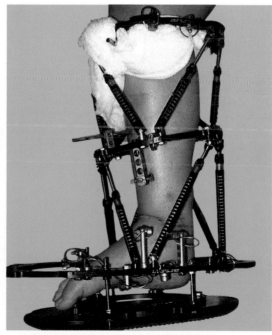

71-4 Taylor Spatial frame on patient. (Courtesy Lynn Scott, Gaston, Oregon.)

ASIF Pelvic Instrument Set*

Possible equipment needed for the procedure includes a soft tissue set.

72-1 *Left to right:* 1 plate bender; 2 pelvic plate-bending templates, long; 1 small hexagonal screwdriver; 1 drill guide, long, 2.5 mm; 1 drill guide, long, 3.5 mm; 1 small hexagonal screwdriver, long, large handle; 1 small hexagonal screwdriver, regular; 1 depth gauge; 4 drill bits, 2.5 × 180 mm; 4 drill bits, 3.5 × 170 mm; 2 taps, 3.5 × 180 mm.

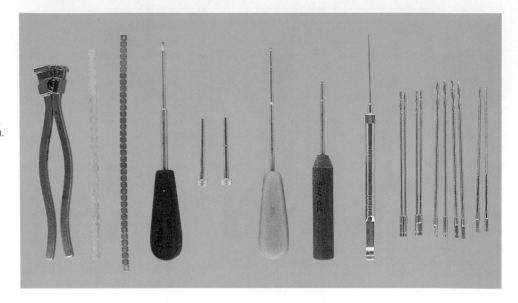

*Additional images are available on the Companion CD.

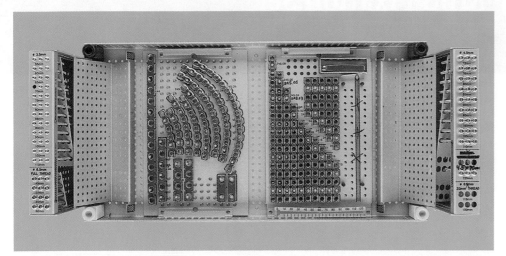

72-2 ASIF pelvic implant set.

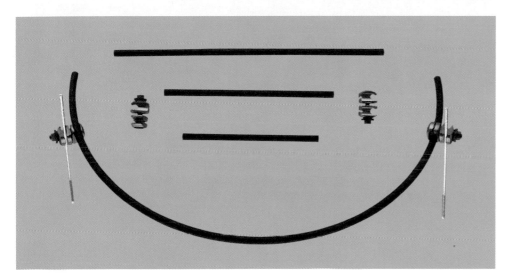

72-3 Pelvic external fixator. *Top to bottom:* 3 straight black carbon tubes with attaching clamps on each side; and one curved black carbon tube with Schanz pins attached on each side.

ASIF Mini Fixation Set

73-1 ASIF external fixator miniset.

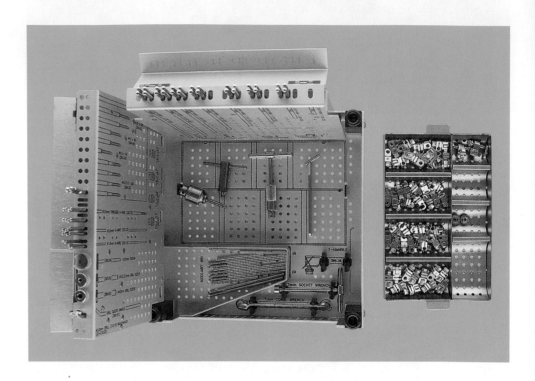

Bone Amputation

A bone amputation is the removal of an extremity or a portion of it.

Possible equipment needed for the procedure includes a soft tissue set.

A brief description of the procedure follows:

1. A Key elevator is used to remove periosteum.
2. A Satterlee saw is used to cut bone.
3. A Liston knife is used to cut soft tissue.
4. A Putti rasp is used to round the edges of bone.
5. Stille-Horsley forceps are used to cut bone.
6. A Stille-Luer rongeur is used to trim bone.
7. A Gigli saw is used to cut bone if there is not enough room to use the Satterlee saw.

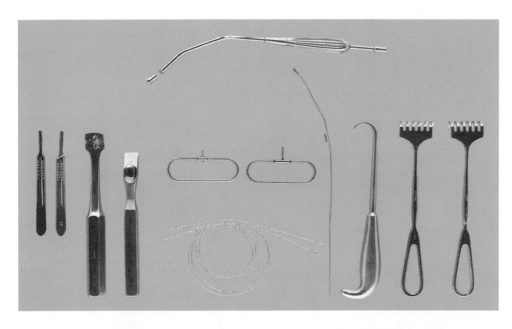

74-1 *Top:* 1 Yankauer suction tube and tip. *Bottom, left to right:* 2 Bard-Parker knife handles #4; 1 Key periosteal elevator, large; Gigli saw: 1 guide, 2 handles, 3 blades; 1 bone hook; 2 Volkmann retractors, 6 prong, sharp.

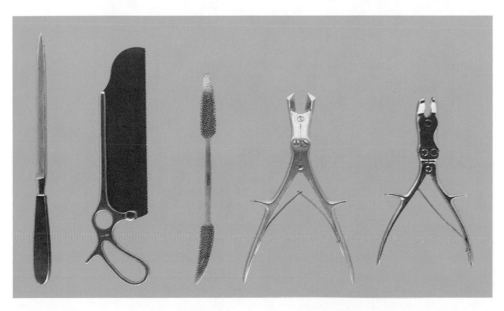

74-2 *Left to right:* 1 Liston amputation knife; 1 Satterlee amputation saw; 1 Putti bone rasp, double ended; 1 Stille-Horsley bone-cutting forceps, double action; 1 Stille-Luer rongeur.

Possible equipment needed for the posterior fusion pan #1 includes a soft tissue set.

It is the surgeons' preference concerning which fixation system they use to provide immobilization and stabilization of the spinal segments as an adjunct to fusion. One type of fixation system is the Stryker Spine, XIA Low Profile Titanium Spine System that can be seen in Figures 75-6 through 75-17.

75-1 *Top, left to right:* 1 Frazier suction tube; and 1 Love nerve retractor, 90-degree angle. *Bottom, left to right:* 2 Bard-Parker knife handles #7, #3 long; 2 bayonet dressing forceps; 2 Gerald tissue forceps without teeth; 1 nerve hook; and 1 Penfield dissector #4.

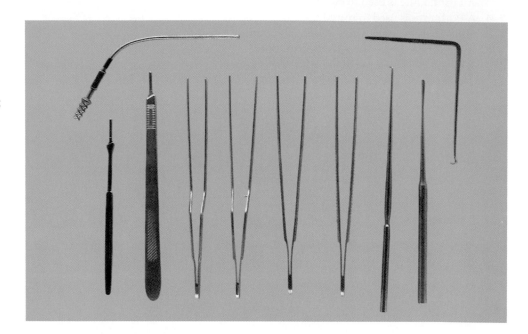

75-2 *Instruments in container, left to right:* 1 pin cutter, double-action; 1 Beyer rongeur, curved; 2 Cobb spinal elevators; 1 French bender; 6 Weitlaner retractors, various sizes; 4 cerebellar retractors, various sizes; 1 mallet; 2 pituitary rongeurs; and 5 Kerrison rongeurs, 1 mm to 5 mm.

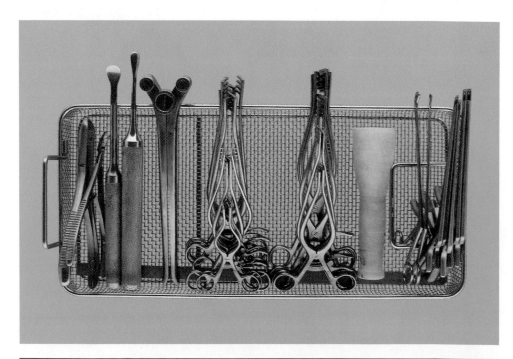

*Additional images are available on the Companion CD.

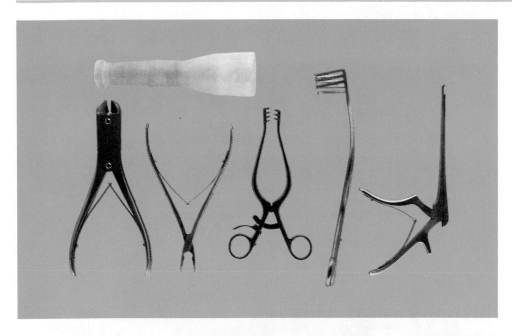

75-3 *Top:* 1 mallet. *Left to right:* 1 pin cutter, double-action; 1 Beyer rongeur, curved; 1 Weitlaner retractor; 1 cerebellar retractor, side view; and 1 Kerrison rongeur.

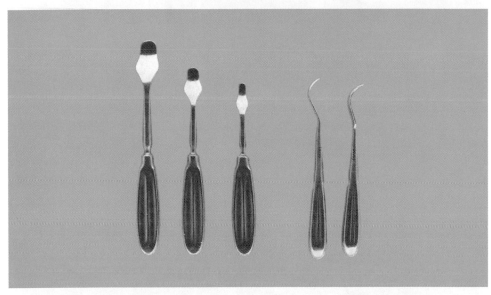

75-4 *Left to right:* 3 Chandler retractors, various sizes; and 2 Crego retractors.

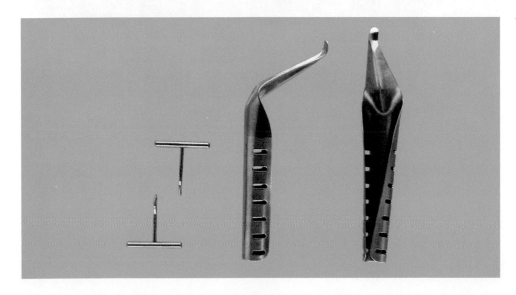

75-5 *Left to right:* 2 Gigli saw handles; and 2 Rang retractors, side view, front view.

75-6 Hook tray. *Top:* rods. Tray contains laminar blades; thoracic laminar blades; lumbar transverse process blades; and large and small pedicle hooks (all marked in tray). *Bottom:* template. *Right:* blockers.

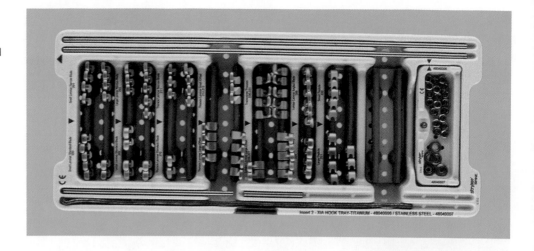

75-7 *Top to bottom:* 3 lamina finders, 2 straight, 1 curved; 4 C-rings; 1 hook forceps; and 1 hook impactor.

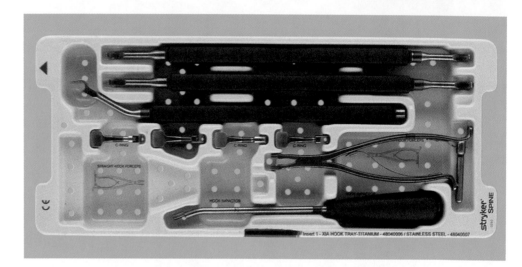

75-8 *Left, top to bottom:* 1 rod rotation forceps; and 2 lamina forceps. *Right, top to bottom:* 2 lateral hook forceps; and 1 rod rotation forceps.

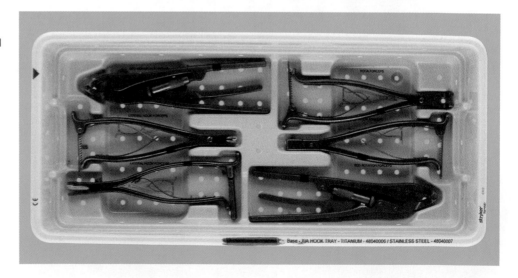

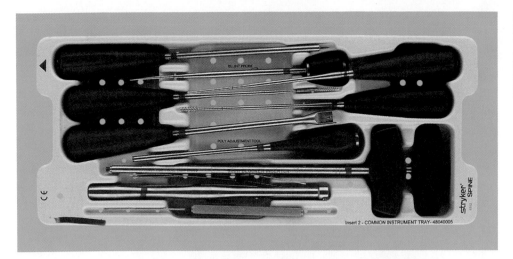

75-9 *Left, top to bottom:* 1 awl; tap, 6.5/7.5; 1 screw head adjustor; 1 pedicle feeler; and 1 ball tip probe. *Right, top to bottom:* 1 blunt probe; 1 curette; 1 tap, 4.5/5.5; 1 poly adjustment tool; and 2 block inserters.

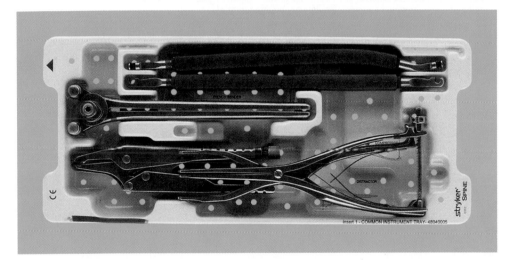

75-10 *Top,* 2 in situ benders. *Left, top to bottom:* 1 French bender; and 1 vice-grip rod holder. *Right, bottom:* 1 compressor (bottom); and 1 distractor (top).

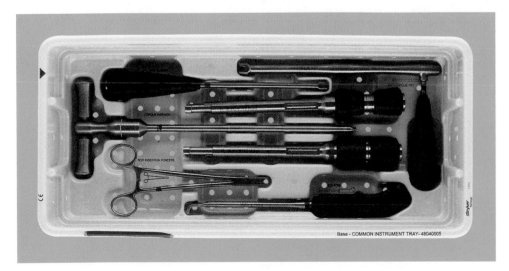

75-11 *Left, top to bottom:* 1 rod pusher; 1 torque wrench; and 1 rod insertion forceps. *Right, top to bottom:* 1 torque; 2 persuaders; and 1 rod fork.

75-12 One tray of polyaxial screws, 6.5; bottom, 2 rods; 5.5 and 7.5 screws also available.

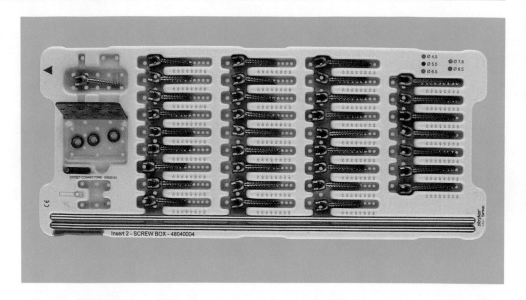

75-13 *Left to right:* polyaxial screwdriver, disassembled and assembled.

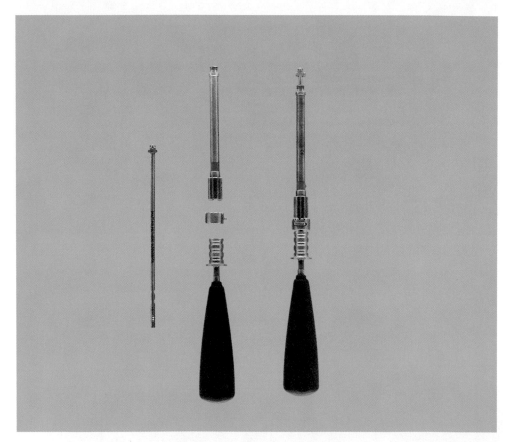

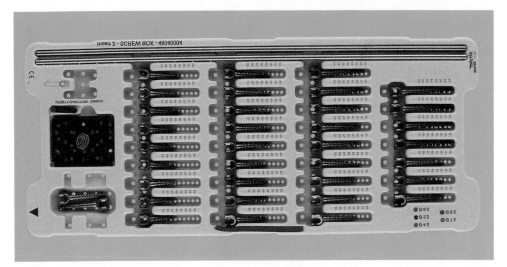

75-14 One tray of monoaxial screws, 6.5; bottom, 2 rods; 5.5 and 7.5 screws also available.

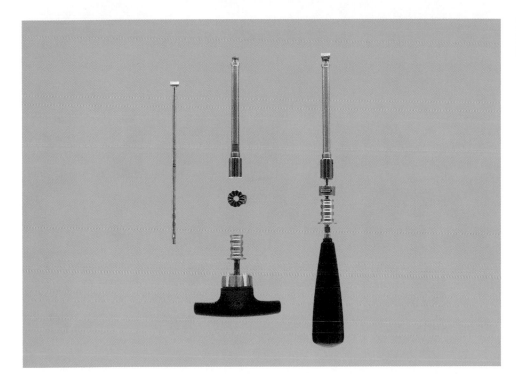

75-15 *Left to right:* monoaxial screwdriver, disassembled and assembled.

75-16 *Left, top to bottom:* 1 set of calipers; and 1 screwdriver, 5 mm. *Right, top to bottom:* 1 screwdriver, 3.5 mm; 1 screwdriver, 3.5 mm, round tip; and 1 forceps.

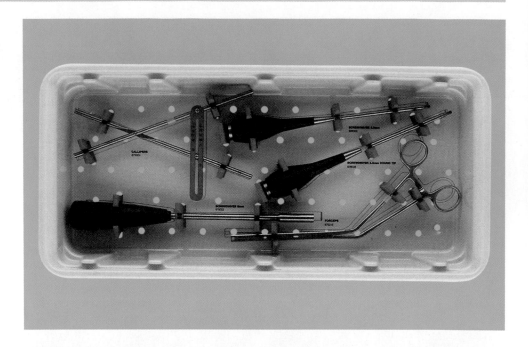

75-17 One tray of various sizes of crosslinks, marked on tray.

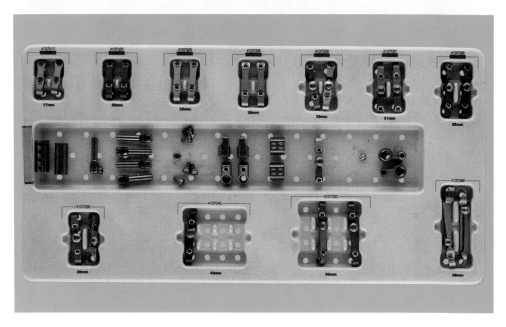

Basic Eye Set

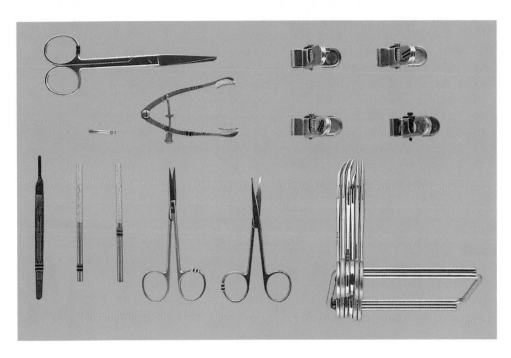

76-1 *Top, left to right:* 1 plastic scissors, straight, sharp, 5½ inch; 1 Lancaster speculum; 4 Edwards holding clips. *Bottom, left to right:* 1 Bard-Parker knife handle #9; 2 Beaver knife handles, knurled, one insert above; 1 iris scissors, straight, 4½ inch; 1 Stevens tenotomy scissors; 4 Halsted mosquito hemostatic forceps, curved; 2 Halsted mosquito hemostatic forceps, straight.

Cataract Removal*

A cataract is the clouding of the lens of the eye.

Possible equipment and instruments needed for the procedure includes an operating microscope, a phacoemulsifier, and a cataract removal set.

A brief description of the procedure follows:

1. A Lieberman speculum is placed to retract the eyelids.
2. A Beaver knife handle with blade is used for sharp dissection of the conjunctiva.
3. Needle cannulas are used for irrigation.
4. Bishop-Harman forceps are used to stabilize the eye.
5. Westcott tenotomy scissors are used to incise into the lens capsule.
6. A Drysdale nucleus manipulator is used to loosen the lens nucleus.
7. A Barraquer spatula is used to divide the nucleus into quadrants.
8. The phacoemulsifier is used to remove the nucleus.
9. The Thornton IOL forceps are used to insert the IOL into the eye.
10. The Sinskey hook is used to position the IOL accurately.
11. The Castroviejo needle holder is used to close the incision, if needed.
12. The McPherson forceps are used to tie the suture.
13. Plastic suture scissors are used to cut the suture.

77-1 *Top, left to right:* 1 Barraquer wire speculum and 1 Lieberman speculum. *Bottom, left to right:* 2 Halsted mosquito hemostatic forceps and 1 drape clip.

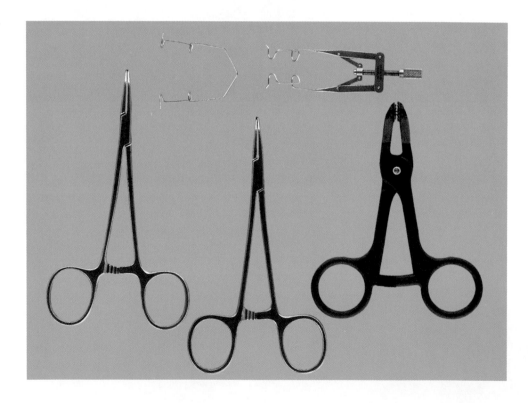

*Additional images are available on the Companion CD.

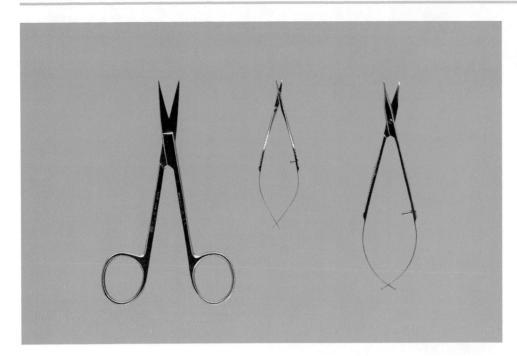

77-2 *Left to right:* 1 suture scissors, straight; 1 Vannas capsulotomy scissors; and 1 Westcott tenotomy scissors.

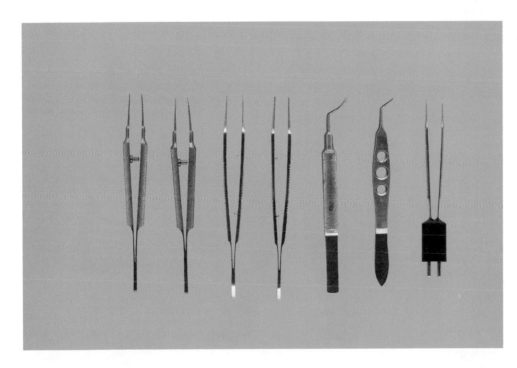

77-3 *Left to right:* titanium tying forceps, 1 straight, 1 curved; 2 Castroviejo suturing forceps, wide handles, 0.12 mm and 0.5 mm; 1 Lehner Utrata forceps; 1 Kelman-McPherson tying forceps, angled; and 1 Codmen cautery forceps.

77-4 *Left to right:* 1 Thornton fixation ring; 1 Nagahara nucleus manipulator; 1 Drysdale nucleus manipulator; 1 Kirby hook and loop; 1 Von Graefe strabismus hook; 1 Sinskey iris and IOL hook; 1 Elschnig cyclodialysis spatula; and 2 Beaver knife handles.

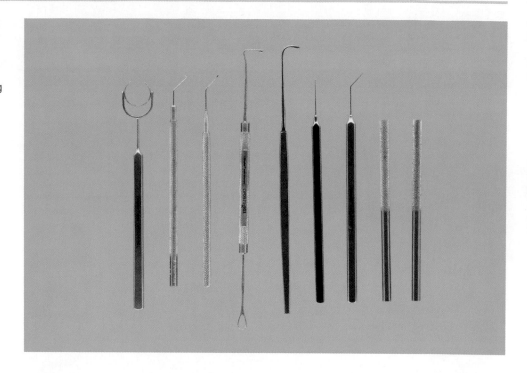

77-5 *Top, left to right:* 1 insert for Beaver knife handle; 5 needle cannulas, 2 27-gauge, 1 Chang, 1 19-gauge, and 1 30-gauge. *Bottom, left to right:* 1 Beaver knife handle; 3 Edwards holding clips; and 1 Castroviejo caliper.

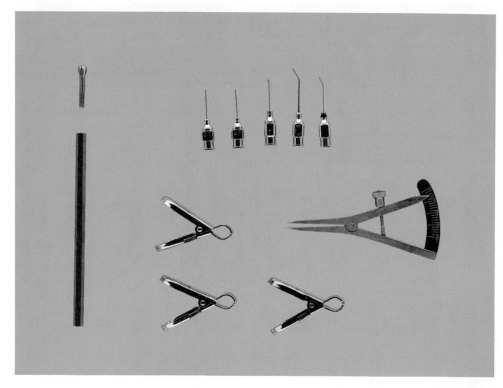

Clear Corneal Set*

The clear corneal cataract procedure that has recently been developed is performed with the use of topical anesthetics, foldable IOLs, and diamond knives. This allows the surgeon to make microincisions that are self healing and may not need stitches. For this procedure to be performed, it is imperative that the patient can hear and is able to follow specific directions. While performing this procedure, the surgeon can usually do full correction of refractive errors at the time of surgery.

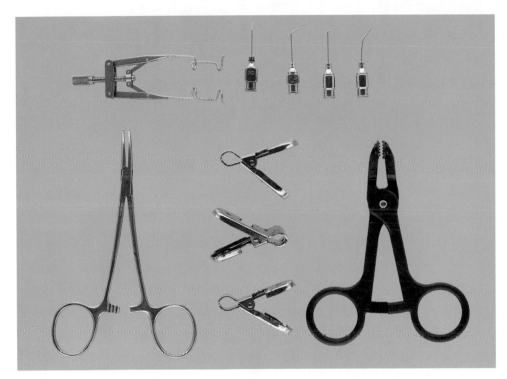

78-1 *Top, left to right:* 1 Lieberman speculum; 4 needle cannulas, 1 30-gauge, 1 27-gauge, 1 Chang, and 1 27-gauge. *Bottom, left to right:* 1 Halstead mosquito hemostatic forceps, fine tip; 3 Edwards holding clips; and 1 paper drape clip.

*Additional images are available on the Companion CD.

78-2 *Left to right:* 1 Kelman-McPherson tying forceps, angled; 1 Castroviejo suturing forceps, 0.12 mm; 1 Utrata forceps; and 1 iris scissors, straight.

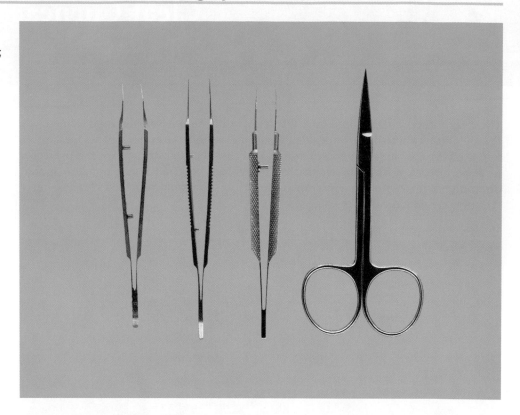

78-3 *Left to right:* 1 Thornton fixation ring; 1 insert and Beaver knife handle; 1 Kirby hook and loop; 1 Sinskey iris and IOL hook; 1 Drysdale nucleus manipulator; 1 Elschnig cyclodialysis spatula; and 1 Nagahara nucleus manipulator.

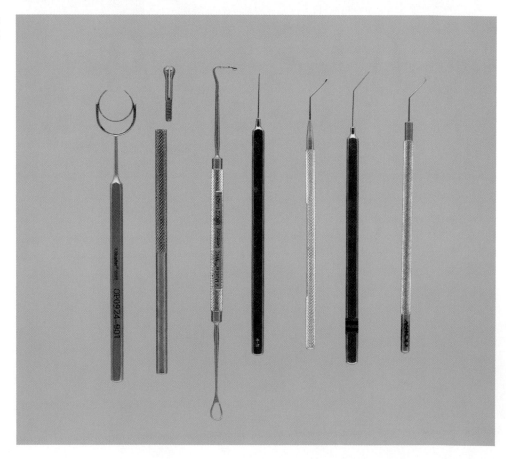

Corneal transplant is the replacement of a damaged cornea with a cornea from a human donor's eye.

Possible equipment and instruments needed for the procedure include an operating microscope, a disposable trephine, and a basic eye set.

A brief description of the procedure follows:

1. The Schott eye speculum is placed to retract the eyelids.
2. The Flieringa fixation ring is placed to stabilize the eyeball.
3. A disposable trephine is used to cut a button from the cornea of the donor's eye.
4. The trephine is used to cut a slightly smaller button from the recipient's eye.
5. The Pollock forceps are used to place the donor's button in the space in the recipient's cornea.
6. The Troutman-Barraquer needle holder with suture and Sinskey tying forceps are used to secure the cornea in place.
7. Irrigating cannulas are used to lubricate the eye with solution as needed.

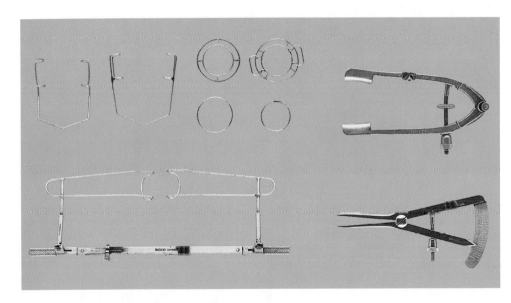

79-1 *Top, left to right:* 2 Barraquer wire speculums, 1 Flieringa fixation ring (double ring); 1 McNeil-Goldman scleral ring (with wings); 2 single-wire Flieringa fixation rings; 1 Lancaster speculum. *Bottom, left to right:* 1 Schott eye speculum; 1 Castroviejo caliper.

*Additional images are available on the Companion CD.

79-2 *Left to right:* 1 jeweler's forceps, straight; 1 Elschnig fixation forceps; 1 Lester fixation forceps; 1 serrated forceps, fine; 1 Castroviejo suturing forceps, 0.5 mm; 1 Castroviejo suturing forceps, 0.12 mm; 1 McPherson tying forceps, angled; 1 Troutman-Barraquer forceps (Colibri type); 1 Polack double-tipped, corneal forceps (Colibri type); 1 Maumenee corneal forceps; 1 Clayman lens-holding forceps.

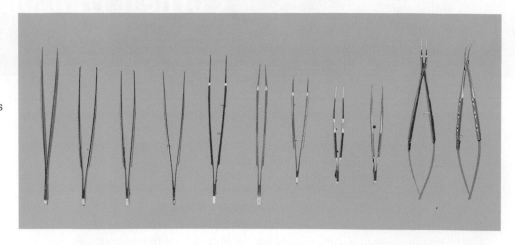

79-3 *Left to right:* enlarged tips: **A,** Jeweler's forceps, straight; **B,** Elschnig fixation forceps; **C,** Lester fixation forceps.

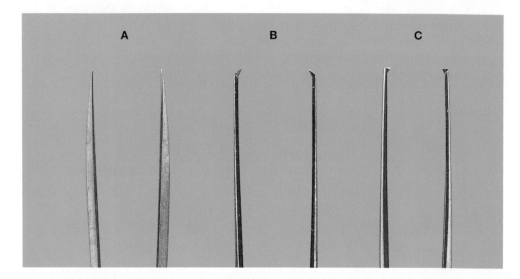

79-4 *Left to right:* enlarged tips: **A,** Castroviejo suturing forceps, 0.5 mm; **B,** Castroviejo suturing forceps, 0.12 mm; **C,** McPherson tying forceps, angled; **D,** Troutman-Barraquer forceps (Colibri type); **E,** Polack double-tipped corneal forceps (Colibri type).

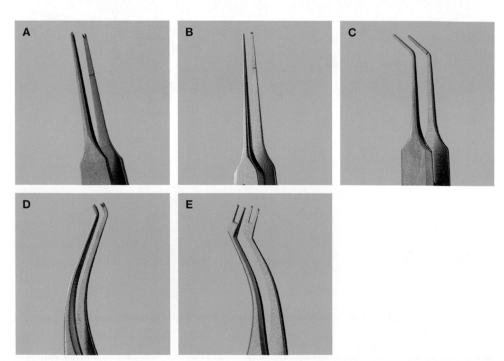

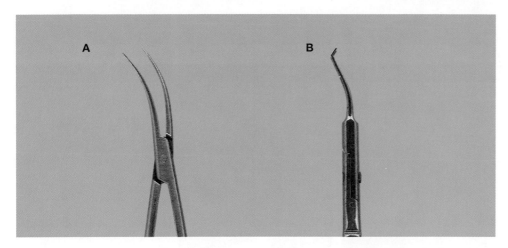

79-5 *Left to right:* enlarged tips: **A**, Clayman lens-holding forceps; **B**, Maumenee corneal forceps, side view.

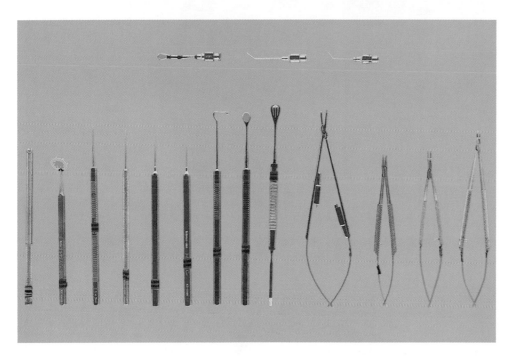

79-6 *Top, left to right:* 1 Sheets irrigating vectis, 27 gauge; 2 irrigating cannulas, 23 and 27 gauge. *Bottom, left to right:* 1 Beaver knife handle, knurled, with insert; 1 corneal scleral marker; 1 Shepard iris hook; 1 Bechert nucleus rotator, Y-shaped tip; 1 Sinskey iris and IOL hook; 1 Culler iris spatula; 1 Jameson muscle hook; 1 lens loop; 1 Paton spatula, double-ended; 1 Castroviejo needle holder with lock, curved; 1 titanium needle holder with stop, no lock, curved; 1 Sinskey tying forceps, straight; 1 Troutman-Barraquer microneedle holder, curved.

79-7 *Left to right:* enlarged tips: **A**, Corneal scleral marker; **B**, Shepard iris hook; **C**, Bechert nucleus rotator, Y shaped tip; **D**, Sinskey iris and IOL hook; **E**, Culler iris spatula.

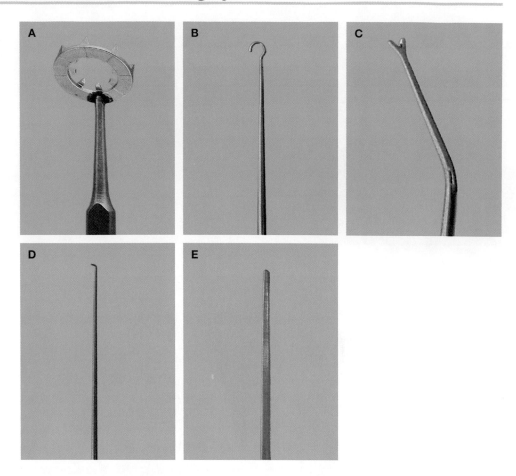

79-8 *Left to right:* enlarged tips: **A**, Jameson muscle hook; **B**, lens loop; **C**, Paton spatula, double-ended.

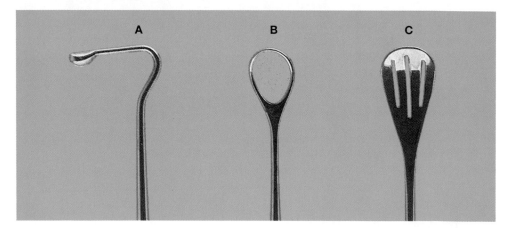

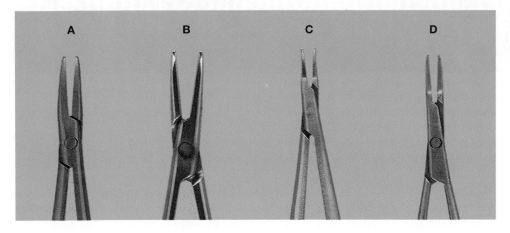

79-9 *Left to right:* enlarged tips: **A**, Titanium needle holder with stop, no lock, curved; **B**, Castroviejo needle holder with lock, curved; **C**, Troutman-Barraquer microneedle holder, curved; **D**, Sinskey tying forceps, straight.

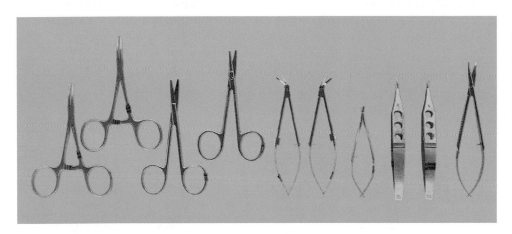

79-10 *Left to right:* 2 Halsted mosquito hemostatic forceps; 2 blunt scissors, straight; 2 Castroviejo corneal section scissors, left and right; 1 Vannas capsulotomy scissors, straight; 2 transplant microscissors, right and left; 1 Westcott tenotomy scissors.

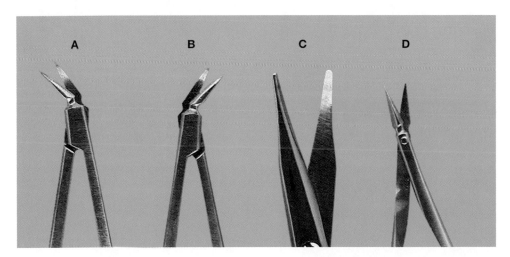

79-11 *Left to right:* enlarged tips: **A**, Castroviejo corneal section scissors, left; **B**, Castroviejo corneal scissors, right; **C**, Westcott tenotomy scissors; **D**, Vannas capsulotomy scissors, straight.

Chapter 80

Deep Lamellar Endothelial Keratoplasty (DLEK)

Deep lamellar endothelial keratoplasty (DLEK) is a split-thickness (lamellar transplant) form of corneal transplantation. When this procedure is performed, a smaller incision is used, and only the diseased tissue is removed. The remainder of the patient's cornea remains intact. This procedure involves the replacement of the back layers of the cornea rather than the front layers. It is performed through a small pocket incision, which avoids any changes in the front surface of the cornea. In the DLEK procedure, one to three tiny sutures are placed, rather than the 16 or one to two long looping sutures in a circle that are used in penetrating keratoplasty (PK). In the DLEK procedure, the cornea has a smoother surface and a clearer transplant, which allows many of the patients to see better in a matter of weeks instead of the months or years in a standard full-thickness corneal transplant.

Possible instruments needed for the procedure include a cataract-removal set.

80-1 *Left to right:* 1 8-mm corneal marker; 1 Charlie insertion forceps; 2 Devers dissectors, curved; 1 Cindy scissors; 1 Cindy 2 scissors; 1 reverse Sinskey hook; 1 Nick pick; and 1 Terry scraper.

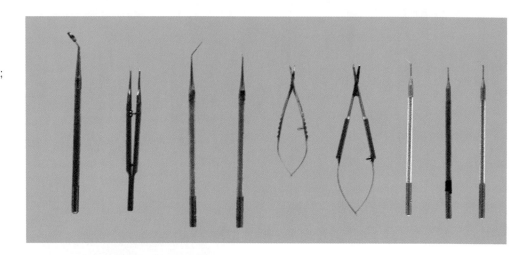

80-2 *Top,* anterior chamber. *Middle,* 2 stopcocks. *Bottom,* 2 blue caps for stopcocks, and top part to the anterior chamber.

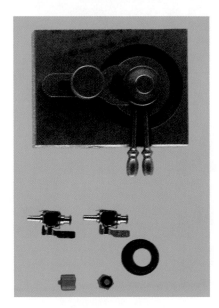

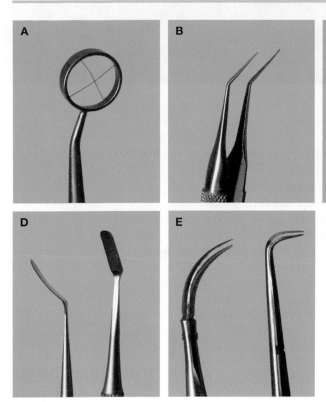

80-3 *Left to right:* Tips: **A**, 8-mm corneal marker; **B**, Charlie insertion forceps; **C**, Terry scraper, Nick pick, and reverse Sinskey hook; **D**, Devers dissectors; **E**, Cindy scissors and Cindy 2 scissors.

Glaucoma

Glaucoma is a condition of increased intraocular pressure because of obstructed aqueous humor outflow.

Possible instruments and equipment needed for the procedure include a basic eye set, an operating microscope, and a shunt.

A brief description of the procedure follows:

1. A Lancaster speculum is placed to retract the eyelids.
2. A Beaver knife handle with blade is used to incise the conjunctiva.
3. A Jameson muscle hook is used to isolate the rectus muscles.
4. The device plate is sutured to the sclera using the Barraquer needle holder and Kelman-McPherson tying forceps.
5. A Kelly-Descemet membrane punch is used to create a tunnel into the anterior chamber.
6. The device tube is inserted into the anterior chamber and anchored with suture.
7. The conjunctiva is closed.

81-1 *Left to right:* 1 Kelman-McPherson tying forceps, straight, front view; 1 Kelman-McPherson tying forceps, angled, side view; 2 McCullough utility forceps, front view and side view; 1 McPherson tying forceps, straight; 1 McPherson tying forceps, curved; 1 Chandler (Gills) forceps; 2 Hoskins forceps, straight and curved.

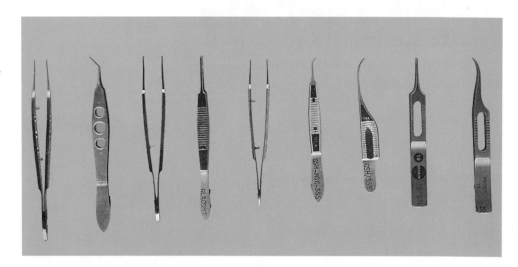

81-2 *Top right:* 1 irrigation cannula, 19 gauge. *Bottom, left to right:* 2 Vannas scissors, straight and curved; 1 Westcott corneal miniscissors, sharp; 1 Westcott tenotomy scissors, blunt; 1 Kelley-Descemet membrane punch; 1 Elschnig cyclodialysis spatula; 2 Halsted mosquito hemostatic forceps, curved.

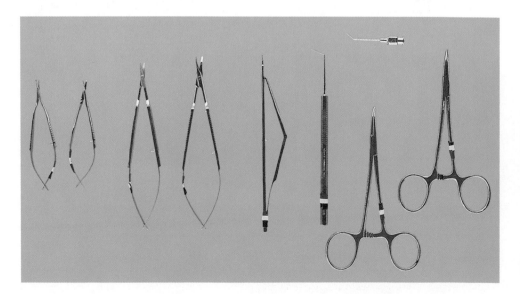

Eye Muscle Surgery*

Eye muscles are released and tucked to treat the condition called strabismus or "cross eyes."

Possible instruments needed for the procedure includes a basic eye set.

A brief description of the procedure to loosen the inferior oblique muscle follows:

1. A Cook speculum is used to retract the lids.
2. Westcott tenotomy scissors are used for incision into the tenon capsule.
3. A Jameson muscle hook is used to isolate and lift the muscle.
4. A Beaver knife with blade is used to bisect the muscle.
5. Jameson recession forceps are used to grasp ends of muscle.
6. A cautery is used for hemostasis.
7. A Castroviejo caliper is used to measure how much to relax the muscle.

A brief description of the procedure to tuck the superior rectus muscle follows:

1. Follow steps 1 through 3 above.
2. A Castroviejo caliper is used to measure how big a tuck to make.
3. Jameson recession forceps are used to grasp the muscle.
4. A Von Graefe strabismus hook is used to elevate the tendon to be doubled into a loop.
5. A Troutman Barraquer needle holder is used for attaching the loop to the sclera.
6. A Titanium needle holder is used for closing the conjunctiva.
7. Kelman-McPherson tying forceps are used to tie the suture.

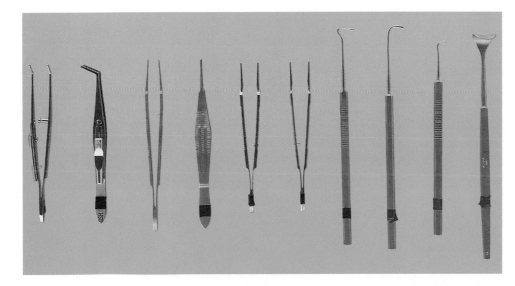

82-1 *Left to right:* 2 Jameson muscle recession forceps, right, front view and side view; 2 Castroviejo suture-tying forceps, wide handles, without tying platforms, 0.5 mm teeth (1 × 2), front view and side view; 2 McCullough utility forceps, cross serrated; 1 Jameson muscle hook; 1 Von Graefe strabismus hook; 1 Stevens tenotomy hook; 1 Desmarres lid retractor.

---

*Additional images are available on the Companion CD.

82-2 *Left to right:* enlarged tips: **A**, Jameson muscle recession forceps, right; **B**, McCullough utility forceps, cross-serrated; **C**, Jameson muscle hook; **D**, Stevens tenotomy hook; **E**, Desmarres lid retractor.

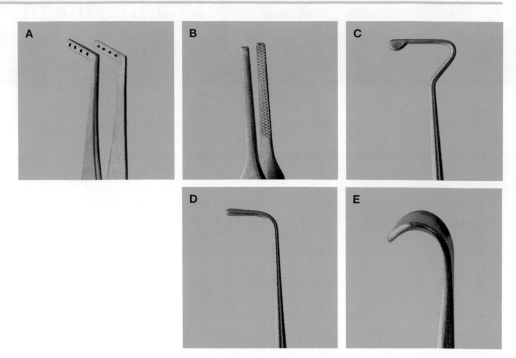

82-3 *Top, left to right:* 1 Castroviejo caliper; 1 Cook eye speculum, child-sized; 1 Lancaster speculum. *Bottom, left to right:* 4 serrefines; 1 strabismus scissors, straight; 1 Westcott tenotomy scissors, curved; 1 Stevens tenotomy scissors, curved; 1 Castroviejo needle holder with lock, curved; 1 Castroviejo needle holder with lock, straight; 1 Erhardt chalazion clamp; 1 metal ruler, small.

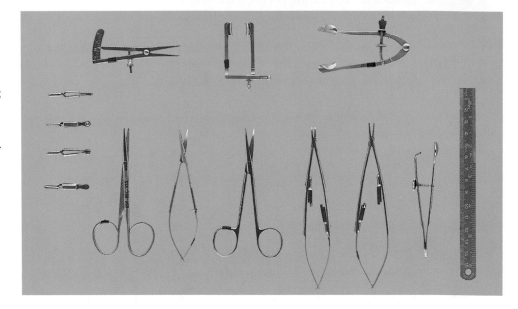

A retinal detachment is the separation of the retina from the internal wall of the eye.

Possible instruments needed for repair of a detachment include a basic eye set.

A brief description of the possible methods of repairing a detached retina follows:

1. Scleral buckling. This procedure places a silicone band, sponge, or other device against the outside of the eye at the area of the detachment. This presses the wall of the eye into the retina to encourage reattachment.

2. Pneumatic retinopexy. This procedure uses gas, which is injected into the posterior chamber. By positioning the patient, the gas bubble is forced against the wall of the eye where the detachment is. The gas used will expand and later diffuse in 7 to 10 or 30 to 50 days, depending on which gas is used.

3. Laser photocoagulation. This procedure uses a laser beam to treat the retinal hole. The laser may be used in conjunction with scleral buckling or pneumatic retinopexy.

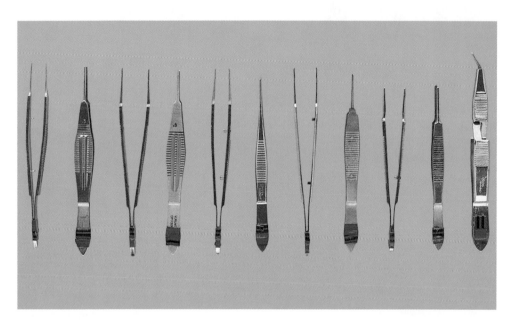

83-1 *Left to right:* 4 Castroviejo suturing forceps, wide handles, with tying platforms: 0.3 mm front view, 0.5 mm side view, 0.12 mm front view, 0.12 mm side view; 1 Bonn suture forceps; 1 Wills Hospital utility forceps, straight; 1 Elschnig fixation forceps; 1 Harms tying forceps; 2 McCullough utility forceps, front view and side view; 1 Watzke sleeve-spreader forceps.

83-2 *Left to right:* enlarged tips: **A**, Bonn suture forceps; **B**, Wills Hospital utility forceps, straight; **C**, Elschnig fixation forceps; **D**, Harms suture-tying forceps, straight; **E**, Watzke sleeve-spreading forceps.

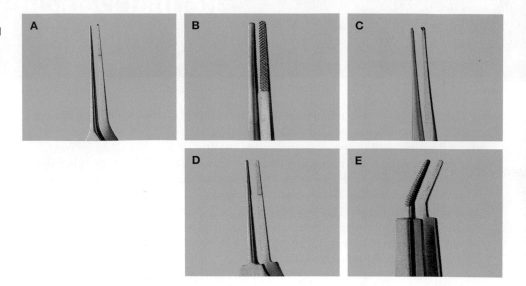

83-3 *Left to right:* 1 Stevens tenotomy scissors; 1 Westcott tenotomy scissors; 1 Green needle holder and forceps; 1 Castroviejo needle holder, straight, without lock; 2 Castroviejo needle holders, straight, with locks; 1 Thorpe calipers; 1 Castroviejo calipers.

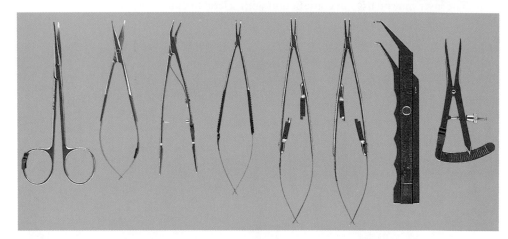

83-4 *Top, left to right:* 2 Barraquer wire speculums; 5 Mira diathermy tips, assorted. *Bottom, left to right:* 4 serrefines; 1 Beaver knife handle, knurled, with insert above; 1 Schepens orbital retractor; 1 Jameson muscle hook; 1 Von Graefe strabismus hook; 1 Gass retinal detachment hook.

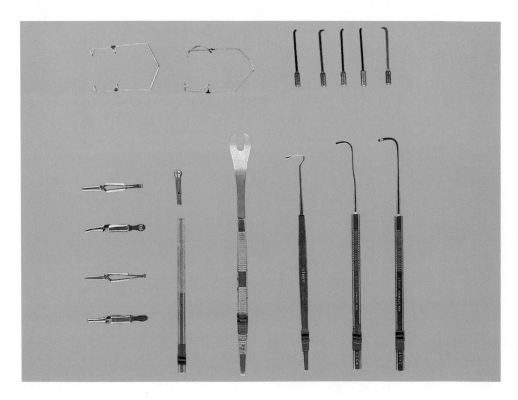

Vitrectomy is the removal of the vitreous humor in the posterior chamber of the eye.

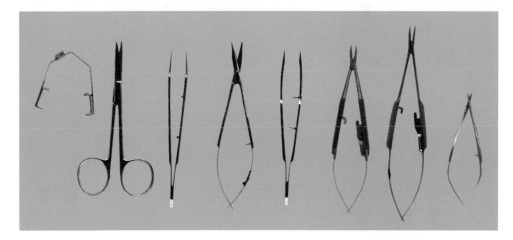

84-1 *Left to right:* 1 Barragaer wire speculum; 1 iris scissors, straight; 1 Castroviejo suturing forceps, 0.12 mm; 1 Westcott tonotomy scissors; 1 Paton forceps; 1 Troutman-Barraquer needle holder with lock; 1 Castroviejo needle holder with lock; and 1 Vannas capsulotomy scissors.

84-2 *Top, left to right:* 1 19-gauge irrigating cannula; white sponge; 1 27-gauge Bishop-Harmon irrigating cannula; 1 20-gauge and 1 19-gauge cannulas. *Bottom, left to right:* 1 Castroviejo caliper; 2 scleral plug forceps; 1 flat Machemer irrigating lens with attached silicone tubing; 1 Minus irrigating lens with attached silicone tubing; 1 Schocket scleral depressor, doubled-ended; 1 Von Graefe strabismus hook; and 2 Castroviejo needle holders, curved, straight.

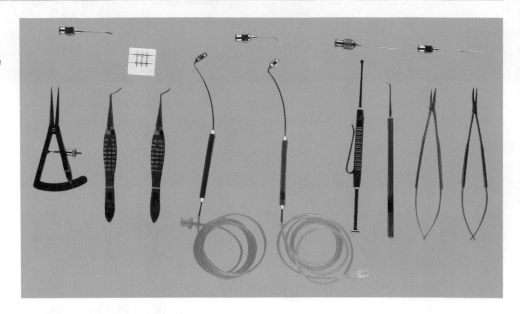

84-3 *Left to right:* Tips: Minus and Machemer irrigating lens.

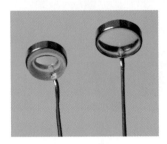

84-4 *Left to right:* Tips: scleral plug forceps, side view, front view.

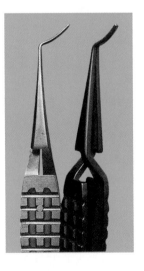

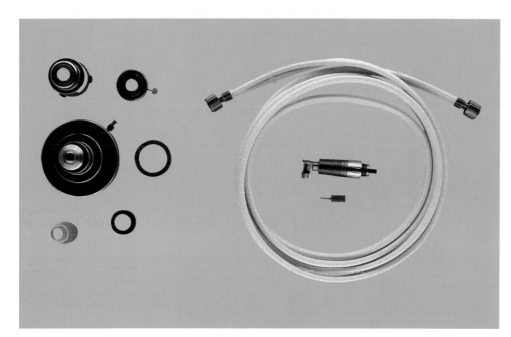

85-1 *Left upper:* 4 parts of a Moira microkeratone. *Left lower:* 2 parts of a tonometer. *Right lower:* white power cord to microkeratone and microkeratone handpiece and tip.

Oculoplastic Instrument Set*

86-1 *Top, left to right:* Lancaster speculum; and 2 Edwards holding clips. *Bottom, left to right:* 1 Castroviejo caliper; 1 Bard-Parker knife handle #3; 1 Mayo dissecting scissors, straight, 6 inch; 1 Westcott tenotomy scissors; 1 Stevens tenotomy scissors; 1 Adson tissue forceps with teeth; (1 × 2); and 2 Halsted mosquito hemostatic forceps, curved, straight.

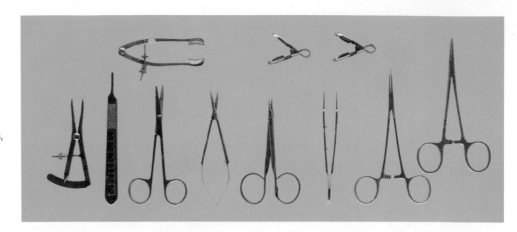

86-2 *Left to right:* 1 Mueller clamp; 1 lacrimal sac retractor, 4 prong, blunt; 1 double fixation hook, 2 prong; 1 iris scissors, sharp; 2 Bishop-Harmon tissue forceps, 0.5 mm; 2 Paufique suture forceps with teeth (1 × 2); 1 Desmarres lid retractor; and 2 Castroviejo needle holders with locks, straight, curved.

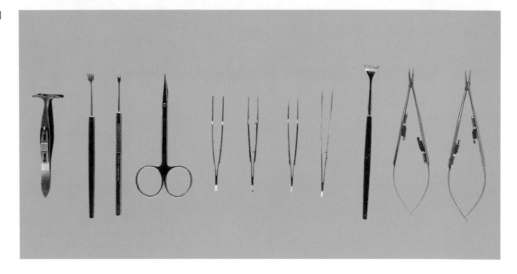

*Additional images are available on the Companion CD.

Dacrocystorhinotomy (DCR) is done to make a new lacrima duct.

A brief description of the procedure follows:
1. A Bard-Parker scalpel handle #3 with a #15 blade is used to make an incision into the medial canthus.
2. A curved Halsted mosquito may be used for blunt dissection to the orbicularis muscle.
3. A Freer elevator is used to separate the orbicularis muscle from the nasal bone.
4. A Freer chisel with a mallet may be used to punch a hole into the lacrimal bone.
5. A Kerrison rongeur can be used to enlarge the hole.
6. A Goldstein lacrimal sac retractor is placed for visualization.
7. A lacrimal dilator is used to dilate the inferior punctum.
8. Bowman lacrimal probes are passed into the lacrimal sac.
9. Stevens tenotomy scissors are used to incise the lacrimal sac and nasal mucosa.
10. Castroviejo needle holder and suture are used to suture the posterior lacrimal sac to the posterior nasal mucosa.
11. Silastic lacrimal duct tubing is passed into the nose (to be removed after healing).
12. A Vienna nasal speculum may be placed in the nares to check the entrance of the tubing.
13. A Castroviejo needle holder with Castroviego suture forceps are used to suture the anterior lacrimal sac flap and the nasal mucosa to form a tunnel for the silastic tubing.

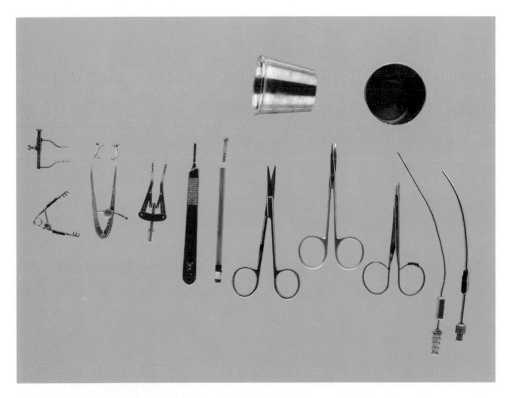

87-1 *Top, right:* 2 metal medicine cups. *Top to bottom, middle left:* 1 Goldstein lacrimal sac retractor and 1 Agrikola lacrimal sac retractor. *Left to right:* 1 Lancaster eye speculum; 1 Knapp lacrimal sac retractor, blunt; 1 Bard-Parker knife handle #3; 1 insert and Beaver knife handle; 1 suture scissors, blunt, straight; 1 stitch scissors, sharp; 1 Stevens tenotomy scissors; 2 Frazier suctions, 7 Fr and 10 Fr.

*Additional images are available on the Companion CD.

87-2 *Top:* 1 19-gauge irrigating cannula. *Middle, left to right:* 2 Bowman lacrimal probes; 1 punctal lacrimal dilator; 1 groove director; 1 probe dilator; 1 lacrimal sac retractor, 4-prong blunt; 1 Von Graefe muscle hook; 1 Desmarres lid retractor; 1 Vienna nasal speculum (2 × 1 inch); 1 Cottle nasal speculum (1 × 1¼ inch); 2 Bishop-Harmon tissue forceps with teeth (1 × 2); 1 Paufique suturing forceps; and 1 Adson tissue forceps with teeth (1 × 2). *Bottom, left to right:* 2 bayonet tissue forceps, 7¼ inch, front view, 6⅜ inch, side view.

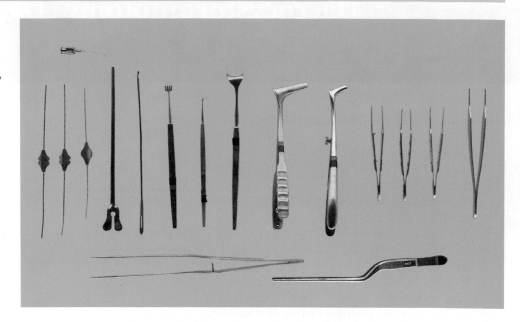

87-3 *Top, left to right:* 1 pituitary rongeur, straight, 5½ inch; and 2 Kerrison rongeurs, 40-degree upbite, 6 inch, 7 inch. *Bottom, left to right:* 1 Belz lacrimal sac rongeur; 1 Kerrison rongeur, 40-degree upbite, micro, 3 mm, 7 inch; and 1 Kerrison rongeur, 40-degree upbite, 6 inch, narrow.

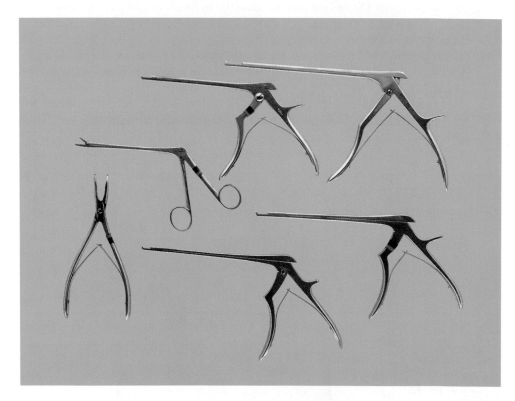

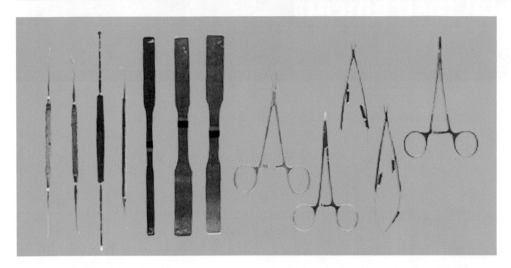

87-4 *Left to right:* 2 Freer elevators, double-ended, straight, curved; 1 Cottle elevator, double-ended; 1 burnisher dental tool; 3 brain spatulas; 2 Halsted mosquito hemostatic forceps, straight, curved; 2 Castroviejo needle holders; and 1 Crile-Wood needle holder, diamond jaw, 5 inch.

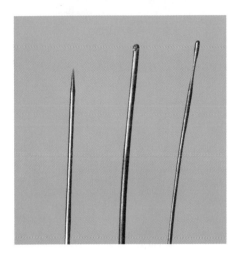

87-5 *Left to right:* Tips: 1 punctal lacrimal dilator and 2 Bowman lacrimal probes.

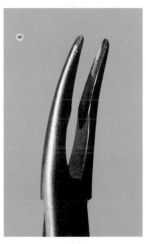

87-6 Tip: Belz lacrimal rongeur.

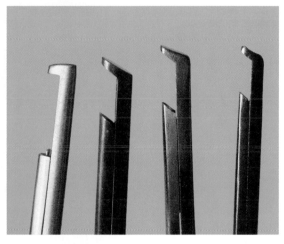

87-7 Tips: 4 Kerrison rongeurs, 40-degree upbite, 7 inch; 6 inch narrow; micro 3-mm / inch.

Orbital Instruments

Possible instruments needed for the procedure includes a basic eye set.

88-1 *Top to bottom:* 1 Cottle septum elevator, double-ended; 2 Freer elevators, double-ended. *Bottom, left to right:* 1 Belz lacrimal sac rongeur; 1 Dingman flexible retractor; 1 Schepens orbital retractor; 1 orbital retractor-elevator; 1 Converse alar retractor, double-ended.

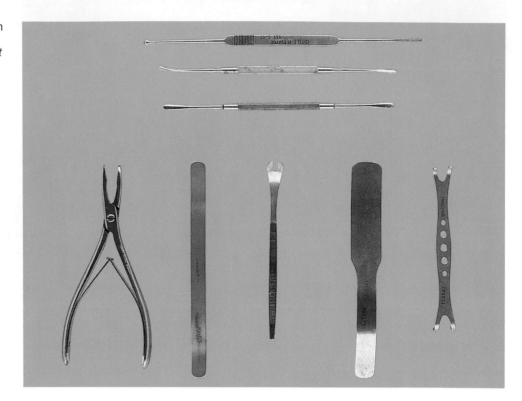

Enucleation is the removal of the eyeball.

Possible instruments needed for the procedure includes a basic eye set.

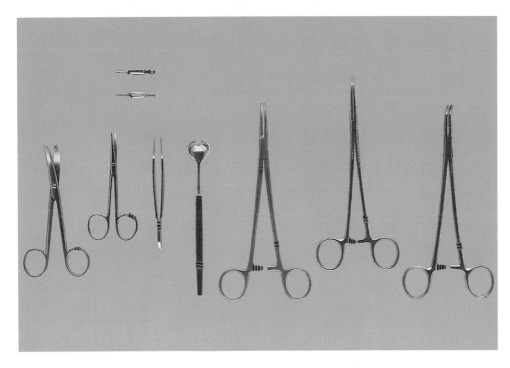

89-1 *Top:* 2 serrefines. *Bottom, left to right:* 1 enucleation scissors, sharp, curved; 1 Stevens tenotomy scissors; 1 Castroviejo suturing forceps with tying platforms, 0.5 mm teeth (1 × 2); 1 Wells enucleation spoon; 2 tonsil hemostatic forceps; 1 Westphal hemostatic forceps.

Myringotomy

Myringotomy is an incision into the tympanic membrane (eardrum).

Possible equipment needed for the procedure includes an operating microscope.

A brief description of the procedure follows:

1. A Boucheron ear speculum is placed in the ear canal.
2. A Frazier suction tip, which is attached to tubing, is used for removal of the secretions.
3. A Crabtree ring curette is used to remove ear wax.
4. A myringotomy knife with a Royce blade is used to incise the drum.
5. House alligator forceps are used to place the prosthetic tube.

90-1 *Left, top to bottom:* 5 Boucheron ear speculums, assorted sizes, top and side views. *Top, left to right:* 1 metal medicine cup, 8 oz; 3 Frazier suction tubes with finger valves. *Bottom, left to right:* 1 ear curette, small; 1 ear curette, large; 1 myringotomy knife in folding handle with straight Royce blade; 1 iris scissors, straight; 1 alligator forceps, straight.

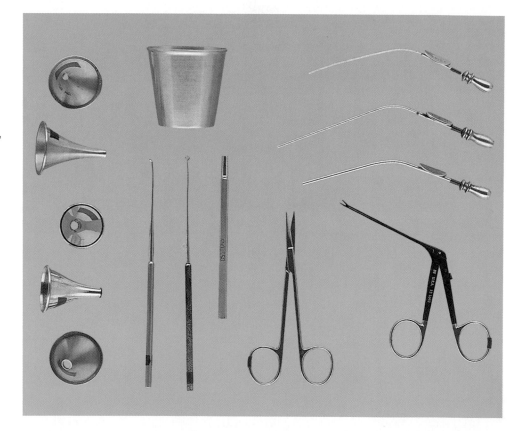

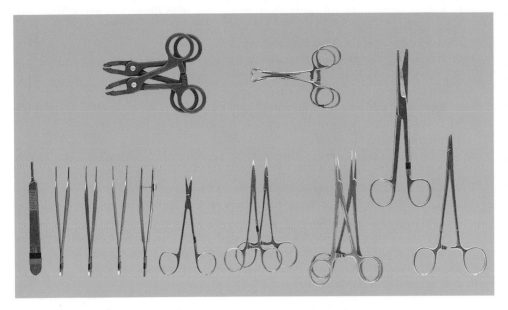

91-1 *Top, left to right:* 2 paper drape clips; 2 Backhaus towel forceps, small. *Bottom, left to right:* 1 Bard-Parker knife handle #3; 1 Adson tissue forceps, without teeth; 1 Adson tissue forceps, with teeth (1 × 2); 1 Brown-Adson tissue forceps with teeth (7 × 7); 1 Sheehy ossicle-holding forceps; 1 strabismus scissors, curved; 2 Halsted mosquito hemostatic forceps, curved; 2 Crile hemostatic forceps; 1 Mayo dissecting scissors, straight; 1 Johnson needle holder, 7 inch.

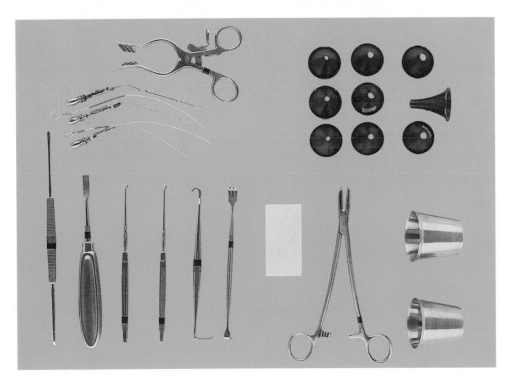

91-2 *Left, top to bottom:* 1 Weitlaner retractor, dull prongs, angled; 3 Baron ear suction tubes with finger valve control: 3, 5, and 7 Fr; 2 stylets. *Right, top to bottom:* 9 Richards ear speculums, assorted sizes, 4 to 8 mm, one side view. *Bottom, left to right:* 1 Cottle elevator, double-ended; 1 Lempert elevator (converse periosteal); 2 Johnson skin hooks; 2 Senn-Kanavel retractors, side view and front view; 1 House Teflon block; 1 House Gelfoam press or Sheehy fascia press; 2 metal medicine cups, 2 oz.

Tympanoplasty

A tympanoplasty is the repair of the tympanic membrane (eardrum).

Possible equipment and instruments needed for the procedure include an operating microscope for visualization, House suction/irrigation and tubing to remove fluid and irrigate, a stylet to keep the tip open, an ototome drill with micro bits and microburrs, and a basic ear set.

A brief description of the procedure follows:

1. A Richards speculum of appropriate size is placed in the ear canal.
2. A Crabtree wax curette is used to remove wax from the canal.
3. A Jordan oval knife may be used to incise the tympanomeatal junction.
4. A Rosen needle is used to elevate the skin of the canal.
5. Richards cup forceps are used to clean all epithelium from the ear drum perforation.
6. An ototome drill with micro burrs may be needed if the perforation is not clearly visible.
7. A House pick is used to explore the middle ear for ossicle mobility.
8. Richards alligator forceps are used to remove any epithelium in the middle ear. To harvest a graft from the temporalis muscle, a Lempert elevator may be used to separate fascia from the temporalis muscle. A strabismus scissors is used to cut the fascia, and a Sheehy fascia press is used to thin the fascia before placement.
9. Richards alligator forceps are used to place the graft over the perforation.
10. A Rosen needle is used to position the graft securely.

If an ossicular reconstruction may be performed; a brief description of the procedure follows:

1. A Bellucci scissors is used to cut soft tissue.
2. A Mueller malleus nipper is used to loosen the bones.
3. A House sickle knife is used to free the incus from the stapes.
4. Richards alligator forceps are used to remove the bones or fragments.
5. A PORP (partial ossicular replacement prosthesis) is needed to replace several bones.
6. A TORP (total ossicular replacement prosthesis) is needed when all middle-ear bones are removed.

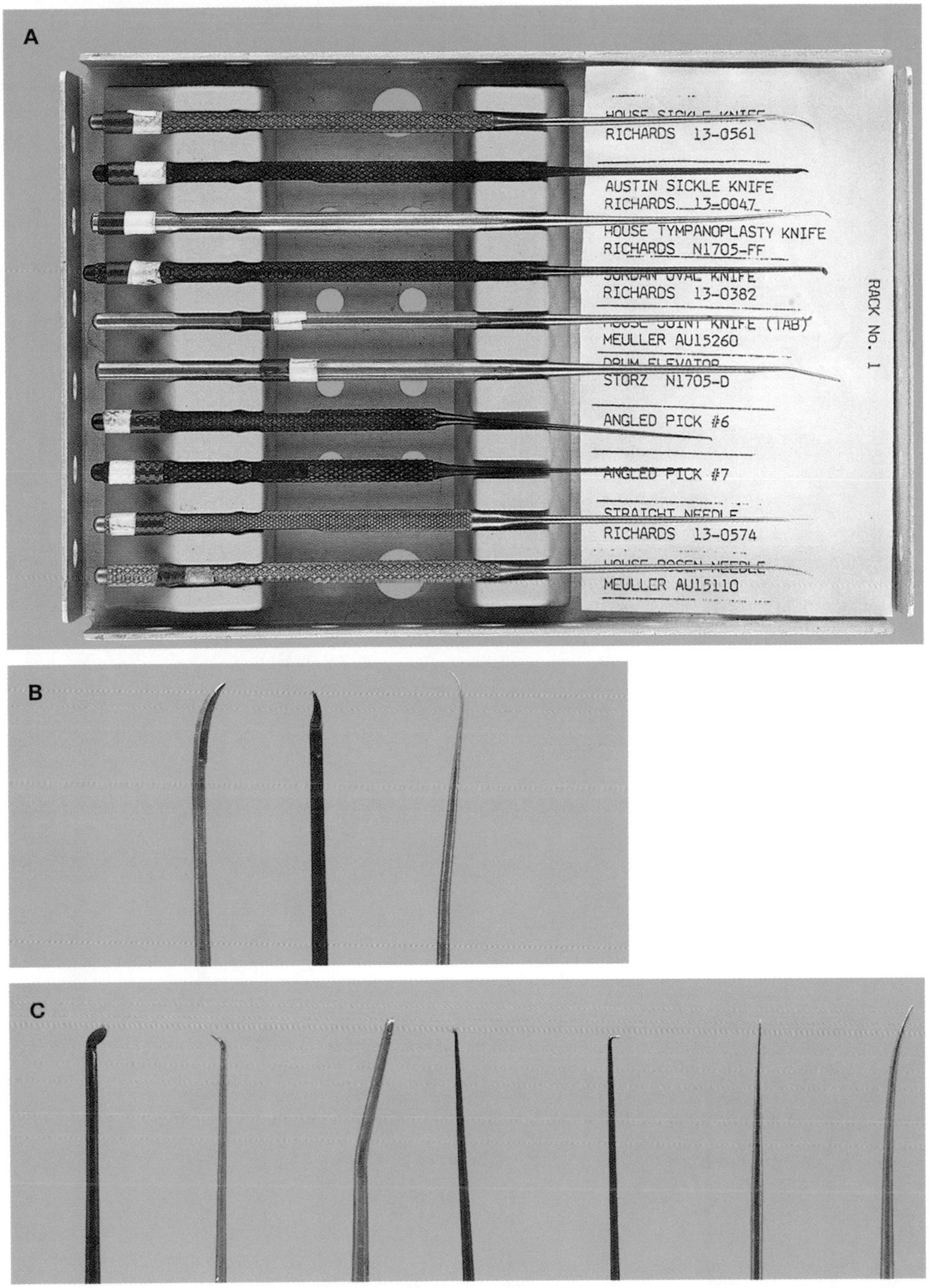
A
RICHARDS 13-0561
AUSTIN SICKLE KNIFE
RICHARDS 13-0047
HOUSE TYMPANOPLASTY KNIFE
RICHARDS N1705-FF
RICHARDS 13-0382
MEULLER AU15260
STORZ N1705-D
ANGLED PICK #6
ANGLED PICK #7
RICHARDS 13-0574
MEULLER AU15110
RACK No. 1
B
C

92-1 **A**, Rack No. 1 of delicate ear instruments with labels. **B**, *Left to right:* tips of delicate ear instruments: House sickle knife; Austin sickle knife; House tympanoplasty knife. **C**, *Left to right:* tips of delicate ear instruments: Jordan oval knife; House joint knife; drum elevator; angled pick #6; angled pick #7; straight needle; House-Rosen needle.

92-2 A, Rack No. 2 of delicate ear instruments with labels. **B,** *Left to right:* tips of delicate ear instruments: curved needle, large curve; curved needle, small curve. **C,** *Left to right:* tips of delicate ear instruments: straight needle; Austin 25-degree pick; House pick, 1 mm; House pick, 3 mm; oval window pick; whirlybird, left; whirlybird, right.

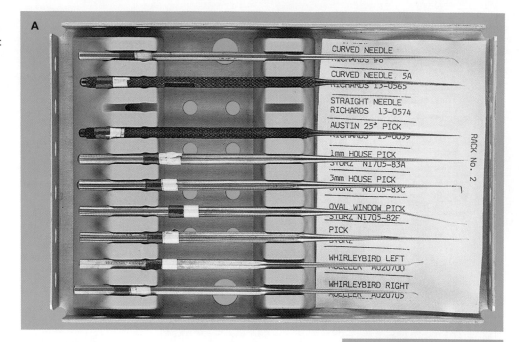

A

CURVED NEEDLE
RICHARDS #6
CURVED NEEDLE 5A
RICHARDS 13-0565
STRAIGHT NEEDLE
RICHARDS 13-0574
AUSTIN 25° PICK
RICHARDS 13-0659
1mm HOUSE PICK
STORZ N1705-83A
3mm HOUSE PICK
STORZ N1705-83C
OVAL WINDOW PICK
STORZ N1705-82F
PICK
STORZ
WHIRLEYBIRD LEFT
MOELLER AU20700
WHIRLEYBIRD RIGHT
MOELLER AU20705

RACK No. 2

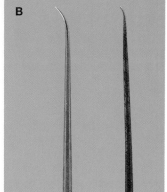

B

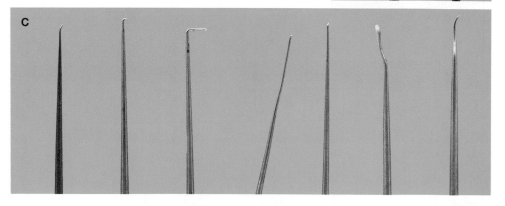

C

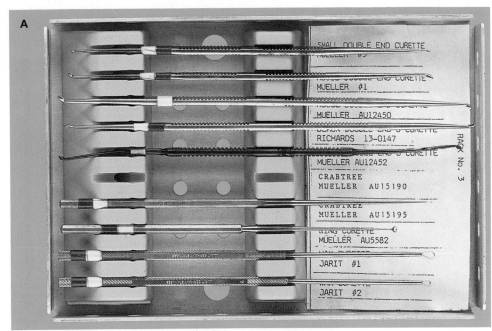

A

SMALL DOUBLE END CURETTE
MUELLER #3

HOUSE DOUBLE END CURETTE
MUELLER #1

HOUSE DOUBLE END CURETTE
MUELLER AU12450

BLACK DOUBLE END J CURETTE
RICHARDS 13-0147

HOUSE DOUBLE END J CURETTE
MUELLER AU12452

CRABTREE
MUELLER AU15190

CRABTREE
MUELLER AU15195

RING CURETTE
MUELLER AU5582

WAX CURETTE
JARIT #1

WAX CURETTE
JARIT #2

RACK NO. 3

92-3 A, Rack No. 3 of delicate ear instruments with labels. **B**, *Left to right:* tips of delicate ear instruments: small double-end curette #3; House double-end curette #1; House double-end curette; Black double-end J curette; House double-end J curette. **C**, *Left to right:* tips of delicate ear instruments: Crabtree; ring curette; wax curette #1; wax curette #2.

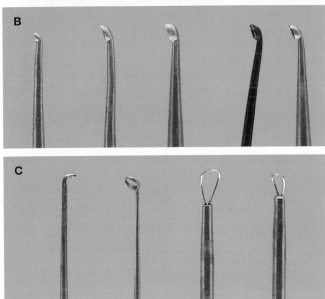

B

C

92-4 A, Rack No. 4 of delicate ear instruments with labels. **B**, *Left to right:* tips of delicate ear instruments: measuring rod; House measuring rod, 4 mm; House measuring rod, 4.5 mm; House measuring rod. **C**, *Left to right:* tips of delicate ear instruments: measuring rod; Derlacki; angled pick. **D**, *Left to right:* tips of delicate ear instruments: delicate hook #14; Buckingham footplate hand drill; Rosen knife.

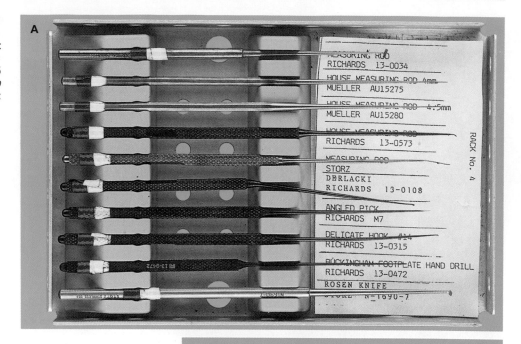

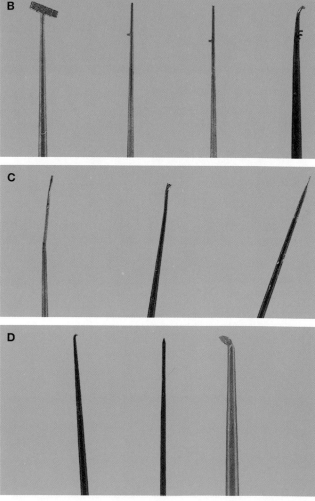

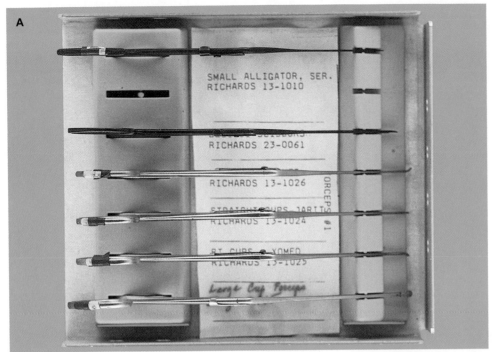

A

SMALL ALLIGATOR, SER.
RICHARDS 13-1010

RICHARDS 23-0061

RICHARDS 13-1026

RICHARDS 13-1024

RICHARDS 13-1025

Large Cup Forceps

92-5 A, Tray No. 1 of delicate ear forceps with labels. **B,** Delicate ear forceps out of tray. **C,** *Left to right:* tips of delicate ear forceps: small alligator, serrated; Bellucci scissors; left cup forceps. **D,** *Left to right:* tips of delicate ear forceps: straight-cup forceps; right-cup forceps; large-cup forceps.

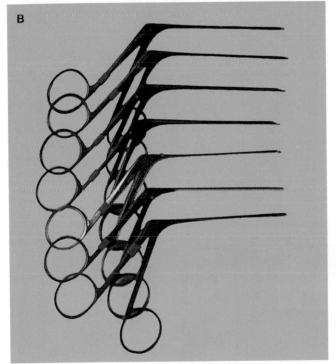

B

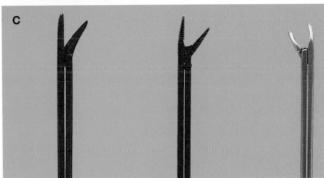

C

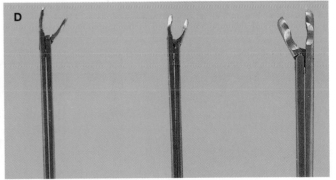

D

92-6 **A**, Tray No. 2 of delicate ear forceps with labels. **B**, *Left to right:* tips of delicate ear forceps: large crimper, small crimper; malleus nipper.

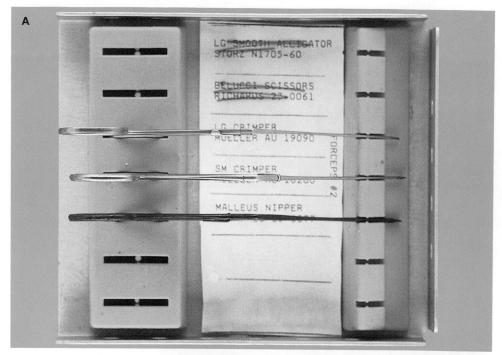

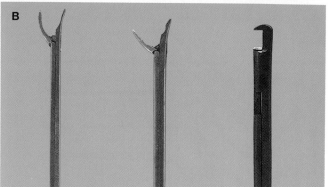

92-7 Blunt needles attached to tubing for suction tips, assorted sizes, 15 to 24 gauge.

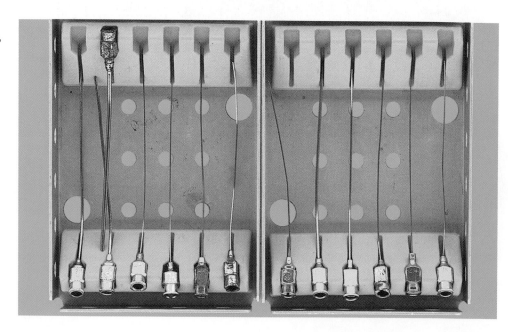

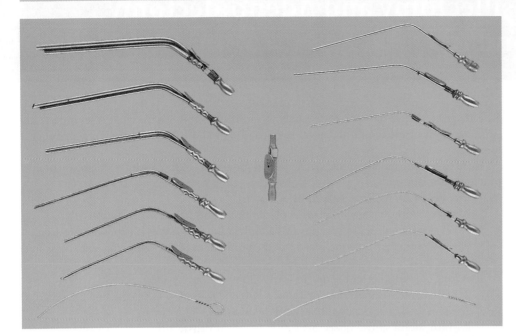

92-8 *Left to right:* 6 House suction/ irrigators with finger valve control and 1 stylet; 1 metal suction connector; 6 Baron ear suction tubes with finger valve control and 1 stylet.

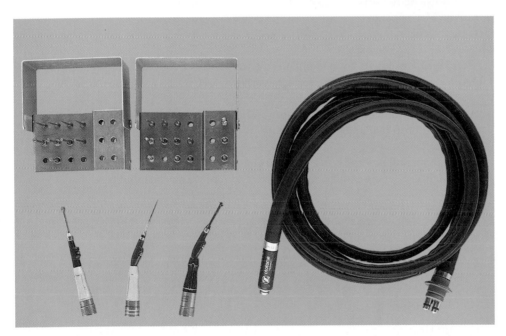

92-9 *Left, top:* Ototome drill bits and burs in cases, diamond, cutting, and air microburs. *Bottom, left to right:* straight high-speed handpiece with bur; angled high-speed handpiece with bit; angled low-speed handpiece with diamond bur; power cord.

Tonsillectomy and Adenoidectomy (T and A)

Tonsillectomy is the removal of the palatine tonsils in the oropharynx. Adenoidectomy is the removal of the lymph tissue on the posterior wall of the nasopharynx (pharyngeal tonsils).

Possible equipment and instruments needed for the procedure include an electrosurgical unit and a tonsil snare.

A brief description of a tonsillectomy follows:

1. A McIvor mouth gag with blade is placed in the mouth for visualization.
2. A Wieder tongue depressor is placed and held on the tongue to expose the tonsils.
3. An Andrews-Pynchon suction tip with tubing is used for removing secretions and blood.
4. A long curved Allis tissue forceps is used to grasp the tonsil.
5. A Bard-Parker scalpel handle #7 with #11 blade is used to incise the tonsil capsule.
6. A Fisher knife may be used to extend the incision.
7. A Hurd spoon (tonsil dissector) is used to bluntly dissect the tonsil.
8. A tonsil hemostatic forceps are used to clamp the main blood supply.
9. The Metzenbaum dissecting scissors are used to excise the tonsil.
10. A Ballenger sponge forceps with tonsil sponge is placed in the tonsil fossa to apply pressure for hemostasis.
11. A Hurd tonsil dissector and pillar retractor may be used to check for bleeding.
12. Electrocautery may be used for hemostasis.

A brief description of an adenoidectomy follows:

1. The Lothrop uvula retractor is placed at the back of the throat for exposure of the adenoids.
2. A LaForce adenotome is inserted and cuts out the adenoid.
3. A Meltzer adenoid punch may be needed to remove any adenoid tags.

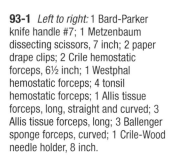

93-1 *Left to right:* 1 Bard-Parker knife handle #7; 1 Metzenbaum dissecting scissors, 7 inch; 2 paper drape clips; 2 Crile hemostatic forceps, 6½ inch; 1 Westphal hemostatic forceps; 4 tonsil hemostatic forceps; 1 Allis tissue forceps, long, straight and curved; 3 Allis tissue forceps, long; 3 Ballenger sponge forceps, curved; 1 Crile-Wood needle holder, 8 inch.

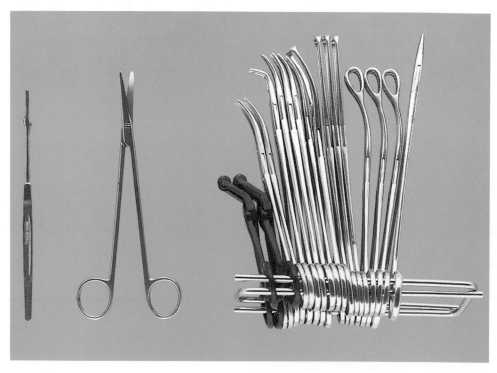

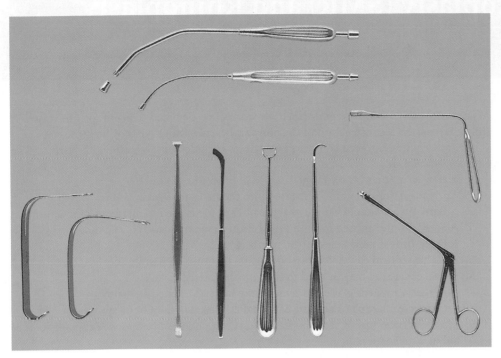

93-2 *Top to bottom:* 1 Andrews-Pynchon suction tube with tip; 1 adenoid suction tube, tip connected. *Bottom, left to right:* 2 Weder tongue depressors; 1 Hurd tonsil dissector and pillar retractor; 1 Fisher tonsil knife and dissector; 1 LaForce adenotome, small, front view; 1 LaForce adenotome, large, side view. *Right, top to bottom:* 1 Lothrop uvula retractor; 1 Meltzer adenoid punch, round, with basket.

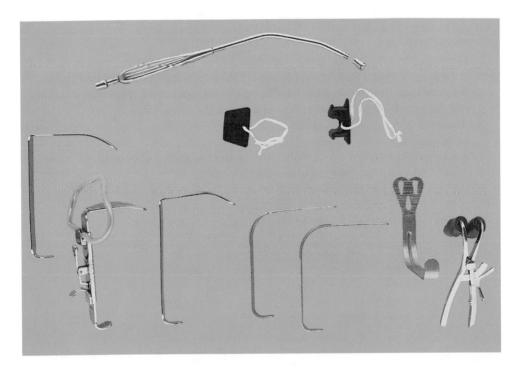

93-3 Mouth set. *Top to bottom:* 1 Andrews-Pynchon suction tube with tip; 2 bite blocks: child and adult. *Left to right:* 1 McIvor blade, long; 1 McIvor mouth gag frame with blade; 1 McIvor blade, medium; 3 Weder tongue depressors, 2 side views and 1 front view; 1 side mouth gag.

Septoplasty (SMR) and Rhinoplasty*

A submucous resection is performed to correct a deviated septum of the nose. A rhinoplasty is the reconstruction of the bony and cartilaginous parts of the nose.

Possible equipment needed for the procedures includes a power drill with burrs and an electrosurgical unit.

A brief description of the septoplasty (SMR) procedure follows:

1. A Vienna nasal speculum is inserted into the nares for visualization.
2. A Bard-Parker scalpel handle #7 with a #15 blade is used to incise into the septum.
3. A Freer elevator is used for blunt dissection to separate and elevate tissue layers.
4. A Freer knife is used to incise the cartilage.
5. A Cottle septum elevator is used to elevate the mucous membrane.
6. A Becker scissors may be used to trim the deviated cartilage.
7. A Kerrison rongeur is used to remove any bony, thickened structures.
8. A Converse guarded osteotome with mallet is used to trim bony spurs.
9. Frazier suction tips of various sizes with tubing are used to remove drainage so as to aid in visualization.

A brief description of the rhinoplasty procedure follows:

1. A Bard-Parker scalpel handle #3 with #15 blade may be used to make an incision in the tip of the nose.
2. Joseph hooks are placed to retract the skin.
3. A McKenty elevator may be used to elevate the skin from underlying structures.
4. A Cottle septum elevator is used to free up the periosteum and perichondrium.
5. A Ballenger chisel with a mallet is used to break the nasal bones.
6. A curved Metzenbaum dissecting scissors may be used to trim the upper lateral cartilage.
7. A Converse osteotome with a mallet may be used to shape the bony dorsal hump.
8. An Aufricht rasp may be used to smooth the hump.
9. A Cottle dorsal angular scissors may be used to remove a cartilaginous hump.
10. A Becker septum scissors may be used to remove the septal cartilage.
11. A Cottle osteotome with a mallet is used to remove bony spurs.

---

*Additional images are available on the Companion CD.

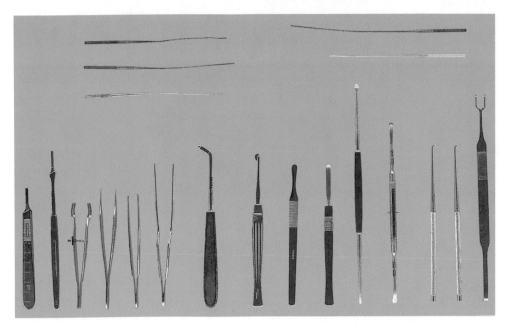

94-1 *Top:* 5 Ludwig wire applicators. *Bottom, left to right:* 1 Bard-Parker knife handle #3; 1 Bard-Parker knife handle #7; 1 Cottle columella forceps; 1 Brown-Adson tissue forceps with teeth (7 × 7); 1 Beasley-Babcock tissue forceps; 1 Jansen thumb forceps, bayonet shaft, serrated tips; 1 Joseph button-end knife, curved; 1 Freer septum knife; 1 Cottle nasal knife; 1 McKenty elevator; 1 Cottle septum elevator; 1 Freer elevator; 2 Joseph skin hooks; 1 Cottle knife guide and retractor.

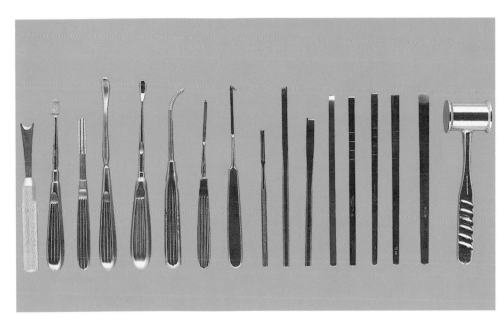

94-2 *Left to right:* 1 Bauer rocking chisel; 1 Lewis rasp; 1 Maltz rasp; 1 Aufricht rasp, large; 1 Aufricht rasp, small; 1 Wiener antrum rasp; 2 Ballenger swivel knives; 1 Ballenger chisel, 4 mm; 2 Converse guarded osteotomes; 1 Cottle osteotome, round corners, curved, 6 mm; 4 Cottle osteotomes, straight: 4, 7, 9, and 12 mm; 1 mallet, lead-filled head.

94-3 *Top, left to right:* 1 Fomon lower lateral scissors; 1 Metzenbaum dissecting scissors. *Bottom, left to right:* 1 Metzenbaum dissecting scissors, 4 inch, straight; 1 Metzenbaum dissecting scissors, 4 inch, curved; 1 Mayo dissecting scissors, straight; 1 Cottle spring scissors; 1 Cottle dorsal angular scissors; 1 Becker septum scissors.

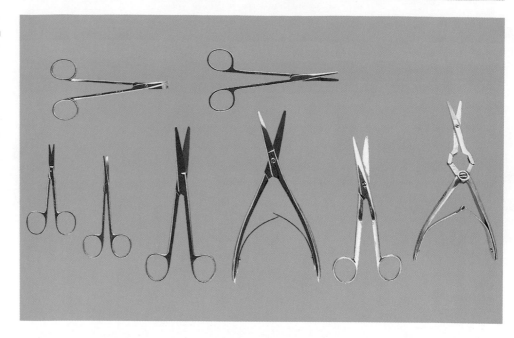

94-4 *Top:* 1 Andrews-Pynchon suction tube with tip. *Bottom, left to right:* 1 Bard-Parker knife handle #3; 1 Bard-Parker knife handle #7; 1 Beasley-Babcock tissue forceps; 1 Brown-Adson tissue forceps with teeth (7 × 7); 2 Frazier suction tubes with stylets, 7 Fr; 2 Frazier suction tubes with stylets, 12 Fr; 2 Backhaus towel forceps, small; 2 paper drape clips; 12 Halsted mosquito hemostatic forceps, curved; 2 Allis tissue forceps; 2 tonsil hemostatic forceps; 1 Johnson needle holder.

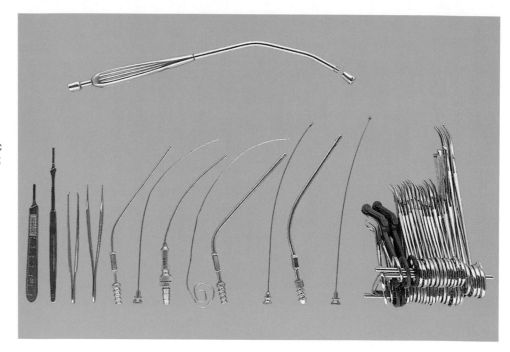

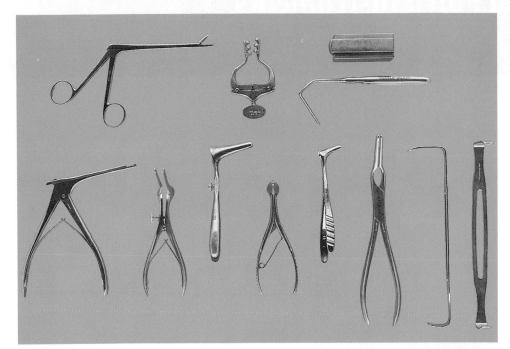

94-5 *Top, left to right:* 1 Ferris-Smith fragment forceps; 1 mastoid articulated retractor; 1 Cottle bone crusher, closed; 1 Aufricht retractor. *Bottom, left to right:* 1 Kerrison rongeur, upbite; 1 Killian nasal speculum, 2 inch, front view; 1 Killian nasal speculum, 3 inch, side view; 1 Vienna nasal speculum, $1^3/_8$ inch, front view; 1 Vienna nasal speculum, $1^1/_8$ inch, side view; 1 Asch septal forceps; 2 Army Navy retractors, side view and front view.

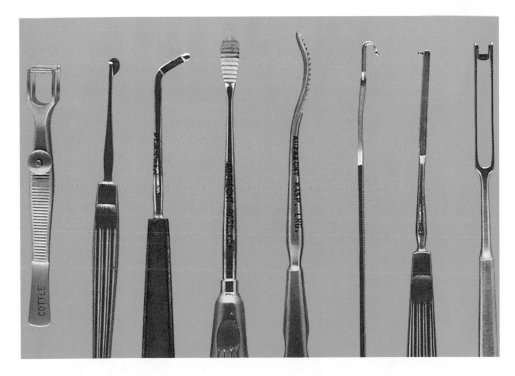

94-6 *Left to right:* Tips: 1 Cottle columella forceps; 1 Freer septum knife; 1 Joseph button-end knife; 1 Aufricht rasp, small, front view; 1 Aufricht rasp, large, side view; 1 Cottle knife guide and retractor, side view; 2 Ballenger swivel knives, side view and front view.

Nasal Polyp Instruments

95-1 *Left to right:* 1 Killian nasal speculum, 3 inch; 1 Druck-Levine antrum retractor with blade (2 parts); 6 Coakley antrum curettes, assorted sizes, #1 to #6; 1 Bruening nasal snare, bayonet (disposable wire).

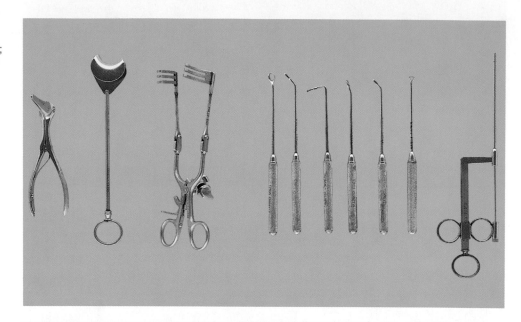

95-2 *Left to right:* **A**, Tips: Coakley antrum curettes, 7.5 mm × 9.5 mm; oval tip #1, 30-degree angle; oval tip #2, 60-degree angle; oval tip #3, 100-degree angle; **B**, Coakley antrum curettes, 6 mm × 7.5 mm, oval tip #4, 30-degree angle; oval tip #5, 60-degree angle; Coakley antrum curette, #6, 6 mm × 6 mm, triangular tip, 30-degree angle.

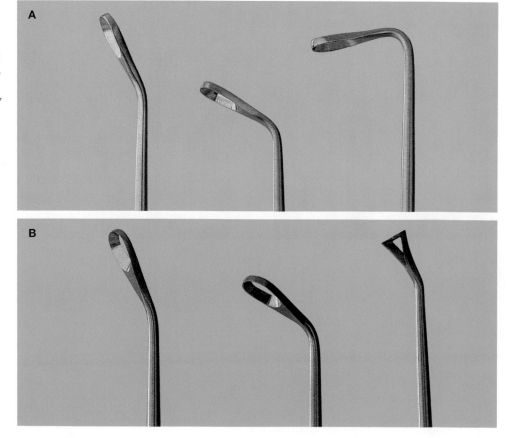

Nasal Fracture Reduction

A brief description of the procedure follows:
1. A Gillies elevator is inserted to align the bones and cartilage.
2. Asch forceps may be inserted to maintain alignment during packing insertion.

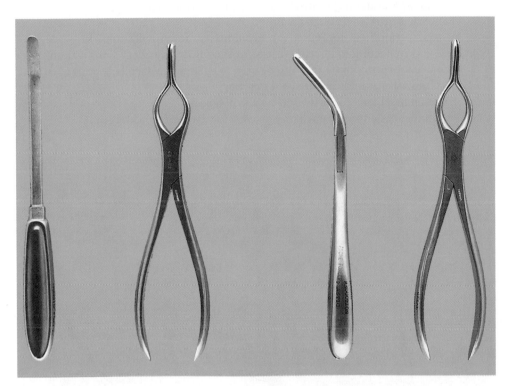

96-1 *Left to right:* 1 Gillies elevator; 3 Asch forceps, assorted angles.

Sinus Surgery*

The paranasal sinuses may need drainage improved or may need diseased membranes removed.

The endoscopy approach may be used. The instruments are introduced along side the scope. Possible equipment and instruments needed for the procedure include a light source and a nasal set. For irrigation, cysto tubing, a bag of normal saline, and suction tubing may be used.

A brief description of the procedure follows:

1. A Vienna speculum may be needed to dilate the nares.
2. The scope is inserted through the nose.
3. An axial suction/irrigator is used for secretions and for visualization.
4. Blakesley-Weil ethmoid forceps are used to enlarge the maxillary sinus ostium.
5. A Coakley antrum curette may also be used to enlarge the maxillary sinus opening.
6. The Grunwals nasal forceps are used to grasp polyps.
7. Struycken nasal forceps are used to cut the polyps.
8. A Stammberger antrum punch may be used to remove diseased tissue.

97-1 A, *Left to right:* pediatric and small nasal Blakesley-Weil forceps: 1 pediatric straight; 1 pediatric 45-degree; 1 45-degree small; and 1 90-degree small. **B**, *Left to right:* tips: pediatric and small Blakesley-Weil nasal forceps, tips: 1 pediatric straight; 1 pediatric 45-degree, 1 45-degree small; and 1 90-degree small.

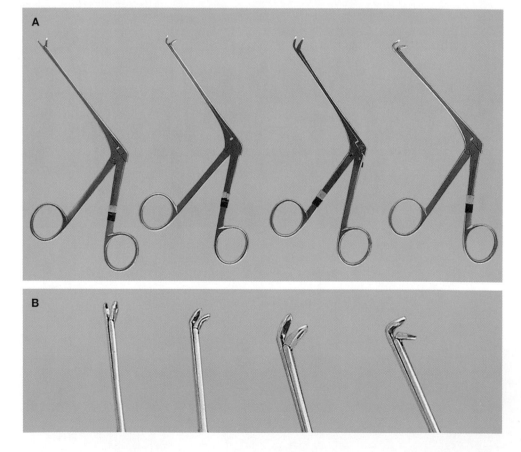

*Additional images are available on the Companion CD.

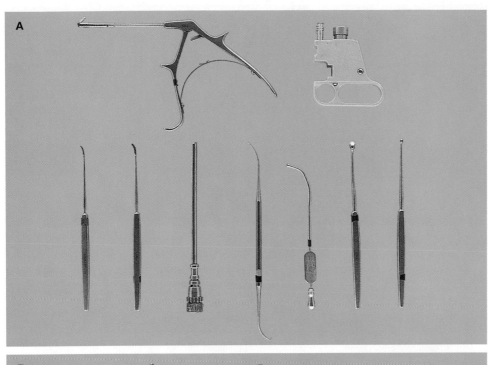

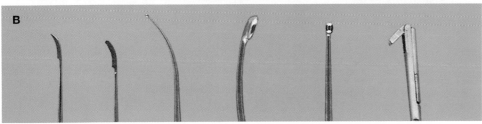

97-2 **A**, *Top, left to right:* 1 Stammberger antrum punch (backbiter); 1 axial suction/irrigation handle. *Bottom, left to right:* 1 sickle knife, sharp; 1 sickle knife, blunt; 1 sheath for 0 and 25 degrees, 4-mm lens; 1 maxillary sinus seeker; 1 Von Eicken antrum wash tube, 11 Fr; 2 antrum curettes, sizes 2 and 1: **B**, *Left to right:* tips: sickle knife, sharp; sickle knife, blunt; maxillary sinus seeker; 2 antrum curettes, sizes 2 and 1; Stammberger antrum punch (backbiter).

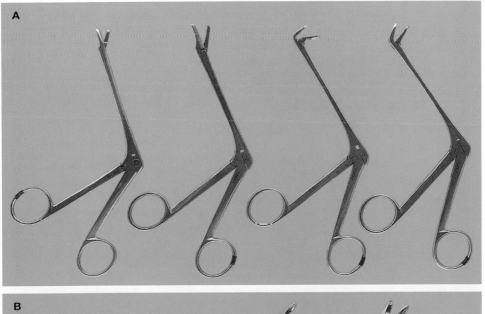

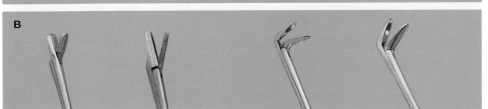

97-3 **A**, *Left to right:* Gruenwald nasal forceps, size 2: 1 straight, cutting; 1 Struycken nasal cutting forceps; 1 90-degree upward-bent; 1 upward-bent. **B**, *Left to right:* Gruenwald nasal forceps, size 2, tips: 1 straight, cutting; 1 Struycken nasal cutting forceps; 1 90-degree upward-bent; 1 upward-bent.

97-4 A, *Left to right:* Blakesley-Weil nasal forceps: 1 straight, size 0; 1 straight, size 1; 1 straight, size 2. **B**, *Left to right:* Blakesley-Weil nasal forceps, tips: 1 straight, size 0; 1 straight, size 1; 1 straight, size 2.

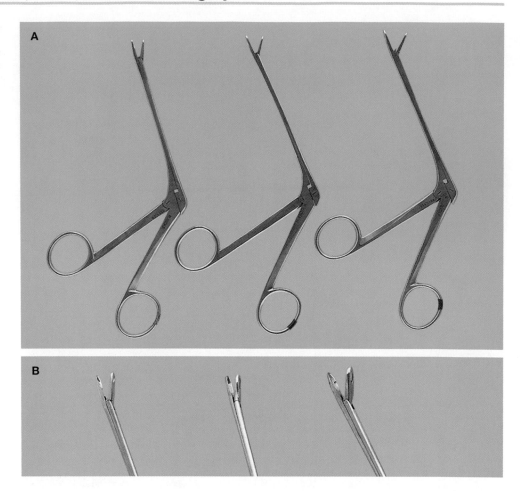

97-5 A, *Left to right:* 1 Kuhn-Bolger giraffe forceps, 90-degree (frontal sinus punch); 1 Kuhn-Bolger giraffe forceps, 110-degree (frontal sinus punch); 1 Stammberger antrum punch, left; 1 Stammberger antrum punch, right. **B**, *Left to right:* tips: 1 Kuhn-Bolger giraffe forceps, 90-degree; 1 Kuhn-Bolger giraffe forceps, 110-degree; 1 Stammberger antrum punch, left; 1 Stammberger antrum punch, right.

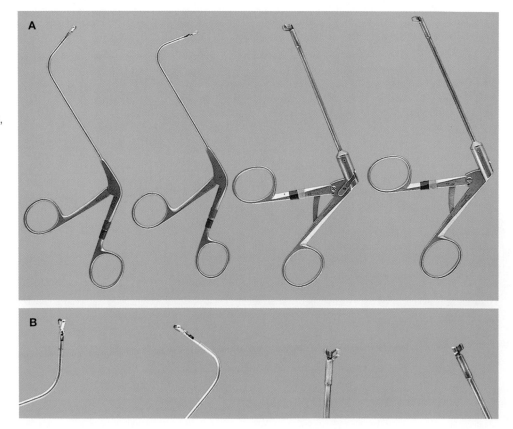

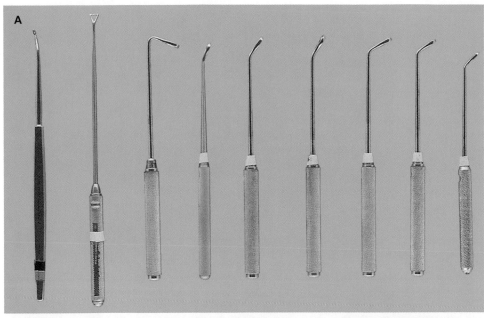

97-6 A, *Left to right:* 1 frontal sinus curette, 90-degree; 1 Coakley antrum curette, straight with triangle tip; variety of Coakley antrum curettes with various angles and sizes 1 to 6. **B,** *Left to right:* tips: frontal sinus curette and a variety of Coakley antrum curettes with various angles and sizes 1 to 6.

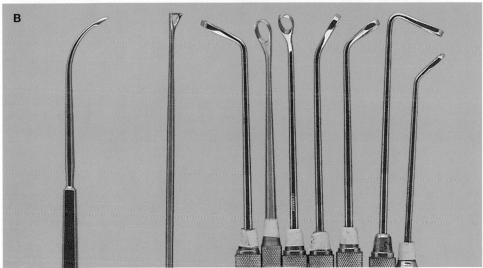

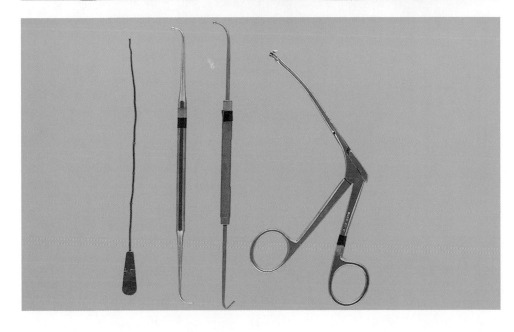

97-7 *Left to right:* 1 beaded measuring probe; 1 maxillary sinus ostium seeker; 1 frontal ostium seeker; 1 Ostrom-Terrier ostium forceps, retrograde.

97-8 *Left to right:* 1 small nasal scissors, straight: Tips: small nasal scissors, curved left; small nasal scissors, curved right.

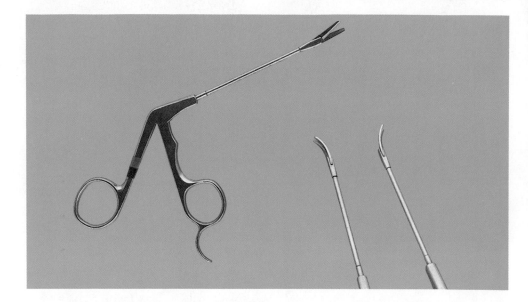

97-9 *Top to bottom:* 3 telescope lenses, 4 mm: 0 degree, 25 degree, 70 degree.

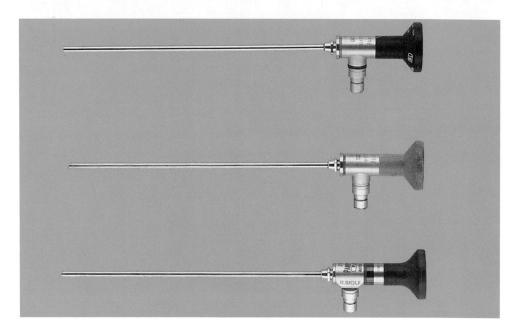

Facial Fracture Set

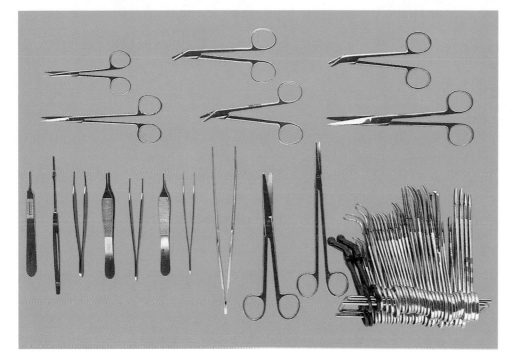

98-1 *Top, left to right:* 1 Stevens tenotomy scissors, curved; 1 plastic scissors, straight, sharp; 3 wire-cutting scissors; 1 Mayo dissecting scissors, straight. *Bottom, left to right:* 1 Bard-Parker knife handle #3; 1 Bard-Parker knife handle #7; 2 Adson tissue forceps with teeth (1×2), front view and side view; 2 Adson tissue forceps without teeth, front view and side view; 1 Brown-Adson tissue forceps with teeth (9×9), front view; 1 bayonet dressing forceps, 7½ inch; 1 Mayo dissecting scissors, curved; 1 Metzenbaum dissecting scissors; 2 paper drape clips; 2 Backhaus towel forceps, small; 2 Backhaus towel forceps; 6 Halsted mosquito hemostatic forceps, curved; 2 Halsted mosquito hemostatic forceps, straight; 2 Providence Hospital hemostatic forceps, curved; 2 Halsted hemostatic forceps, straight; 4 Crile hemostatic forceps, curved; 2 Allis tissue forceps; 2 Webster needle holders, 4 inch; 2 Crile-Wood needle holders, 6 inch; 2 Johnson needle holders, 6 inch.

98-2 *Left to right:* 1 Weder tongue retractor, large, side view; 1 Weder tongue retractor, small, front view; 2 University of Minnesota cheek retractors, front view and side view; 3 ribbon retractors, assorted sizes; 2 Senn-Kanavel retractors, side view and front view.

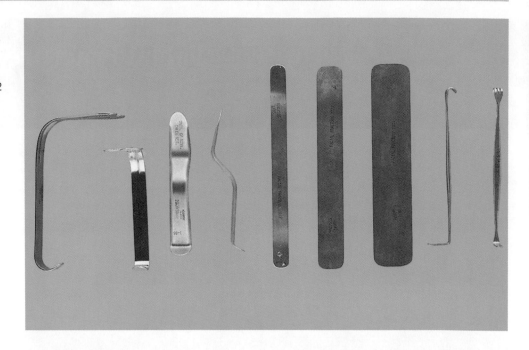

98-3 *Left to right:* 1 Cottle nasal speculum, #1, side view; 1 Cottle nasal speculum, #2, front view; 1 Cottle nasal speculum, #3, side view; 1 Friedman rongeur, single action; 1 Asch forceps; 2 Rowe disimpaction forceps, left and right.

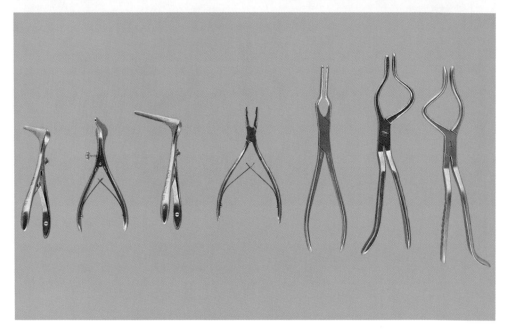

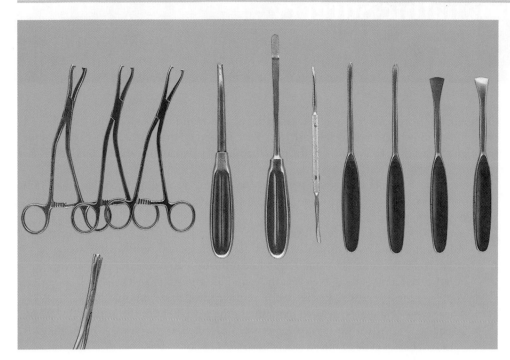

98-4 *Top, left to right:* 3 Dingman bone-holding forceps; 1 Dingman zygoma elevator; 1 Gillies malar elevator; 1 Freer elevator; 2 Langenbeck elevators; 1 Langenbeck periosteal elevator, straight; 1 Langenbeck periosteal elevator, angled. *Bottom left:* tip of Dingman bone-holding forceps.

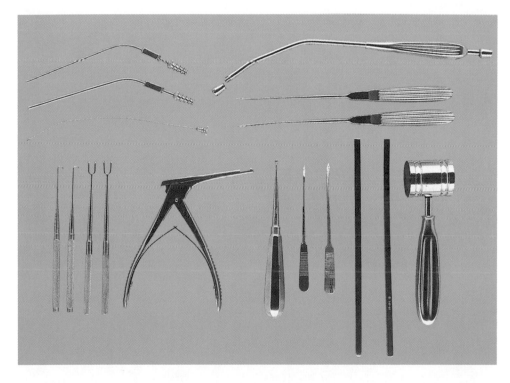

98-5 *Top, left to right:* 2 Frazier suction tubes with stylets; 1 Yankauer suction tube with tip; 2 zygomatic arch awls. *Bottom, left to right:* 2 Joseph skin hooks, single; 2 Joseph skin hooks, double; 1 Kerrison rongeur, 90-degree upbite; 1 Lucas curette #0, short; 2 mandibular awls; 1 Cottle osteotome, curved; 1 Cottle osteotome, straight; 1 crane mallet.

Orthognathic Surgery

Orthognathic surgery is bony reconstruction of the mandible and/or the maxilla. The procedure can be classified as Le Fort I, Le Fort II, or Le Fort III. Le Fort I is a fracture through the maxilla. Le Fort II is a fracture through the zygomatic arches. Le Fort III is a fracture through the bony orbits of the eye.

Possible instruments and equipment needed for the procedure includes small bone instruments, small saws and a drill, arch bars, stainless steel wires, wire cutters, and a mini-fracture fixation system.

A brief description of the procedure follows:

1. A Petri pterygoid retractor is used to retract the cheek and stabilize the jaw.
2. A Weitlaner retractor is used to retract the mucous membrane over the jaw.
3. A Bauer retractor is used to elevate the mandible and stabilize it.
4. A pterygomasseteric stripper is used to remove soft tissue from mandible.
5. Mini screws and plates are used to maintain the placement of the bones.
6. Arch bars with wires are applied to prevent movement of the jaw during healing. The arch bars will be removed at a later time.

99-1 *Top right:* 1 Burton retractor, double. *Left to right:* 2 Bauer retractors, left and right; 1 Joseph coronoid self-retaining retractor; 1 Petri pterygoid retractor; 1 channel retractor; 2 general-purpose retractors; 1 Kent-Wood adjustable retractor.

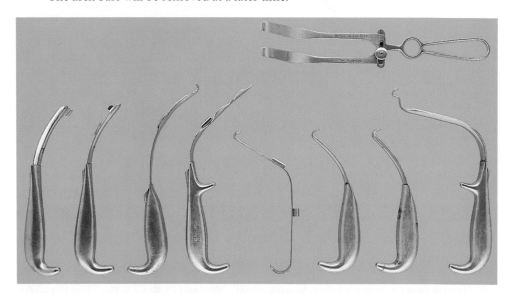

99-2 *Left to right:* 1 piriform rim retractor; 2 Langenbeck retractors, front view and side view; 2 Langenbeck retractors, up-curved tip, front view and side view; 1 pterygomasseteric sling stripper, small; 1 pterygomasseteric sling stripper, medium; 1 Gillies malar elevator; 1 Weitlaner retractor, 5 inch, blunt prong.

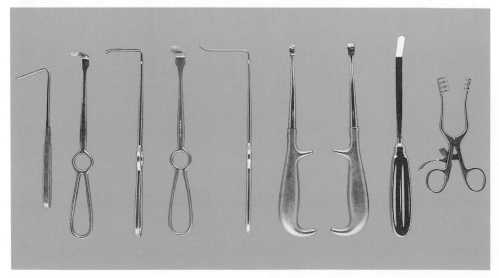

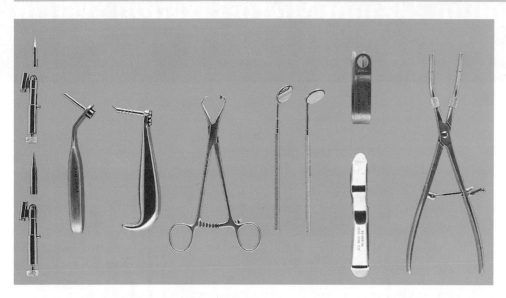

99-3 *Left to right:* 2 roller compressions with metal trocar points, above: small and large; 1 trocar cannula (with trocar); 1 trocar with handle; 1 holding forceps; 2 dental mirrors #5; 2 cheek retractors; 1 mandibular reduction forceps.

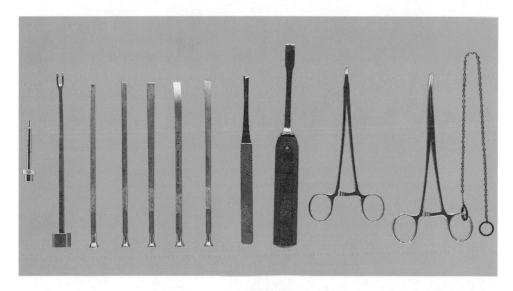

99-4 *Left to right:* 1 drill guide; 1 nasal ball-end osteotome; 3 osteotomes, straight: 4, 6, and 8 mm; 1 osteotome, angled, 6 mm; 1 osteotome, curved, 8 mm; 1 Parkes osteotome; 1 sagittal splitting osteotome; 1 Crile-Wood needle holder, curved, 6 inch; 1 coronoid match retractor.

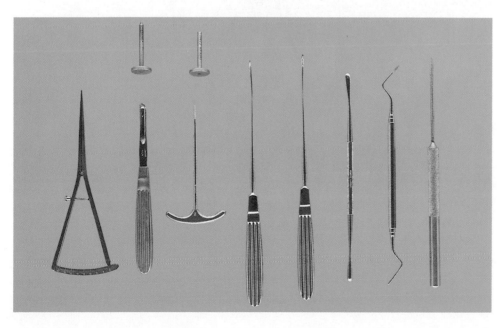

99-5 *Top:* 2 trocar cannulas. *Bottom, left to right:* 1 caliper; 1 condylar stripper; 1 Byrd screw; 2 zygomatic arch awls; 1 Freer elevator, double-ended; 1 periosteal elevator; 1 chisel.

Titanium 2.0-mm Micro-Fixation System

100-1 Titanium 2.0-mm micro–fixation system instrumentation, trays 1 and 2 of 3 (labeled).

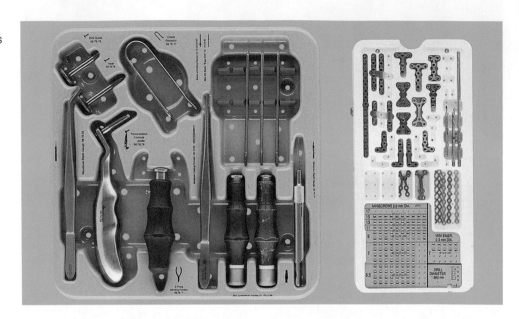

100-2 Titanium 2.0-mm micro–fixation system instrumentation, tray 3 of 3 (labeled).

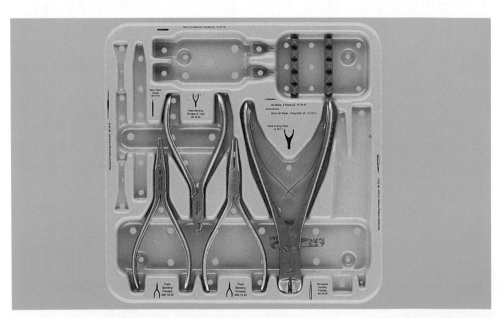

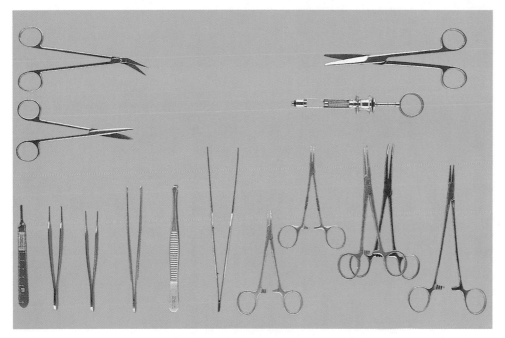

101-1 *Top to bottom, left to right:* 1 Locklin scissors; 1 Metzenbaum scissors, 5 inch; 1 Mayo dissecting scissors, straight; 1 Astra aspirating syringe. *Bottom, left to right:* 1 Bard-Parker knife handle, No. 3; 1 Adson tissue forceps (1 × 2), with teeth; 1 Adson tissue forceps (1 × 2), without teeth; 2 Russian tissue forceps, short, front view and side view; 1 bayonet dressing forceps; 2 Halsted mosquito hemostatic forceps, curved; 2 Crile hemostatic forceps, 6½ inch; 1 Crile-Wood needle holder, 7 inch.

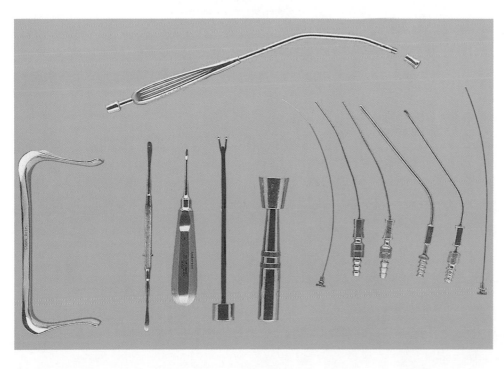

101-2 *Top:* I Yankauer suction tube with tip. *Bottom, left to right:* 1 double-ended retractor; 1 Freer elevator, double ended; 1 Lucas curette, short, straight, No. 0; 1 ball-end nasal osteotome; 1 Gardner mallet; 2 Frazier suction tubes, No. 6, with stylet; 2 Frazier suction tubes, angled, with stylet.

101-3 *Left to right:* 1 single-action rongeur, small; 1 root and splinter forceps; 1 upper incisor and cuspid forceps; 2 Routurier lower third molar forceps: left and right; 1 Molt mouth gag.

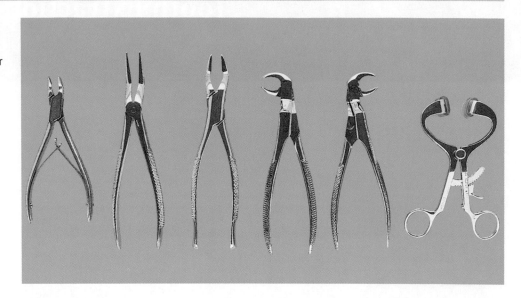

101-4 *Left to right:* 1 cotton pliers; 1 Crane pick elevator; 1 Lucas curette, No. 10; 1 Seldin periosteal elevator; 1 Freer elevator, double ended; 1 bi-beveled carbide chisel; 1 single-beveled carbide chisel; 2 bone files (rasps), side view and front view.

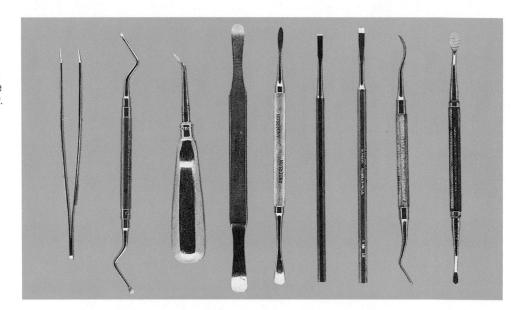

101-5 *Left to right:* 1 laryngeal mirror, No. 5; 1 laryngeal mirror, No. 4; 4 elevators: Nos. 1, 34, 190, and 191; 2 Miller elevators: Nos. 71 and 72; 1 Davis root teaser, No. 11.

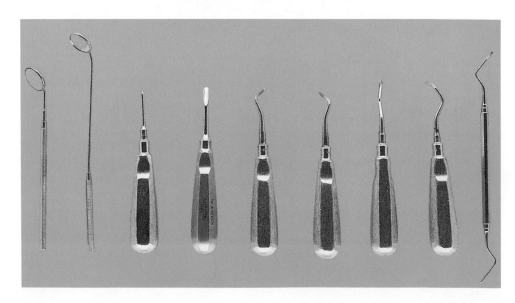

Minor Plastic Set

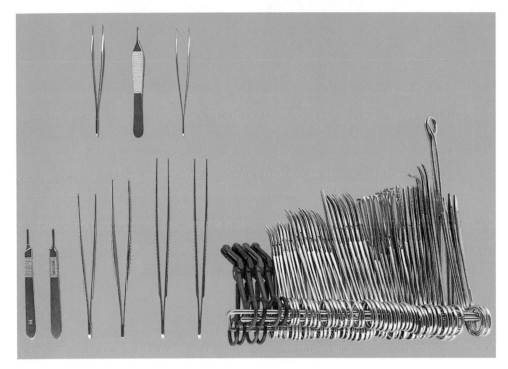

102-1 *Top, left to right:* 2 Adson tissue forceps with teeth (1 × 2), front view and side view; 1 Brown-Adson tissue forceps with teeth (9 × 9), front view. *Bottom, left to right:* 2 Bard-Parker knife handles #3; 2 DeBakey vascular Autraugrip tissue forceps, short; 2 Cushing tissue forceps with teeth (1 × 2); 4 paper drape clips; 6 Halsted mosquito hemostatic forceps, curved; 1 Halsted mosquito hemostatic forceps, straight; 8 Crile hemostatic forceps, curved, 5½ inch; 1 Halsted hemostatic forceps, straight; 6 Crile hemostatic forceps, curved, 6½ inch; 4 Allis tissue forceps; 4 Dabcock tissue forceps; 4 Ochsner hemostatic forceps, straight; 1 Westphal hemostatic forceps; 2 tonsil hemostatic forceps; 1 Foerster sponge forceps; 1 Johnson needle holder, 6 inch; 2 Crile-Wood needle holders, 6 inch.

102-2 *Top, left to right:* 2 Army Navy retractors, front view and side view; 2 Miller-Senn retractors, side view and front view. *Bottom, left to right:* 1 Mayo dissecting scissors, straight; 1 Mayo dissecting scissors, curved; 1 Metzenbaum scissors, 7 inch; 1 Metzenbaum scissors, 5 inch; 2 Goelet retractors, front view and side view; 2 Richardson retractors, small, side view and front view.

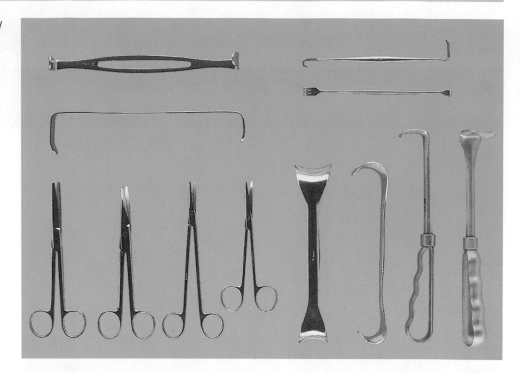

102-3 *Left, top to bottom:* 1 metal medicine cup, 2 oz; 1 Weitlaner retractor, small. *Right, top to bottom:* 1 Yankauer suction tube with tip; 1 Poole abdominal suction tube with shield; 1 Ochsner malleable retractor, medium; 1 Ochsner malleable retractor, narrow; 1 Deaver retractor, medium.

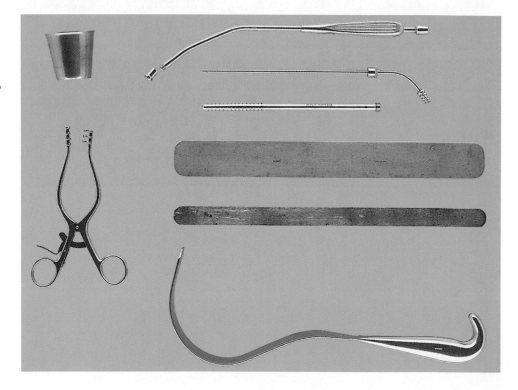

A skin graft is performed when the full thickness of skin has been lost.

Possible instruments needed for the procedure include a minor plastic set.

A brief description of the procedure follows:

1. An electric dermatome is used to harvest skin.
2. Disposable dermatome blades are used in various widths, depending on the size of the graft needed.
3. A Dermamesh graft expander is used to enlarge the piece of skin so it will cover a larger area.

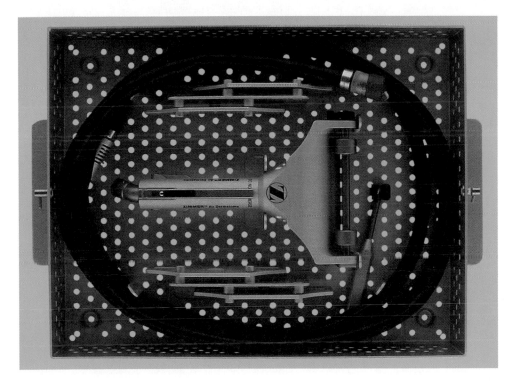

103-1 Zimmer electric air dermatome in sterilizing tray.

103-2 Head of Zimmer electric air dermatome.

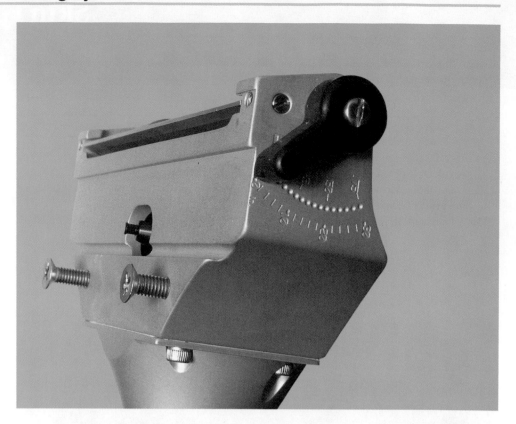

103-3 Blade of Zimmer electric air dermatome.

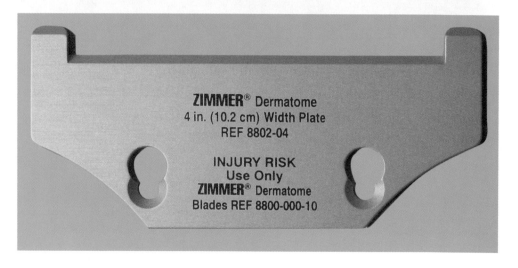

ZIMMER® Dermatome
4 in. (10.2 cm) Width Plate
REF 8802-04

INJURY RISK
Use Only
ZIMMER® Dermatome
Blades REF 8800-000-10

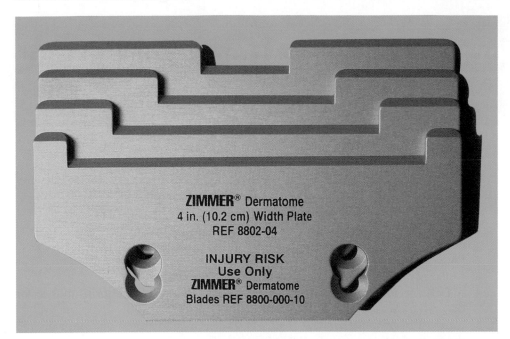

103-4 4 sizes of blades of Zimmer electric air dermatome.

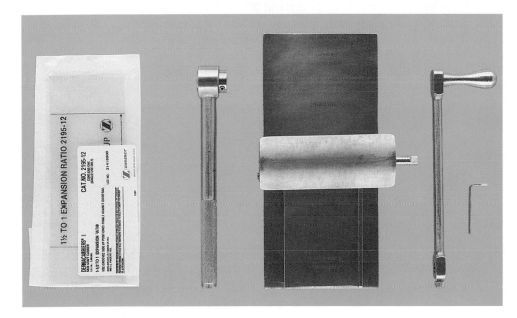

103-5 Mesh graft dermatome (skin expander) with dermacarrier (*left*, in package).

Chapter 104

Femoral to Popliteal Artery Bypass Graft

Possible equipment needed for the procedure includes a DeBakey tunneler, 2 Cooley coarctation clamps, 1 Hollman tunneling forceps, and a synthetic graft.

A brief description of the procedure follows:

1. A Bard-Parker scalpel handle #3 with #11 blade is used to incise into the popliteal artery.
2. Potts-Smith scissors (45 degrees) are used to extend the incision in the artery.
3. DeBakey vascular forceps are used to clamp the popliteal artery.
4. A DeBakey tunneler is used to make a passage beneath the sartorius muscle for the graft from the popliteal artery to the femoral artery.
5. A Bard-Parker scalpel handle #7 with #11 blade is used to make a small incision into the femoral artery.
6. Potts-Smith scissors are used to extend the incision.
7. A Cooley coarctation clamp is used to occlude the femoral artery.
8. Hollman tunneling forceps are used to pull the graft into position.
9. An Ayers needle holder is used for the suturing of the graft.
10. DeBakey tissue forceps are used to help with the suturing.

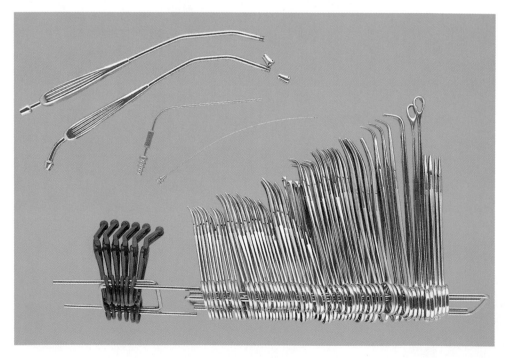

104-1 *Top to bottom:* 2 Yankauer suction tubes with tips; 1 Frazier suction tube with stylet. *Bottom, left to right:* 6 paper drape clips; 10 Halsted mosquito hemostatic forceps, curved; 6 Crile hemostatic forceps, curved, 5½ inch; 6 Providence Hospital hemostatic forceps (delicate tip), curved 5½ inch; 4 Crile hemostatic forceps, curved 6½ inch; 4 Allis tissue forceps; 4 Westphal hemostatic forceps; 6 tonsil hemostatic forceps; 2 Mayo-Péan hemostatic forceps, long, curved; 2 Carmalt hemostatic forceps, long; 2 Adson hemostatic forceps, long; 2 Mixter hemostatic forceps, long, fine and heavy tips; 2 Foerster sponge forceps; 2 Crile-Wood needle holders, 7 inch; 2 Ayers needle holders, 7 inch, fine tips.

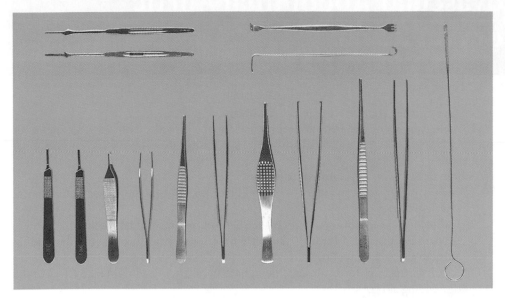

104-2 *Top, left to right:* 2 Bard-Parker knife handles #7; 2 Miller-Senn retractors. *Bottom, left to right:* 2 Bard-Parker knife handles #3; 2 Adson tissue forceps with teeth (1 × 2), side view and front view; 2 DeBakey vascular Autraugrip tissue forceps, short, side view and front view; 2 Ferris Smith tissue forceps, side view and front view; 2 DeBakey vascular Autraugrip tissue forceps, medium, side view and front view; 1 eyed obturator (stylet) for Rumel tourniquet.

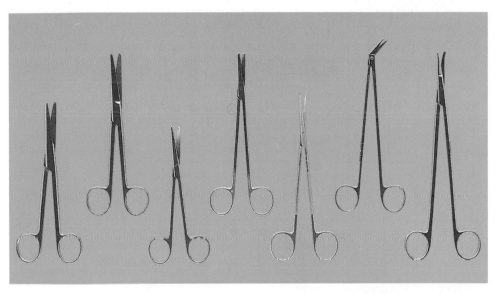

104-3 *Left to right:* 1 Mayo dissecting scissors, straight; 1 Mayo dissecting scissors, curved; 1 Metzenbaum scissors, 5 inch; 1 Metzenbaum scissors, 7 inch; 1 Lincoln-Metzenbaum scissors; 1 Potts-Smith cardiovascular scissors, 45-degree angle; 1 Strully scissors, probe tip.

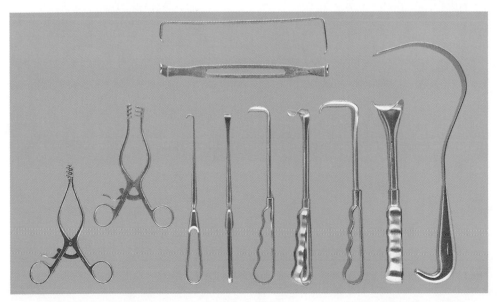

104-4 *Top:* 2 Army Navy retractors, side view and front view. *Bottom, left to right:* 2 Weitlaner retractors, sharp, medium; 2 vein retractors, side view and front view; 2 Richardson retractors, small, side view and front view; 2 Richardson retractors, medium, side view and front view; 1 Deaver retractor, small, side view.

Endovascular Abdominal Aortic Aneurysm Repair*

An aneurysm is the abnormal bulging of an artery.

Possible equipment and instruments needed for the procedure includes an angiocath for an arteriogram, an endolumenal synthetic graft, a small dissection set, 2 Rummel tourniquets, and a skin stapler.

A brief description of the procedure follows:

1. A Bard-Parker scalpel handle #7 with #11 blade for small incisions over both femoral arteries in the groins.
2. Halsted mosquito hemostatic forceps for hemostasis and blunt dissection.
3. A snare is introduced through the left femoral artery up through the descending aorta to above the aneurysm.
4. A pull wire is introduced through the right femoral artery and right iliac artery to the descending aorta.
5. The pull wire is snared and pulled into the left iliac artery to the femoral artery.
6. The endolumenal graft is introduced through the right femoral artery above the bifurcation.
7. The graft is inflated which secures it to the walls of the descending aorta and the iliac arteries.
8. The small incisions are closed with staples with the aid of Adson tissue forceps with teeth.

---

*Endolumenal descending graft designed and patented by Dr. Edward B. Diethrich, Arizona Heart Institute, Phoenix, Arizona.

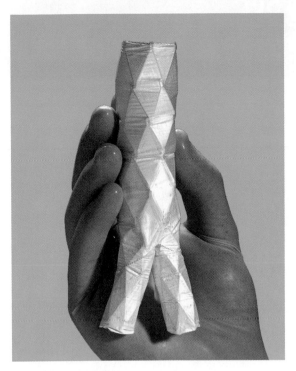

105-1 Endolumenal graft: demonstrating size compared to an adult hand. (Courtesy VAS Communications, Phoenix, Arizona.)

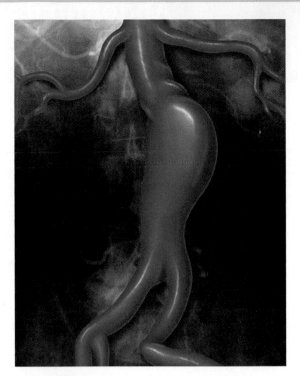

105-2 Graphic diagram of a descending aortic aneurysm. (Courtesy VAS Communications, Phoenix, Arizona.)

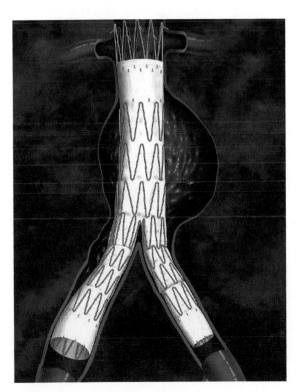

105-3 Graphic diagram of an endolumenal graft in place: descending aorta and iliac arteries. (Courtesy VAS Communications, Phoenix, Arizona.)

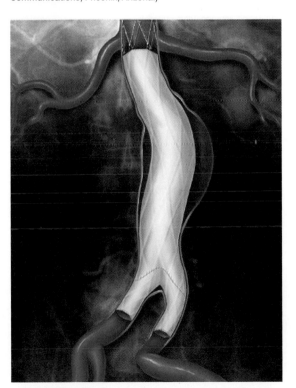

105-4 Graphic diagram of an endolumenal graft postoperatively. (Courtesy VAS Communications, Phoenix, Arizona.)

106-1 *Top, left to right:* 2 Backhaus towel forceps; 6 paper drape clips. *Bottom, left to right:* 2 Ochsner hemostatic forceps, straight, long; 2 Mayo-Péan hemostatic forceps, long; 4 tonsil hemostatic forceps; 1 Westphal hemostatic forceps; 4 Providence Hospital hemostatic forceps (delicate tip), 5½ inch, curved; 4 Crile hemostatic forceps, 5½ inch, curved; 4 Halsted mosquito hemostatic forceps, curved. *Second stringer:* 4 Halsted mosquito hemostatic forceps, curved; 6 Crile hemostatic forceps, 5½ inch, curved; 1 Westphal hemostatic forceps; 4 tonsil hemostatic forceps; 4 Carmalt hemostatic forceps, long; 2 Adson hemostatic forceps, long; 2 Allis tissue forceps, long; 4 Ochsner hemostatic forceps, long, straight; 3 Mixter hemostatic forceps, long, heavy tip; 2 Mixter hemostatic forceps, long, fine tip; 4 Foerster sponge forceps; 2 Ayers needle holders, 8 inch; 2 Crile-Wood needle holders, 8 inch.

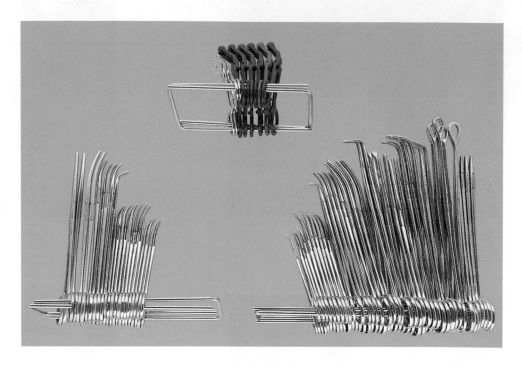

*Laparoscopic vascular instrument images are available on the Companion CD.

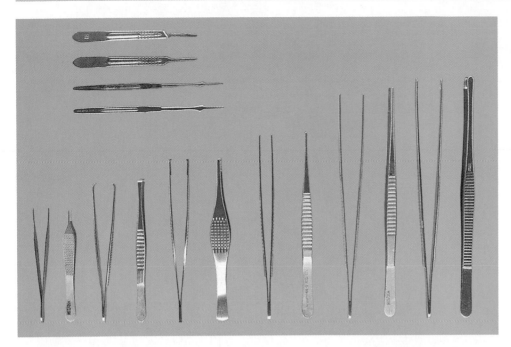

106-2 *Top to bottom:* 2 Bard-Parker needle holders #4; 2 Bard-Parker needle holders #7. *Bottom, left to right:* 2 Adson tissue forceps with teeth (1 × 2), front view and side view; 2 Hayes Martin tissue forceps with multiteeth, short, front view and side view; 2 Ferris Smith tissue forceps, front view and side view; 2 DeBakey vascular Autraugrip tissue forceps, medium, front view and side view; 2 DeBakey vascular Autraugrip tissue forceps, long, front view and side view; 2 Russian tissue forceps, long, front view and side view.

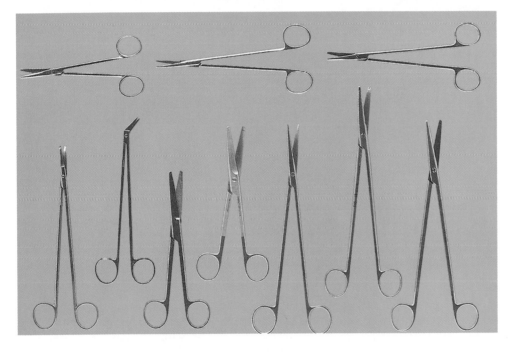

106-3 *Top, left to right:* 1 Metzenbaum scissors, 5 inch; 1 Lincoln-Metzenbaum scissors; 1 Metzenbaum scissors, 7 inch. *Bottom, left to right:* 1 Strully scissors, probe tip; 1 Potts-Smith cardiovascular scissors, 45-degree angle; 2 Mayo dissecting scissors, straight; 1 Metzenbaum scissors, long, sharp; 1 Snowden-Pencer scissors, curved; 1 Snowden-Pencer scissors, straight.

106-4 *Top to bottom:* 2 vein retractors; 1 metal ruler. *Bottom, left to right:* 1 eyed obturator (stylet) for Rumel tourniquet; 2 Weitlaner retractors, sharp, medium; 2 Army Navy retractors, side view and front view; 1 Poole abdominal suction tube with shield; 2 Yankauer suction tubes with tips.

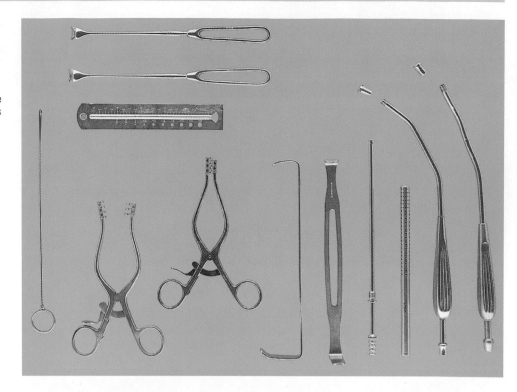

106-5 *Top:* 2 Ochsner malleable retractors: large and small. *Bottom, left to right:* 1 Richardson retractor, small; 1 Richardson retractor, medium, 2 Richardson retractors, large, side view and front view; 3 Deaver retractors: small, medium, and large.

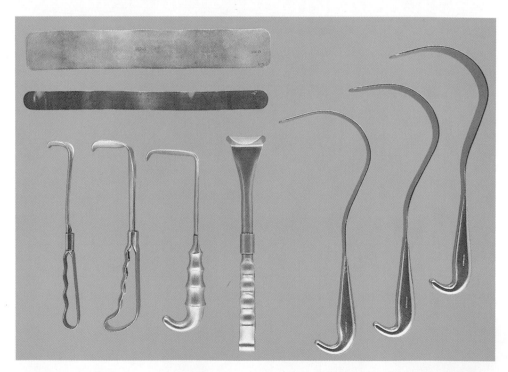

106-6 *Left to right:* Tips: **A**, Adson hemostatic forceps, curved, 8½ inch; **B**, Mixter forceps, delicate, longitudinal serrations, 10¾ inch; **C**, Mixter forceps, full curve, heavy, 10½ inch; **D**, comparison of the three tips of the above instruments.

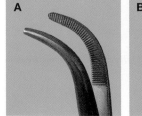
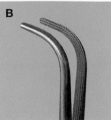
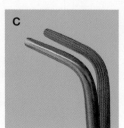
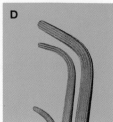

A tracheotomy is an incision into the trachea below the cricoid cartilage in the anterior neck.

A brief description of the procedure follows:

1. A Bard-Parker scalpel handle #3 with a #15 blade is used to make a small incision above the suprasternal notch.
2. Halsted mosquito hemostatic forceps are used to clamp bleeders.
3. A Senn retractor is placed to hold the skin edges.
4. Short curved Metzenbaum dissecting scissors is used to extend the incision to the trachea.
5. A mastoid retractor is placed for exposure.
6. A Bard-Parker scalpel handle #7 with #11 blade is used to incise between the cartilaginous rings of the trachea.
7. A News tracheal hook holds the trachea.
8. A Trousseau dilator is inserted to enlarge the opening for placement of the tracheostomy tube.

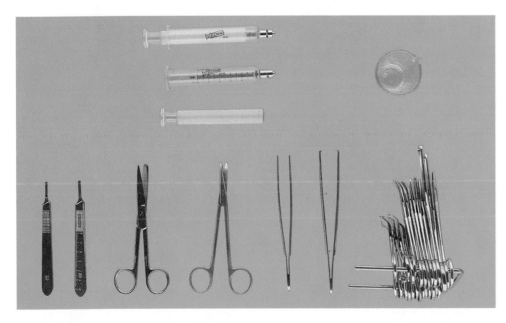

107-1 *Top, left to right:* 2 glass 10-ml syringes, together and separate; 1 glass medicine cup. *Bottom, left to right:* 2 Bard-Parker knife handles, #3; 1 plastic suture scissors, 5½ inch; 1 Metzenbaum dissecting scissors, 5 inch; 2 thumb tissue forceps, without teeth and with teeth (1 × 2); 4 Backhaus towel clips; 3 Halsted mosquito hemostatic forceps, curved; 3 Halsted mosquito hemostatic forceps, straight; 2 Allis tissue forceps; 1 Johnson needle holder, 5 inch.

107-2 *Left to right:* 2 News tracheal hooks, side view and front view; 2 Senn retractors, double-ended, sharp, side view and front view; 1 articulated mastoid retractor; 1 Trousseau tracheal dilator, adult; 2 Army Navy retractors, front view and side view.

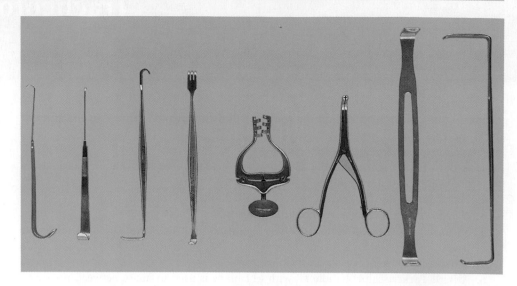

107-3 *Left to right:* Tips: **A**, tracheal hook; **B**, sharp tip of Senn retractor, double-ended; **C**, Trousseau tracheal dilator, adult.

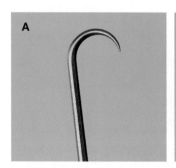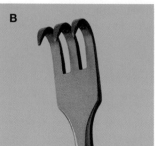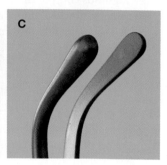

Thoracoscopy

A thoracoscopy visualizes inside the chest cavity via a laparoscope.

Possible instruments needed for the procedure include a laparoscope, an MIS adult set, and a minor instrument set.

A brief description of the procedure follows:

1. Thoracoports include obturators and cannulas and are used for scope insertion.
2. A fan retractor is used for visualization.
3. Roticulating Babcock forceps are used to handle tissue gently.
4. A Duval lung clamp is used to stabilize tissue that is being removed.
5. Roticulating Metzenbaum dissecting scissors are used to excise the tissue.

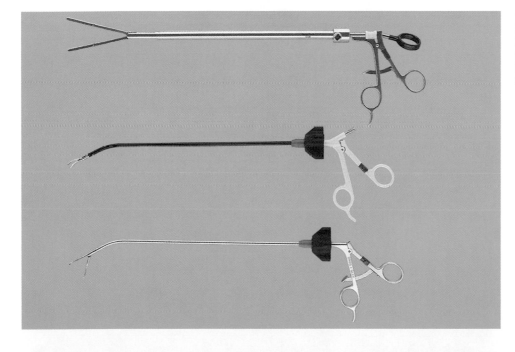

108-1 *Top to bottom:* 1 articulating lung grasper, 10 mm; 1 roticulating Metzenbaum scissors, 5 mm × 33 cm, angled shaft; 1 roticulating Babcock forceps, 5 mm × 33 cm, angled shaft.

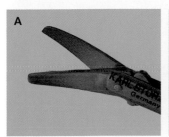
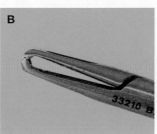
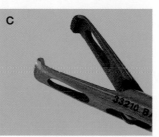

108-2 *Left to right:* Tips: **A**, roticulating Metzenbaum scissors, 5 mm, 33 cm length, angled shaft; roticulating Babcock forceps, 5 mm, 33 cm length, angled shaft; **B**, closed; **C**, open.

108-3 *Top to bottom:* Duval clamp, 10 mm, opened; Duval clamp, 10 mm, closed; fan retractor, 10 mm (two parts, together).

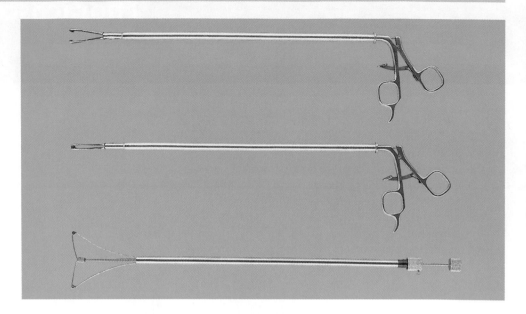

108-4 A, Tip of Duval clamp, 10 mm, closed; **B,** tip of Duval clamp, 10 mm, opened.

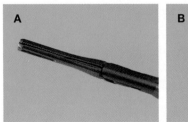
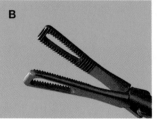

A

B

108-5 Top: 2 5-mm Thoracoports; includes 1 blunt obturator, 1 cannula. *Middle:* 2 10-mm Thoracoports; includes 1 blunt obturator, 1 cannula. *Bottom:* 1 12-mm Thoracoport; includes 1 blunt obturator, 1 cannula; 1 15-mm Thoracoport; includes 1 blunt obturator, 1 cannula.

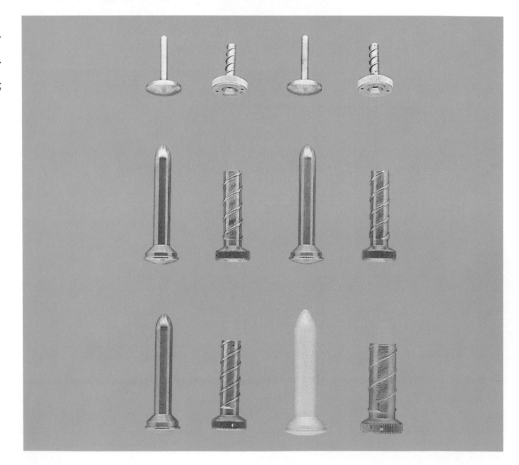

Surgery Blebs, Resectable Tumor, instill sterile talc   **108-6** Position for thoracoscopy.

THORACOSCOPY (LEFT)

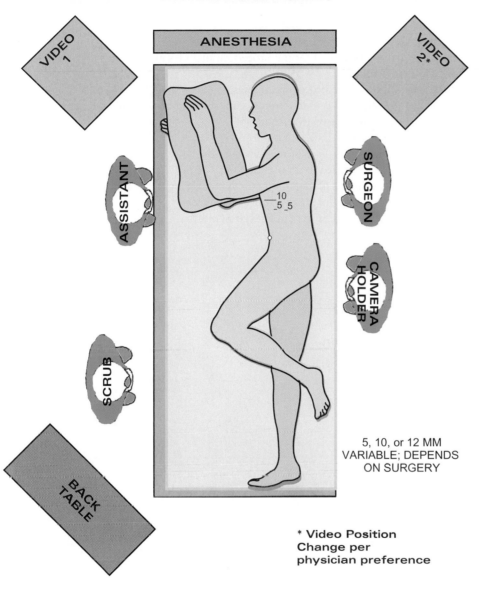

5, 10, or 12 MM
VARIABLE; DEPENDS
ON SURGERY

* **Video Position
Change per
physician preference**

Thoracic Instruments

A thoracotomy is an incision into the chest cavity.

Possible instruments needed for the procedure includes an abdominal vascular set and cardiovascular instruments.

A brief description of the procedure follows:

1. A Matson rib stripper is used to remove muscle and periosteum from ribs.
2. A Giertz rib cutter is used to resect a rib.
3. A Semb rongeur is used to trim bone ends.
4. A Burford retractor is placed to retract the ribs.
5. A Semb retractor is used to expose the lung.
6. A Duval lung clamp is placed for gentle maneuvering of the lobes of the lungs.
7. A Sarot clamp is used for clamping the bronchus.
8. A Bailey rib contractor is used during chest closure.

109-1 *Top, left to right:* 1 malleable T retractor; 1 Giertz (first rib) (rib guillotine) rongeur; 1 Matson rib stripper and elevator. *Bottom left:* Burford rib spreader with shallow blade attached; 1 shallow blade; 2 deep blades.

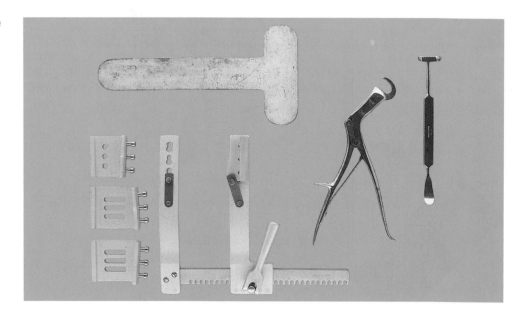

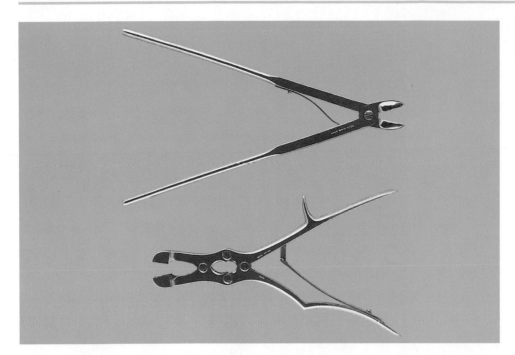

109-2 *Top to bottom:* Bethune (rib) rongeur; 1 Sauerbruch (rib) rongeur, double-action.

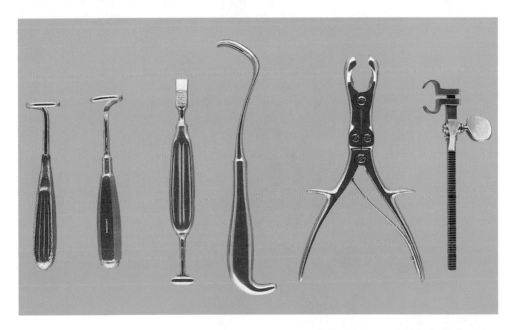

109-3 *Left to right:* 2 Doyen rib elevators and raspatories, left and right; 1 Alexander rib raspatory (periosteotome), double-ended; 1 Semb lung retractor; 1 Semb gouging rongeur, double-action; 1 Bailey rib contractor.

109-4 *Top:* 2 Crile-Wood needle holders, 11 inch. *Bottom, left to right:* 1 Sarot bronchus clamp, angled; 1 Lee bronchus clamp, angular; 4 Allis tissue forceps, long; 3 Duval lung forceps, 2 front views and 1 side view.

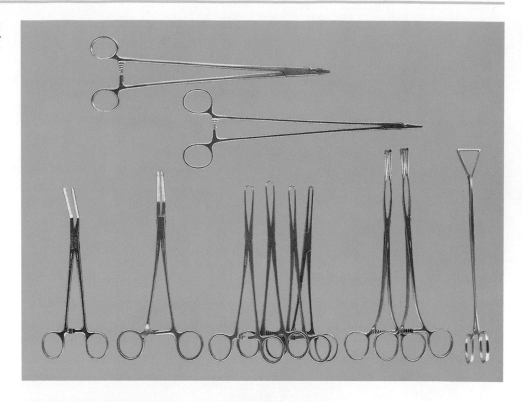

109-5 *Left to right:* Tips: **A**, Sarot bronchus clamp, angled; **B**, Lee bronchus clamp, angled; **C**, Duval lung forceps; **D**, Semb lung retractor.

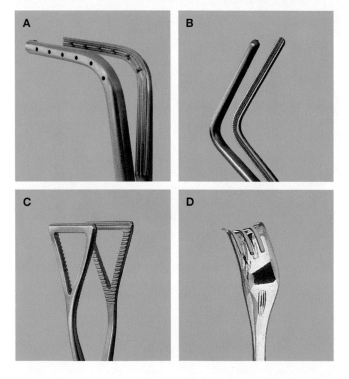

Cardiac surgery relates to surgery of the heart. Some heart surgeries include a coronary artery bypass graft, or CABG; replacement of the heart valves, or valvular annuloplasty; or repair of the wall between the chambers of the heart, also known as a septal repair.

Possible instruments needed for the procedure include sternal saws and open-heart extras.

A brief description of the procedure follows:

1. A Hall sternal saw with blade is used to open the chest.
2. A Himmelstein retractor is used to elevate the chest wall to expose the mammary artery if the patient needs a coronary artery bypass graft.
3. A Cooley clamp is used when retrieving vessels for the grafts.
4. An octopus retractor with stabilizing blades is used to immobilize the area of the heart that is being sutured.

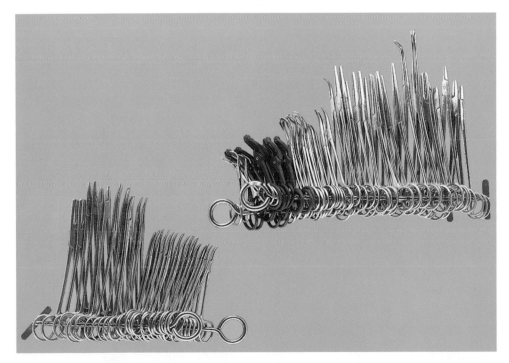

110-1 *Bottom, right to left:* 5 Halsted mosquito hemostatic forceps, curved; 10 Crile hemostatic forceps, 5½ inch; 4 tonsil hemostatic forceps, blunt tip; 2 Mayo-Péan hemostatic forceps, long; 2 Ayers needle holders, 8 inch; 1 DeBakey needle holder, 8 inch; 1 Crile-Wood needle holder, 8 inch; 2 Vorse-Webster tube-occluding clamps. *Top, left to right:* 2 Backhaus towel forceps, small; 8 paper drape clips; 3 Edna towel clamps, nonperforating tips; 3 Backhaus towel forceps, 4 Providence Hospital hemostatic forceps, delicate tip; 3 Crile hemostatic forceps, 5½ inch; 1 Adson hemostatic forceps, curved; 2 Ochsner hemostatic forceps, straight, short jaw; 10 Ochsner hemostatic forceps, straight, medium jaw; 1 Mixter hemostatic forceps, long; 1 Foerster sponge forceps; 2 Jarit (Vorse) tube-occluding forceps; 1 Jarit sternal needle holder and wire twister (short jaw), 7 inch; 1 Crile-Wood needle holder, 8 inch; 2 Crile-Wood needle holders, 7 inch.

110-2 *Top, left:* 2 Bard-Parker knife handles #7; 1 Bard-Parker knife handle #4; 1 Bard-Parker knife handle #3. *Bottom, left to right:* 1 Adson tissue forceps with teeth (1 × 2); 2 Hayes Martin tissue forceps with multiteeth, front view and side view; 1 Ferris Smith tissue forceps; 3 DeBakey vascular Autraugrip tissue forceps with post, long, 2 front views and 1 side view; 2 Russian tissue forceps, long, front view and side view.

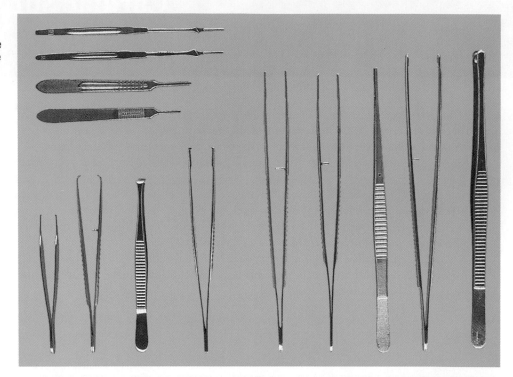

110-3 *Top:* 3 Hegar dilators: 7 and 8, 5 and 6, 3 and 4. *Bottom, left to right:* 1 Mayo dissecting scissors, curved; 3 Mayo dissecting scissors, straight; 2 Metzenbaum scissors, 7 inch, straight, curved; 1 Metzenbaum scissors, 8 inch, straight; 1 Strully scissors with probe tip.

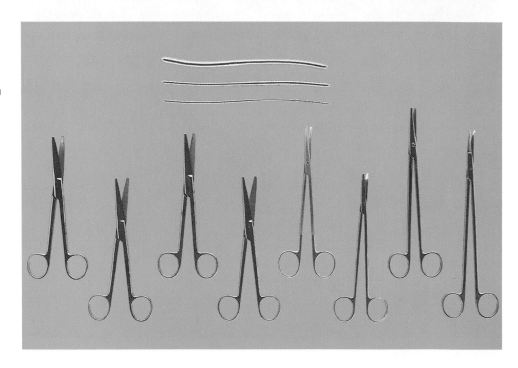

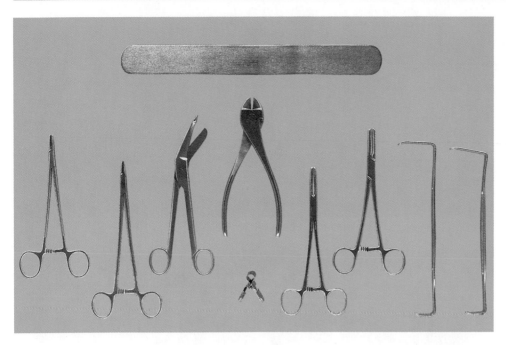

110-4 *Top:* 1 Ochsner malleable retractor, medium. *Bottom, left to right:* 1 Jarit sternal needle holder, 7 inch; 1 Jarit sternal needle holder, 8 inch; 1 bandage scissors, heavy; 1 wire cutter, heavy; 1 Edwards holding clip; 2 Jarit (Vorse) tubing occluding clamps; 2 Army Navy retractors.

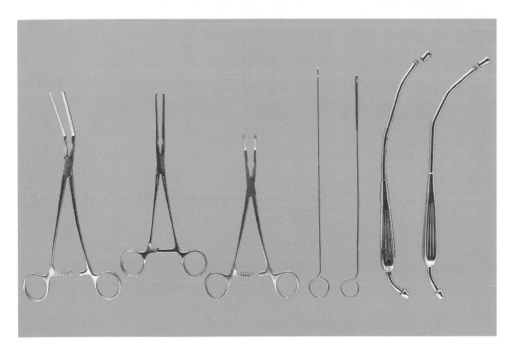

110-5 *Left to right:* 1 DeBakey multipurpose vascular clamp, obtuse angle, 60 degrees, jaw length 4 cm, overall length 9 inches; 1 Glover patent ductus clamp, straight; 1 Beck aorta clamp; 2 eyed obturators (stylets) for Rumel tourniquet; 2 Yankauer suction tubes with tips.

110-6 *Left to right:* Providence Hospital hemostatic forceps, curved, delicate tip; Edna towel clamp, nonperforating; Backhaus towel forceps; Jarit sternal needle holder and wire twister (short jaw); Jarit (Vorse) tube-occluding forceps.

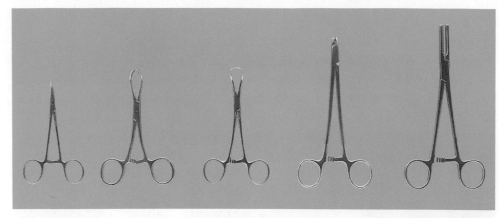

110-7 *Left to right:* Tips: **A**, Providence Hospital hemostatic forceps, curved, delicate tip; **B**, Edna towel clamp, nonperforating; **C**, Backhaus towel forceps; **D**, Jarit sternal needle holder and wire twister (short jaw), 7 inch; **E**, Jarit (Vorse) tube-occluding clamp.

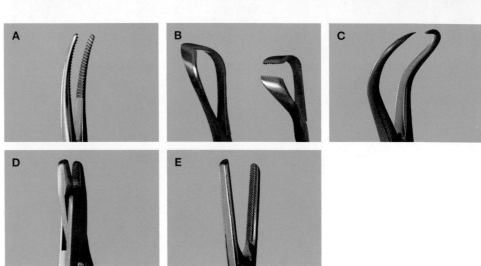

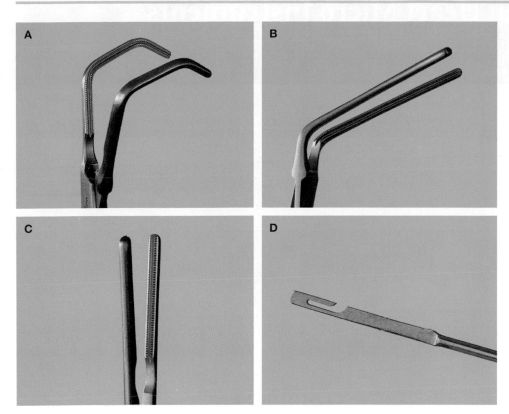

110-8 *Left to right:* Tips: **A**, Beck aorta clamp, jaw length 3 cm; **B**, DeBakey multipurpose vascular clamp, obtuse angle, 60 degrees, jaw length 5 cm; **C**, Glover patent ductus clamp, straight, jaw length 3 cm; **D**, eyed obturator (stylet) for Rumel tourniquet.

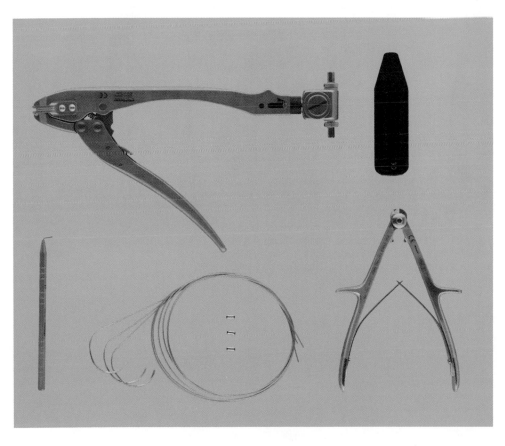

110-9 *Top, left to right:* 1 sternal crimper; and 1 tensioning handle. *Bottom, left to right:* 1 crimp passer; 3 sternal cables with needles attached and 2 crimpers in the middle; and 1 cable cutter.

Open Heart Micro Instruments

Possible instruments needed for the procedure include a basic open heart set and open heart extras.

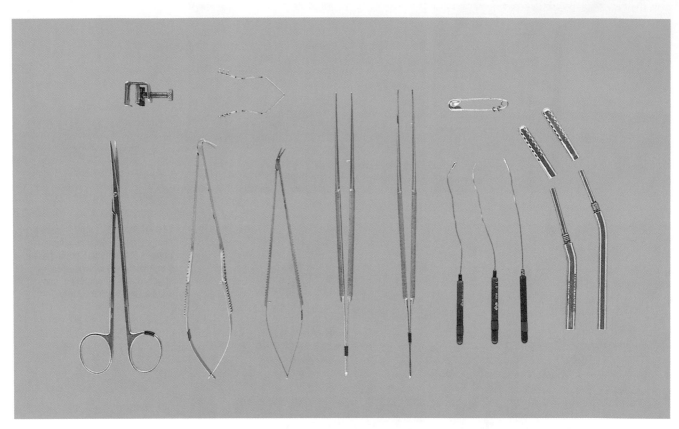

111-1 *Top, left and right:* 1 tubing clamp; 1 Parsonnet epicardial (self-retaining spring) retractor, sharp, 3 × 3 prongs; 1 safety pin with rings. *Bottom, left to right:* 1 Snowden-Pencer scissors, straight; 1 Yasargil scissors, bayonet handle, 125-degree angle; 1 You-Potts scissors, fine, thin 10-mm blades, 45-degree angle; 2 Snowden-Pencer dressing forceps, 8 inch; 3 Garrett dilators: 2.0 mm, 1.0 mm, and 1.5 mm; 2 metal coronary suction tubes with tips.

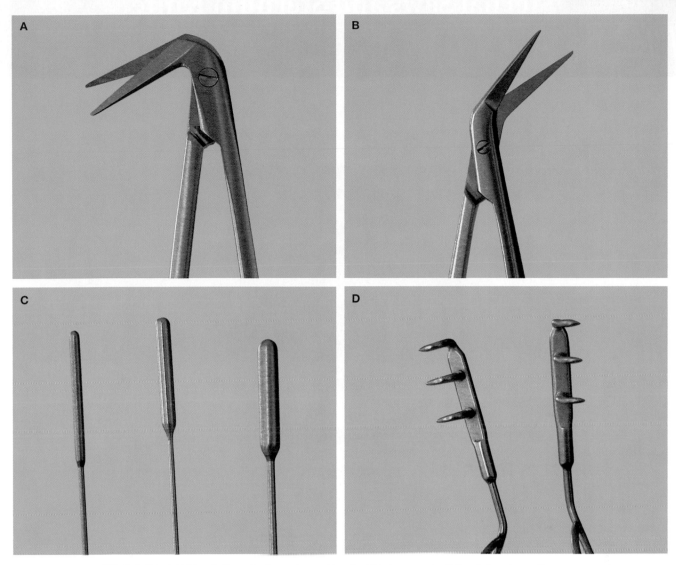

111-2 *Left to right:* Tips: **A**, Yasargil scissors, bayonet handle, 125-degree angle; **B**, You-Potts scissors, fine, thin 10-mm blades, 45-degree angle; **C**, Garrett dilators: 1.0 mm, 1.5 mm, and 2.0 mm; **D**, Parsonnet epicardial retractor, 1⁷/₈ inch, 3 × 3 sharp prongs.

Sternal Saws and Sternum Knife

112-1 *Left to right:* power cord; Hall sternum saw. *Right, top to bottom:* 1 saw blade; 1 saw guide; 1 wrench.

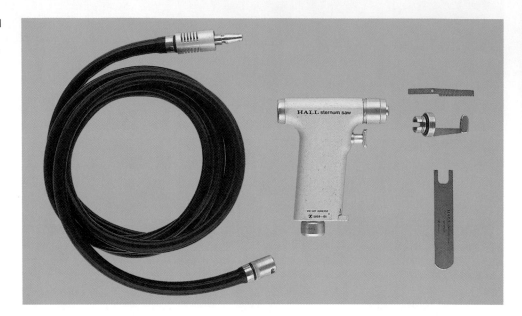

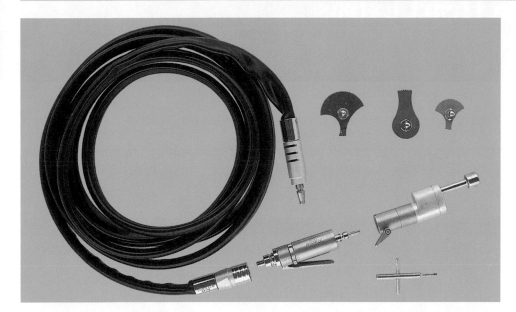

112-2 *Left:* power cord. *Right, top to bottom:* 3 saw blades; Aesculap oscillating sternal saw (2 parts); 1 wrench.

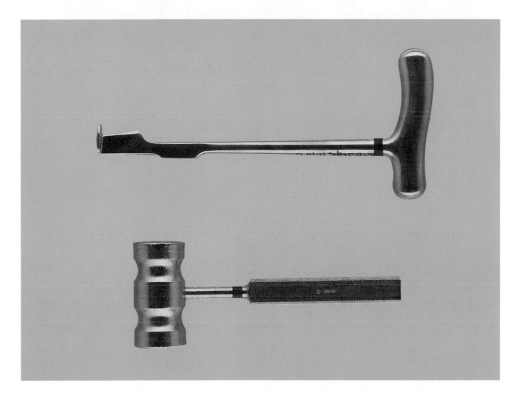

112-3 Surgeons' preference instead of sternal saw. *Top to bottom:* Lebsche sternum knife and mallet.

Open Heart Extras

Possible instruments needed for the procedure include a basic heart set and a sternal saw.

113-1 *Left to right:* 1 Ankeney sternal retractor; 1 Himmelstein sternal retractor.

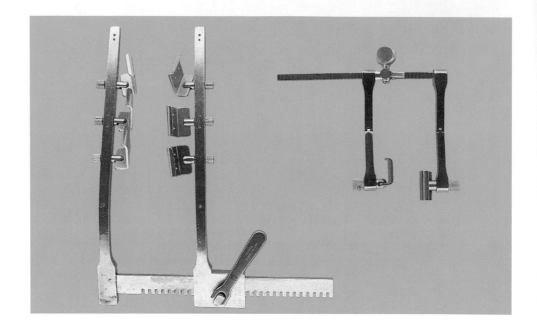

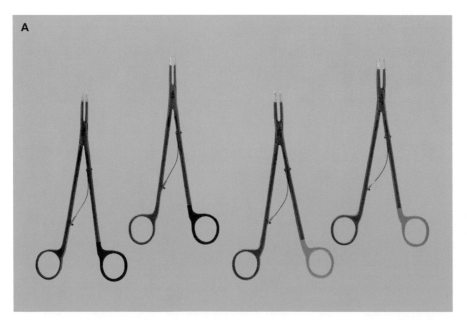 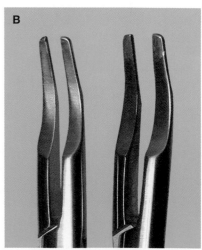

113-2 *Left to right:* **A**, Horizon clip appliers, 2 small, 2 medium; **B**, enlarged tips of Horizon clip appliers, small, medium.

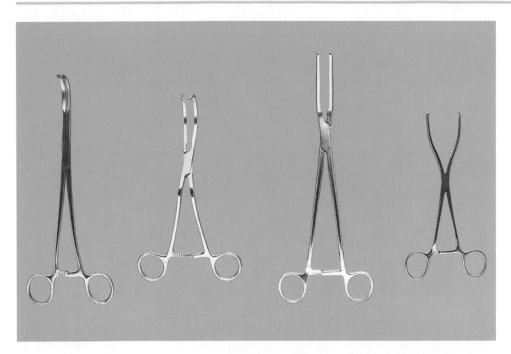

113-3 *Left to right:* 1 Semb ligature-carrying forceps, 9 inch; 1 Lambert-Kay aortic clamp; 1 Fogarty clamp-applying forceps, angled; 1 bulldog clamp applier.

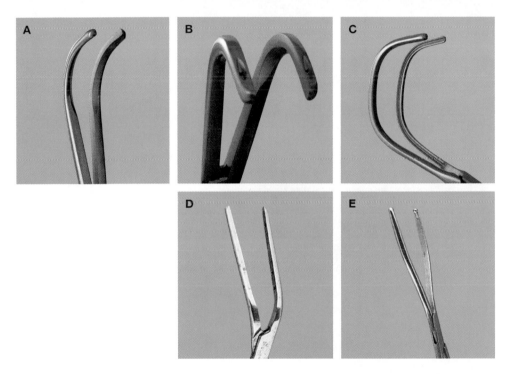

113-4 *Left to right:* Tips: **A** and **B**, Semb ligature-carrying forceps, 9 inch, close-up of the top of the tip; **C**, Lambert-Kay aortic clamp; **D**, Fogarty clamp-applying forceps, angled; **E**, bulldog clamp applier.

113-5 *Top:* 1 Frazier suction tube with stylet, long. *Bottom, left to right:* 1 blunt hook, 2-mm round tip; 2 Reul coronary tissue forceps, delicate, 8 inch; 2 Jarit microsurgical needle holders with locks; Carb-Bite jaws, smooth, 7 inch; 1 Penfield dissector, single-ended, #4; 1 Beaver knife handle, knurled, 6 inch, without insert.

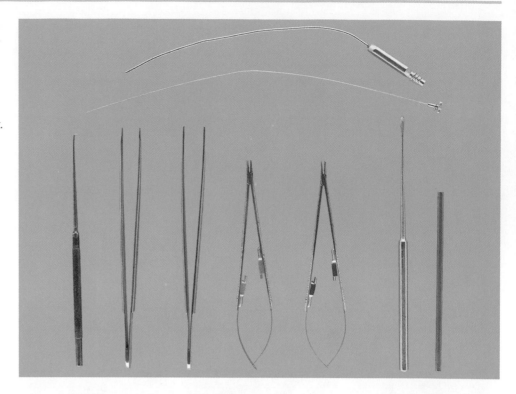

113-6 *Left to right:* Tips: **A**, blunt hook, 2-mm round tip; **B**, Reul coronary tissue forceps, delicate, 8 inch; **C**, Jarit microsurgical needle holder with lock, Carb-Bite jaws, smooth, 7 inch.

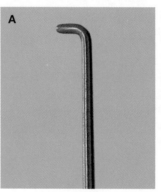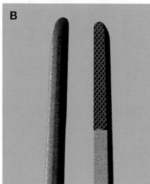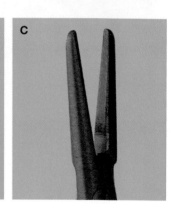

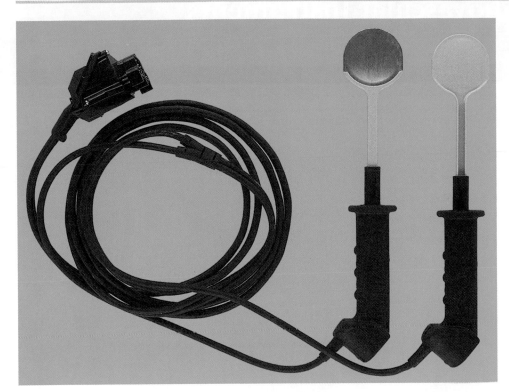

113-7 Internal defibrillator paddles with power cord.

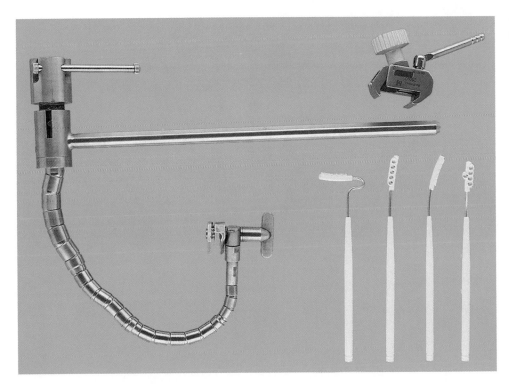

113-8 Octopus retractor with disposable tissue stabilizers.

Cardiovascular Instruments

Possible instruments needed for the procedure include a basic open heart set.

114-1 *Left to right:* **A**, Cooley clamp, angled jaw, straight shank, 5¼ inch, front view and tip; **B**, DeBakey bulldog clamp, ring handle, 45-degree angle, 4¾ inch, front view and tip; **C**, DeBakey peripheral vascular clamp, angular, 7 inch, front view and tip.

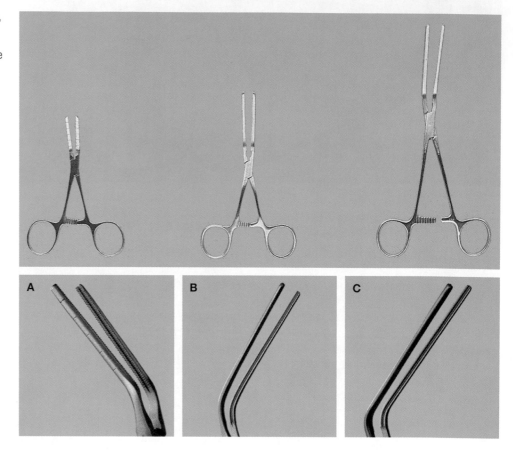

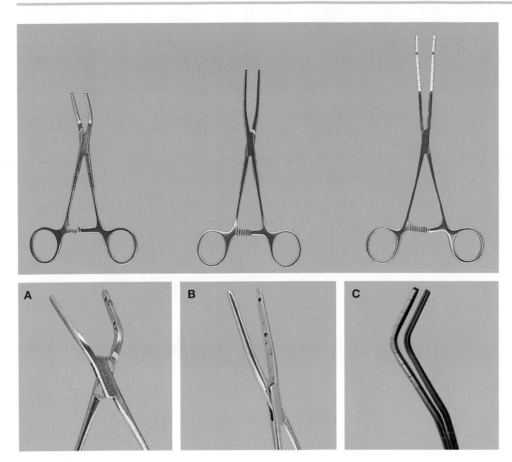

114-2 *Left to right:* **A**, Fogarty clamp-applying forceps, angled, front view and tip; **B**, Fogarty clamp-applying forceps, straight, front view and tip; **C**, renal artery clamp, 7¼ inch, front view and tip.

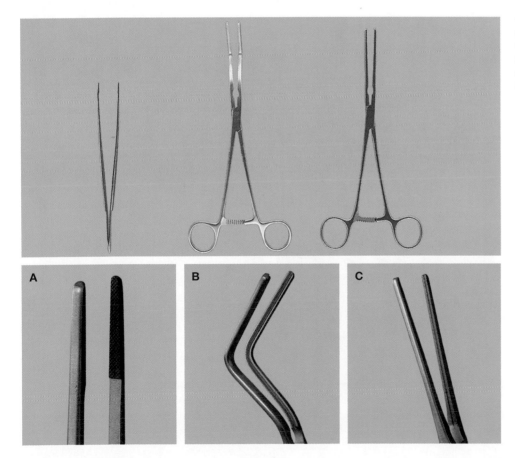

114-3 *Left to right:* **A**, Potts-Smith tissue forceps, Carb-Bite tip, front view and tip; **B**, Lec bronchus clamp, 9¼ inch, front view and tip; **C**, Cooley coarctation clamp, straight handle, 8¾ inch, front view and tip.

114-4 *Left to right:* 1 DeBakey aortic exclusion clamp, acute S-shape, medium, 7¼ inch; 1 DeBakey aortic exclusion clamp, acute S shape, long; 1 DeBakey multipurpose vascular clamp, obtuse angle, 60 degrees, 8¼ inch; 1 Semb ligature-carrying forceps, 9 inch.

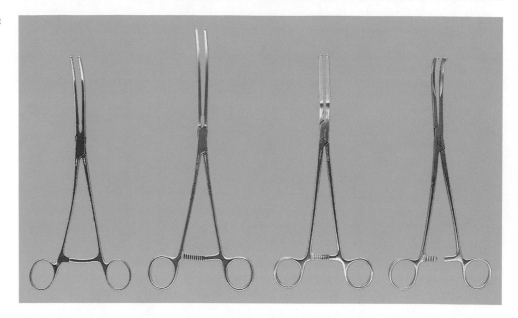

114-5 *Top:* 1 Andrews-Pynchon suction tube. *Bottom, left to right:* 1 metal ruler, 6 inch; 1 Freer double-ended elevator; 1 Penfield dissector, single ended, #4; 1 Hoen nerve hook; 1 Adson hemostatic forceps, angled, fine tip; 2 Ryder needle holders, 7 inch, fine tip.

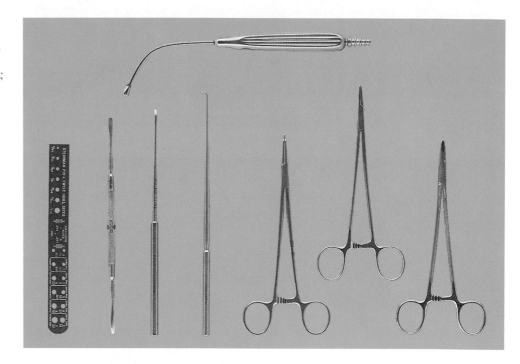

114-6 *Left to right:* Tips: **A**, DeBakey aortic exclusion clamp, S-shape; **B**, Hoen nerve hook, straight.

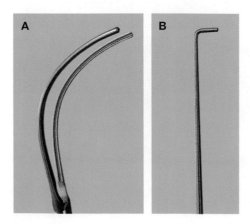

Possible instruments needed for the procedure include a basic open heart set and open heart extras.

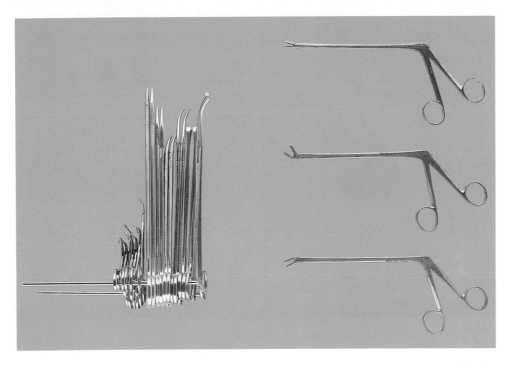

115-1 *Left to right:* 6 Backhaus towel forceps, small; 1 Providence Hospital hemostatic forceps; 2 Ayers needle holders, 11 inch; 2 Heaney needle holders; 2 tonsil hemostatic forceps; 2 tonsil hemostatic forceps, long; 2 Allis tissue forceps, long; 1 Allis tissue forceps, long, curved. *Right, top to bottom:* 1 pituitary rongeur, straight bite, 7 inch; 1 pituitary rongeur, upbite, 7 inch; 1 pituitary rongeur, downbite, 7 inch.

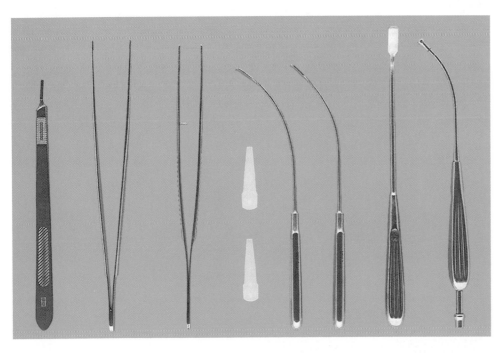

115-2 *Left to right:* 1 Bard-Parker knife handle, #3, long; 1 Cushing-Brown tissue forceps with teeth (9 × 9); 1 Cushing tissue forceps with teeth (1 × 2); 2 Teflon Bardic plugs; 3 leaflet retractors: 2 side view and 1 front view; 1 grafting suction tube.

*Additional images are available on the Companion CD.

115-3 Tips: **A**, leaflet retractor; **B**, Cushing-Brown tissue forceps with teeth (9 × 9); **C**, Heaney needle holder; **D**, Allis tissue forceps, curved.

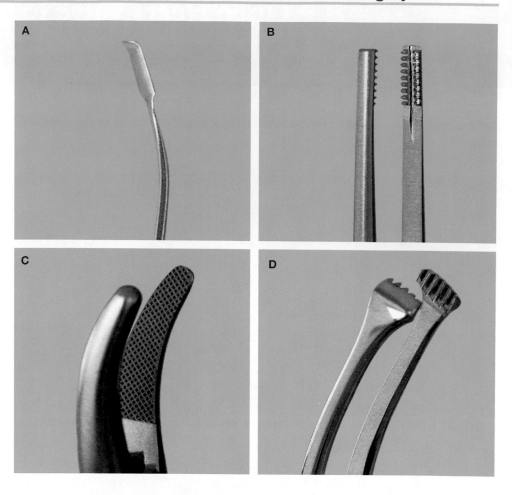

115-4 *Left to right:* 3 pituitary rongeur tips: straight bite, downbite, upbite.

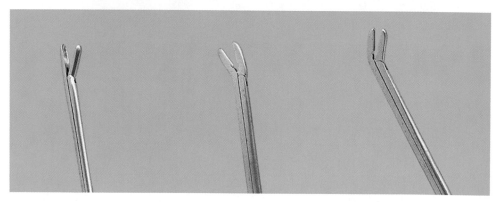

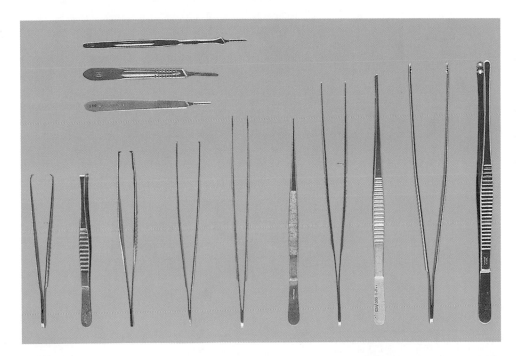

116-1 *Top left:* 3 Bard-Parker knife handles: #7, #4, and #3. *Bottom, left to right:* 2 Hayes Martin tissue forceps with multiteeth, front view and side view; 1 Ferris Smith tissue forceps; 1 Cushing tissue forceps with teeth (1 × 2), 7 inch; 2 Reul dressing forceps, front view and side view; 2 DeBakey vascular Autraugrip tissue forceps, long, front view and side view; 2 Russian tissue forceps, long, front view and side view.

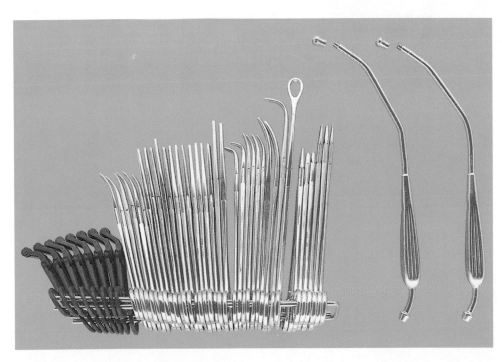

116-2 *Left to right:* 8 paper drape clips; 6 Crile hemostatic forceps, 6½ inch; 12 Ochsner hemostatic forceps, medium jaw; 2 Ochsner hemostatic forceps, long jaw; 2 Westphal hemostatic forceps, short; 4 tonsil hemostatic forceps; 2 Mayo-Péan hemostatic forceps, long, curved; 1 Adson hemostatic forceps, long; 1 Foerster sponge forceps; 1 Crile-Wood needle holder, 7 inch; 2 Jarit sternal needle holders, 7 inch; 2 Crile-Wood needle holders, 8 inch; 1 Ayers needle holder, 8 inch; 2 Yankauer suction tubes with tips.

116-3 *Left to right:* 2 Volkmann retractors, 4 prong, dull, front view and side view; 1 Richardson retractor, small; 1 Ochsner malleable retractor, medium; 2 Army Navy retractors, front view and side view; 1 wire cutter, heavy.

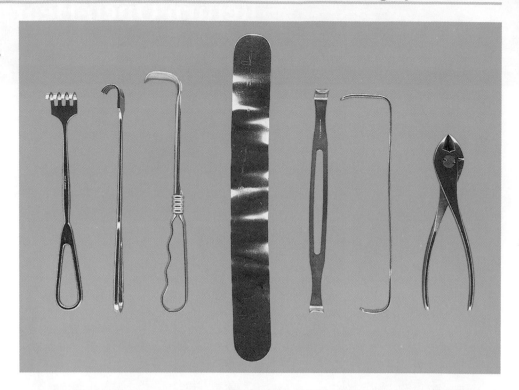

116-4 *Left to right:* 1 Himmelstein sternal retractor; 1 Ankeney sternal retractor.

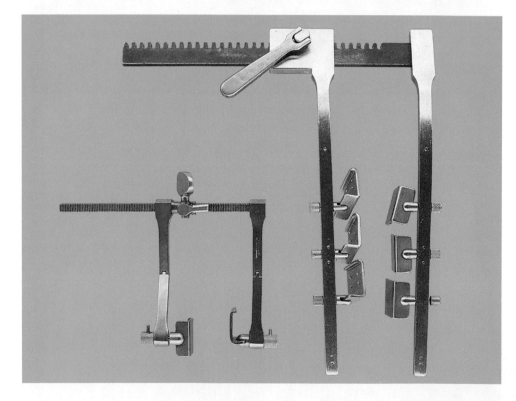

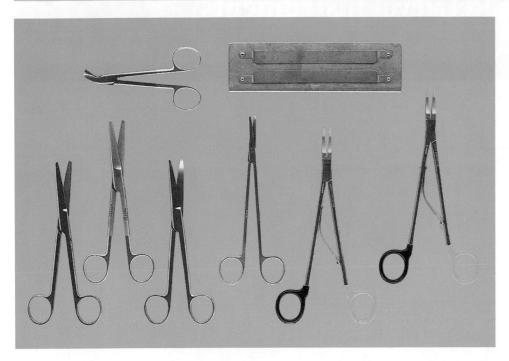

116-5 *Top, left to right,* 1 wire cutter, small; 1 hemoclip cartridge base. *Bottom, left to right,* 2 Mayo dissecting scissors, straight; 1 Mayo dissecting scissors, curved; 1 Metzenbaum scissors, 7 inch; 2 Weck EZ load hemoclip appliers.

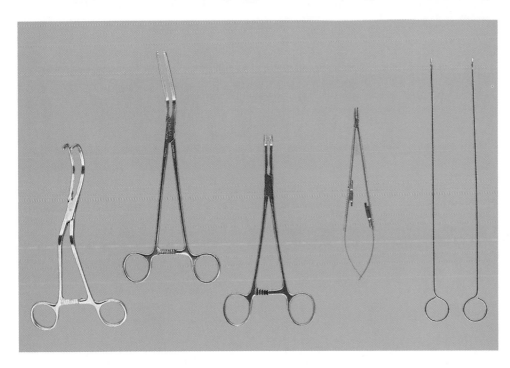

116-6 *Left to right,* 1 Lambert-Kay aortic clamp; 1 DeBakey multipurpose vascular clamp, obtuse angle, 60 degrees; 1 Beck aorta clamp; 1 Jarit microsurgical needle holder with lock, 7 inch; 2 eyed obturators (stylets) for Rumel tourniquet.

117-1 *Top to bottom:* 1 hemoclip cartridge base; 2 Miller-Senn retractors. *Top right:* 1 Weitlaner retractor, sharp, small. *Bottom, left to right:* 2 Adson tissue forceps with teeth (1 × 2); 2 DeBakey vascular Autraugrip tissue forceps, short; 1 Metzenbaum dissecting scissors, 5 inch; 10 Providence Hospital hemostatic forceps; 4 Halsted mosquito hemostatic forceps, curved; 1 Westphal hemostatic forceps, short; 1 Johnson needle holder, 5 inch; 1 Crile-Wood needle holder, 7 inch; 2 Weck EZ load hemoclip appliers, medium; 1 Army Navy retractor; 1 Richardson retractor, small.

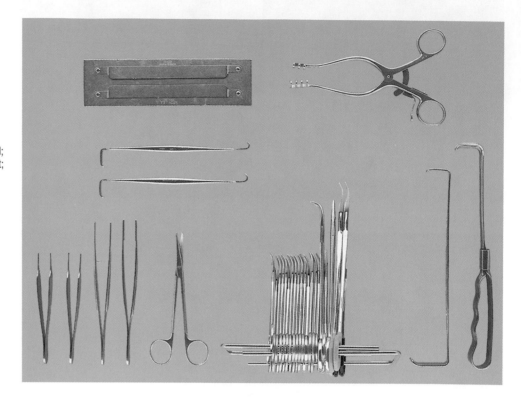

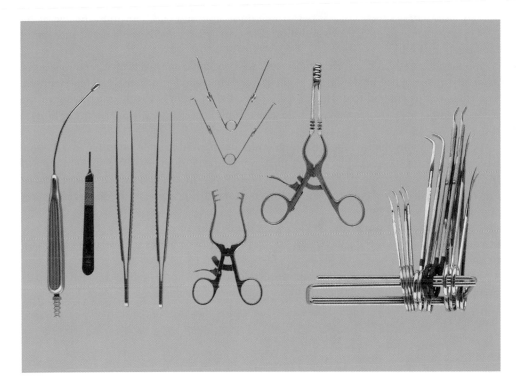

118-1 *Left to right:* 1 Andrews-Pynchon suction tube; 1 Bard-Parker knife handle #3; 2 DeBakey vascular Autraugrip tissue forceps, medium. *Top:* 2 Brawley scleral wound retractors; *bottom,* 1 Weitlaner retractor; and 1 cerebellar retractor, small. *On instrument stringer:* 4 Halsted microline artery forceps; 2 Adson hemostatic forceps, fine, right-angle; 1 Crile-Wood needle holder, 5 inch (difficult to see); 2 Horizon clip appliers, small; and 2 Metzenbaum dissecting scissors, 7 inch, 5 inch.

*Additional images are available on the Companion CD.

Chapter 119

Pediatric Neonatal/Infant Laparotomy Set*

Pediatric surgery is surgery that is performed on infants and children up to the age of 20. Pediatric instruments are smaller and shorter but otherwise exactly the same as those used for surgery in adults.

Esophageal atresia and pyloric stenosis are two congenital anomalies that require surgery in an infant. In esophageal atresia, the esophagus ends in a blind pouch or is severely stenosed. The chest wall is entered to correct the anomaly. Pyloric stenosis is the narrowing of the pyloric sphincter of the stomach. A pyloromyotomy is performed to incise the sphincter muscle.

Bowel conditions that require surgery in an infant or child include intestinal obstruction, which may be atresia (partial lacking of the bowel) or stenosis (narrowing of the lumen of the bowel); intussusception (the telescoping of one section of the bowel into another); or Hirschsprung disease (a congenital anomaly in which the colon lacks the innervation that stimulates peristalsis).

A Wilms tumor (a tumor of the kidney) and a cleft lip or palate (a congenital anomaly in which the lip and/or the palate are separated) are also problems that require surgery in infants and children.

Possible instruments and equipment needed for the procedure include a pediatric laparoscope and an operating microscope.

---

*Additional images are available on the Companion CD.

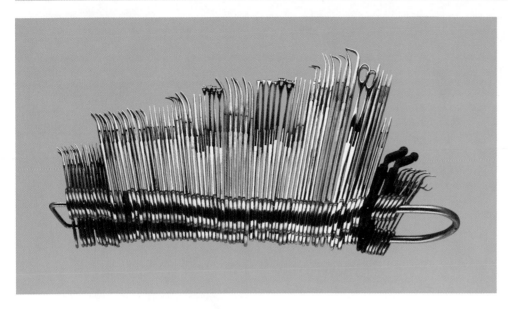

119-1 *Left to right:* 6 Hartmann mosquito hemostatic forceps, curved; 6 Hartmann mosquito hemostatic forceps, straight; 12 Halsted mosquito hemostatic forceps, curved; 6 Halsted mosquito hemostatic forceps, straight; 2 pediatric Jackson forceps, right angle; 2 Halsted hemostatic forceps, curved, 5½ inch; 2 Kocher clamps, straight, 5½ inch; 4 Babcock tissue forceps, delicate, 5¾ inch; 6 Crile hemostatic forceps, curved, 6½ inch; 4 Allis tissue forceps; 2 Babcock tissue forceps; 4 Crile hemostatic forceps, straight, 6½ inch; 2 Westphal hemostatic forceps, 7 inch; 3 tonsil hemostatic forceps, delicate tip; 2 Diethrich hemostatic forceps, right-angle; 1 tonsil hemostatic forceps; 1 Mixter hemostatic forceps, fine point; 2 Foerster sponge forceps, 7 inch; 2 Sarot needle holders, vascular, 7 inch; 2 Ayers needle holders, 7 inch; 2 Johnson needle holders, 5 inch; 2 paper drape clips; and 6 Backhaus towel clips, small.

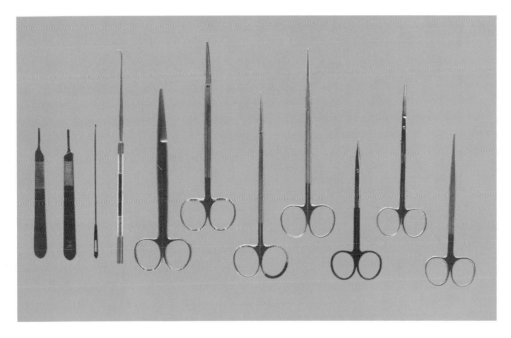

119-2 *Left to right:* 2 Bard-Parker knife handles #3; 1 probe dilator; 1 Hoen nerve hook; 1 Mayo dissecting scissors, straight; 3 Metzenbaum dissecting scissors, 7 inch, 1 curved, 1 Prince, and 1 straight; 1 Stevens tenotomy scissors, 5 inch; 1 Cooley neonatal scissors; and 1 Metzenbaum dissecting scissors, straight, 5 inch.

119-3 *Left to right:* 1 Andrew-Pynchon suction tube; 1 Poole suction tube, 16 Fr; 1 Poole suction tube with valve, 23 Fr; 1 Frazier suction tube, 8 Fr; 2 Adson tissue forceps, 1 with teeth (1 × 2), 1 without teeth; 2 Cushing tissue forceps, without teeth; and 1 Russian tissue forceps, medium.

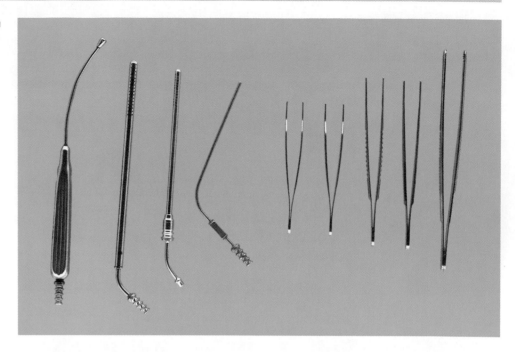

119-4 *Top, left to right:* 3 silicone-coated brain retractors, small, medium, large; 1 infant retractor, double-ended; 1 Ragnell retractor, double-ended; 1 Senn retractor; 1 Love nerve retractor, straight, 9 inch; 1 Little retractor; 2 baby Deaver retractors, $\frac{3}{8}$ inch, $\frac{5}{8}$ inch; 1 Army Navy retractor; and 2 Richardson-Eastman retractors, double-ended, small, large. *Bottom, left:* pediatric Balfour retractor and blade.

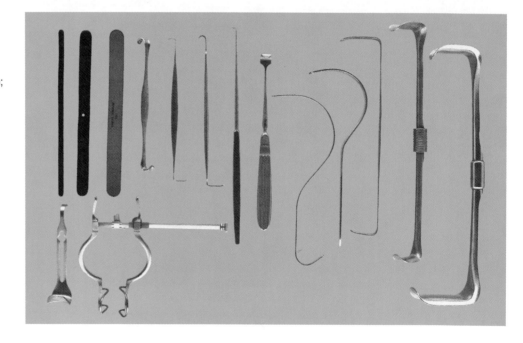

Pediatric Chest Instruments*

Possible instruments needed for the procedure includes a pediatric neonatal/infant laparotomy set.

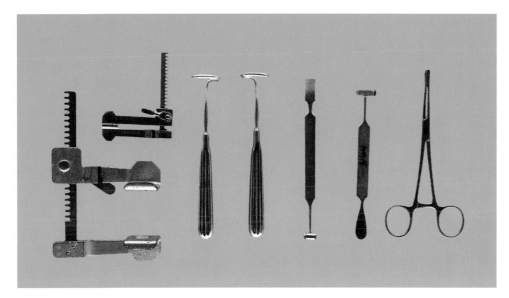

120-1 *Left to right:* 2 Cooley neonatal sternal retractor, pediatric, infant; 2 Doyen rib elevators and raspatories, right, left; 1 Alexander rib raspatory (periosteotome), double-ended, child; 1 Matson rib stripper and elevator, child; 1 Pennington hemostatic forceps.

*Refer to Chapter 109 (Thoracic Instruments) for close-up photos of instrument tips. Additional images are available on the Companion CD.

Pediatric Vascular Instruments*

Possible instruments needed for the procedure include a pediatric neonatal/infant laparotomy set.

121-1 *Left to right:* 12-inch ruler showing the size of the neonatal vascular clamps. 1 Satinsky neonatal vascular clamp; 1 DeBakey neonatal vascular clamp, straight; 1 Cooley neonatal multipurpose clamp, angled; 1 Cooley neonatal peripheral vascular clamp, angled; and 1 Cooley neonatal vascular clamp.

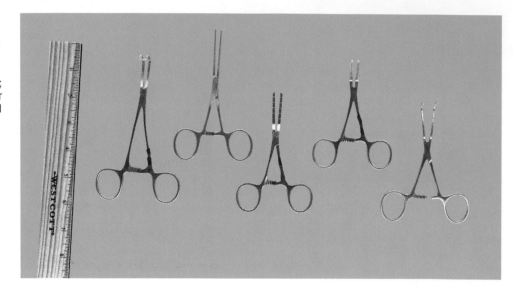

---

*Refer to Chapter 110 (Cardiac Surgery), Chapter 113 (Open Heart Extras), and Chapter 114 (Cardiovascular Instruments) for close-up photos of instruments tips. Additional images are available on the Companion CD.

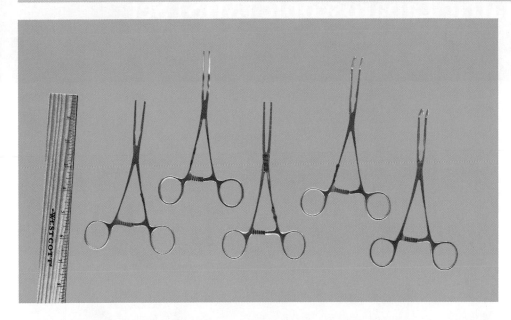

121-2 *Left to right:* 1 Cooley pediatric vascular clamp, straight; 1 Cooley pediatric vascular clamp, angled; 1 Cooley pediatric patent ductus clamp, straight; 1 Cooley-Satinsky pediatric clamp; and 1 Cooley pediatric anastomosis clamp.

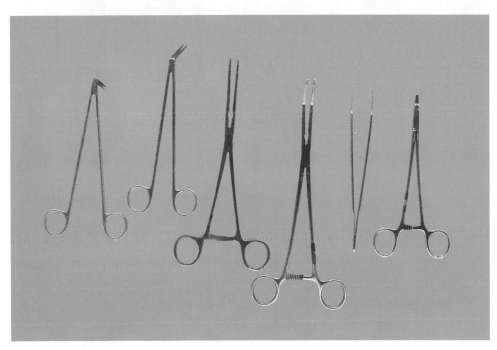

121-3 *Left to right:* 1 reverse Potts cardiovascular scissors; 1 Potts cardiovascular scissors; 2 DeBakey coarctation and peripheral vascular clamps, 9 inch, straight, angled; 1 Gerald tissue forceps without teeth, 7 inch; and 1 Ryder needle holder, 7 inch.

Pediatric Laparoscopic (MIS) Set[*]

122-1 *Top to bottom:* 2 Stryker laparoscopic lens, 2.7 mm, 30 degree, 70 degree. *Left to right,* 1 3-mm Ethicon disposable needle; 2 Verres needles, 100 mm, 70 mm; 1 obturator, 3.5 mm, sharp; 1 3.5-mm × 40 mm cannula with port; 1 obturator, 3.5 mm, blunt; 1 5-mm × 40 mm cannula with port; 1 obturator, 5 mm, blunt; 1 5-mm × 50 mm cannula with port; and 1 obturator, 5 mm, sharp.

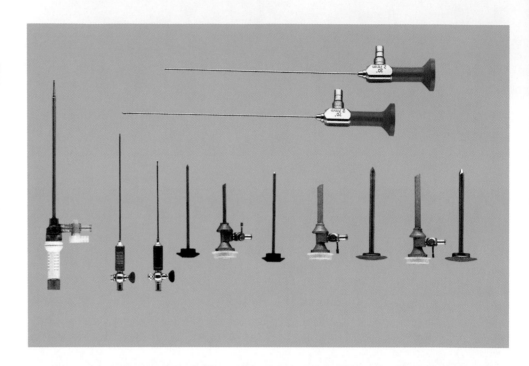

122-2 *Left to right:* Endoflex liver retractor; 1 3.5-mm suction/irrigator; 1 5-mm suction/irrigator, disposable; 1 spatula cautery, 5 mm, disposable; 1 hook cautery, 5 mm, disposable; 1 hook, 3.5 mm, disposable; 1 spatula, 3.5 mm, disposable; and 1 monopolar cord.

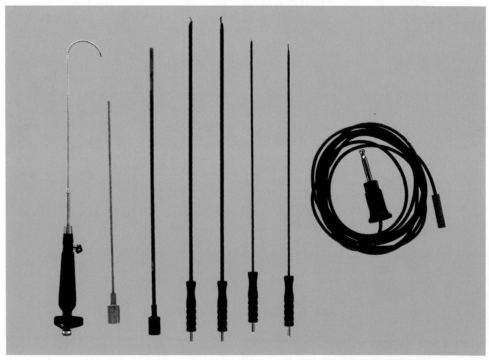

*Refer to Chapter 10 (Laparoscopic Adult MIS Set) for close-up photos of instrument tips.

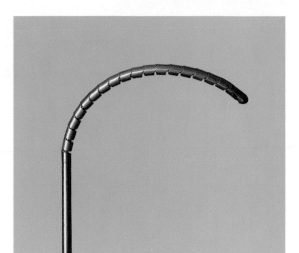

122-3 Tip of endoflex liver retractor.

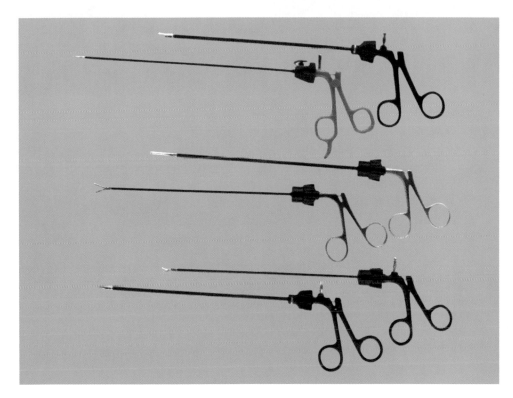

122-4 *Top to bottom:* 1 3.5-mm × 24 cm Hook scissors; 1 3.5-mm × 24 cm Babcock forceps; 1 3.5-mm × 24 cm Hunter bowel grasper; 1 3.5-mm × 24 cm grabber forceps; 1 3.5-mm × 24 cm monopolar Metzenbaum dissecting scissors; and 1 3.5-mm × 24 cm Maryland dissector.

122-5 *Top to bottom:* 1 5-mm ×
24 cm Maryland dissector; 1 5-mm
× 24 cm monopolar Metzenbaun
dissecting scissors; 1 5-mm × 24 cm
Swanstrom grasper; 1 5-mm × 24 cm
Hunter bowel grasper; and 2 5-mm
× 24 cm Jarit needle holders, open,
closed.

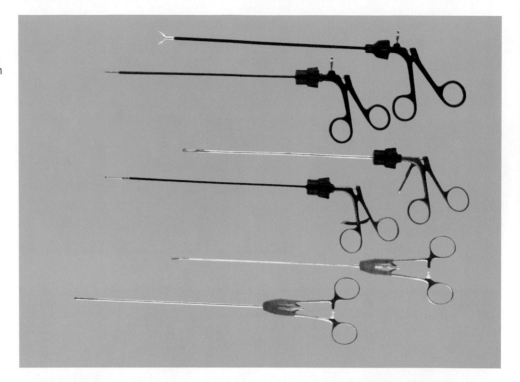

122-6 *Top to bottom:* 1 3-mm
double-ended knot pusher; 1 5-mm
Ranfac knot pusher; and 1 5-mm
Marlow knot pusher.

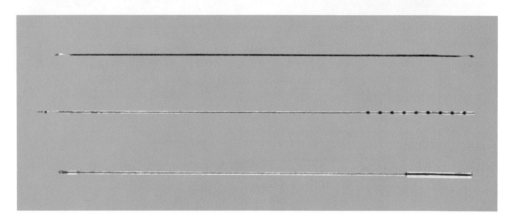

Pediatric Pyloromyotomy Laparoscopic Set (MIS)

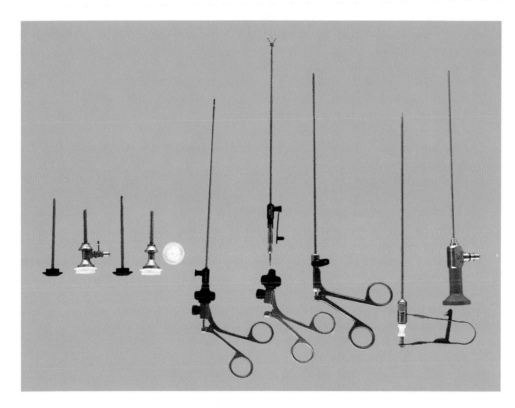

123-1 *Left to right:* 1 obturator, 3 mm, sharp; 1 3-mm cannula with port; 1 obturator, 3 mm, blunt; 1 3-mm cannula without port; 1 port cap; 2 Tan spreaders, tapered; 1 Tan spreader, blunt; 1 Tan endoknife, retractable; and 1 Stryker laparoscopic lens, 2.7 mm × 18 cm, 30 degrees.

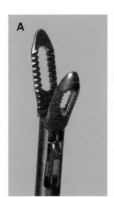
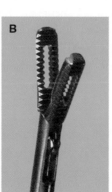
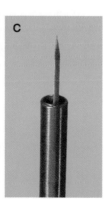

123-2 A, Tan spreader, tapered; **B**, Tan spreader, blunt; and **C**, Tan endoknife, retractable.

Chapter

124

Craniotomy

Craniotomy is an incision made in the head through the skull that allows the performance of surgery on the brain.

Possible equipment needed for the procedure includes:
1. A Midas Rex drill with craniotome blades, used to open the skull.
2. A Cavitron ultrasonic surgical aspirator (CUSA), used for tumor removal.
3. An operating microscope, used for visualization.
4. An electrosurgical unit, used for hemostasis.
5. A neuroplating set of screws and plates, used to repair fractures and to replace the bone flap.
6. Bur-hole covers, used to cover the bur holes.

A brief description of the procedure follows:
1. Raney clip appliers and clips are placed on the skin flaps for hemostasis.
2. Strully scissors are used to incise the scalp muscle.
3. An Adson periosteal elevator is used to strip periosteum from the bone and enlarge the bur holes.
4. A craniotome is used to turn a bone flap.
5. A Penfield dissector is used to remove dura mater from the bone.
6. A Ruskin double-action rongeur is used to remove jagged bone edges.
7. Cushing tissue forceps with teeth are used to grasp and elevate the dura.
8. An Adson dura hook is used to elevate the dura.
9. Metzenbaum dissecting scissors are used to incise the dura.
10. A Leyla retractor is used to expose the brain.
11. Cushing bipolar cautery forceps are used for hemostasis.

To clip an intracranial aneurysm, Yasargil clip appliers and clips are needed. A Delta shunt tool is used to shunt cerebral spinal fluid from the cerebral ventricles to the peritoneum, and a Salmon passer is used to tunnel subcutaneously from a bur hole to a peritoneal catheter.

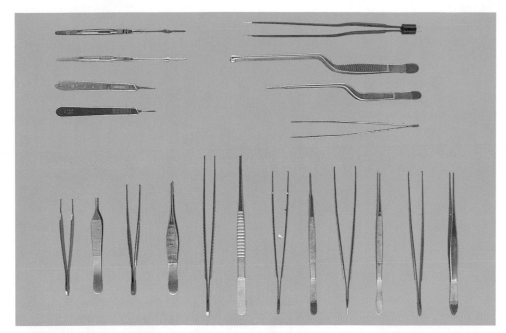

124-1 *Top to bottom, left to right:* 2 Bard-Parker knife handles #7; 2 Bard-Parker knife handles #3; 1 Cushing bipolar cautery forceps, microtip, insulated bayonet shaft; 1 Adson hypophyseal forceps, bayonet shaft, round-cup tip; 1 Gerald dressing forceps, bayonet shaft, narrow tips, serrated; 1 Adson dressing forceps, bayonet shaft. *Bottom, left to right:* 2 Adson tissue forceps with teeth (1 × 2); 2 Gillies tissue forceps with teeth (1 × 2); 2 DeBakey vascular Autraugrip tissue forceps, medium; 2 Gerald tissue forceps with teeth (1 × 2); 2 Cushing tissue forceps with teeth (1 × 2); 2 Cushing tissue forceps with teeth (1 × 2), Gutsch handle.

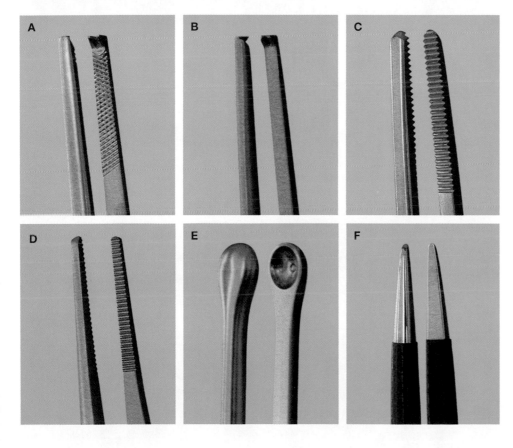

124-2 *Left to right:* Tips: **A**, Gillies tissue forceps with teeth (1 × 2); **B**, Gerald tissue forceps with teeth (1 × 2); **C**, Adson dressing forceps, bayonet shaft; **D**, Gerald dressing forceps, bayonet shaft, narrow tips, serrated; **E**, Adson hypophyseal forceps, bayonet shaft, round-cup tip; **F**, Cushing bipolar cautery forceps, microtip, insulated bayonet shaft.

124-3 *Top to bottom, left to right:* 1 Mayo dissecting scissors, straight; 1 Metzenbaum dissecting scissors, 7 inch; 1 Metzenbaum dissecting scissors, 5 inch; 1 Strully scissors, 8 inch; 1 Adson ganglion scissors, straight, 6¼ inch. *Bottom, left to right:* 2 Raney scalp clip appliers; 3 paper drape clips; 2 Ligaclip appliers, small/short; 4 Backhaus towel forceps; 6 Backhaus towel forceps, small; 6 Cairns hemostatic forceps; 6 Crile hemostatic forceps, curved; 2 Allis tissue forceps; 2 Ochsner tissue forceps; 2 Ligaclip appliers, medium/medium; 1 Westphal hemostatic forceps; 1 Adson hemostatic forceps, fine tip; 2 DeBakey needle holders, 7 inch; 2 Webster needle holders, 6 inch; 2 Crile-Wood needle holders, 7 inch.

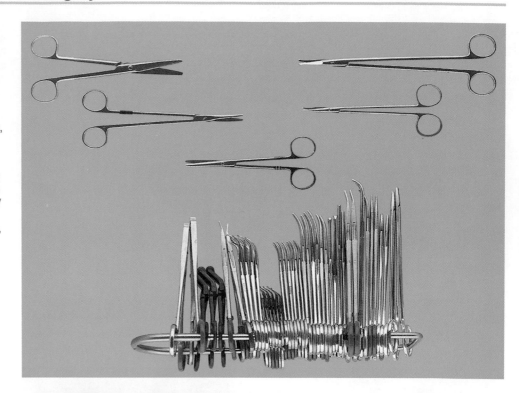

124-4 *Left to right:* Tips: **A**, Strully scissors; **B**, Adson ganglion scissors, straight.

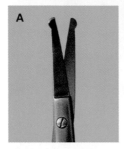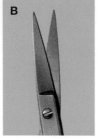

124-5 *Top, left to right:* 6 Frazier suction tubes, sizes 6 to 12. *Bottom, left to right:* 5 silicone spatula retractors, 6, 9, 13, 16, and 22 mm; 1 metal ruler; 5 Davis brain spatulas, various widths.

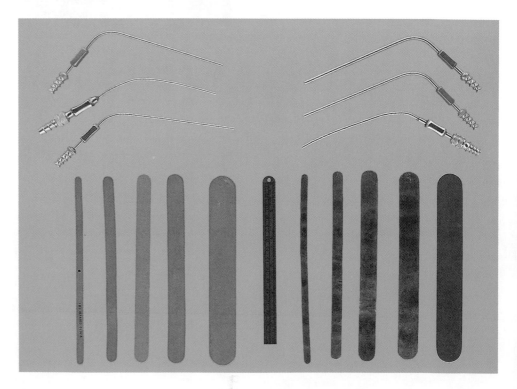

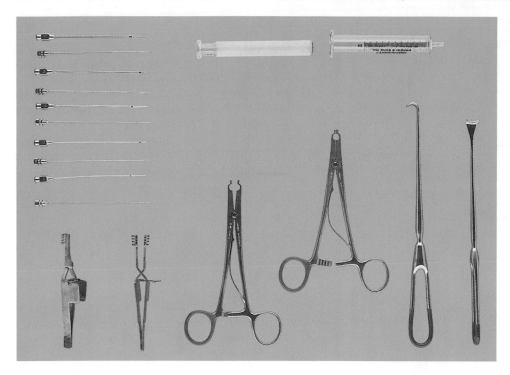

124-6 *Top to bottom, left to right:* 5 ventricular needles with stylets, 3½ inch, 12, 14, 16, 18, and 20 gauge; 1 10-ml glass-tipped syringe (2 parts). *Bottom, left to right:* 2 Jarit crossing-action retractors, 4 inch, blunt prongs; 2 Raney scalp clip appliers, side view; 2 vein retractors, side view and front view.

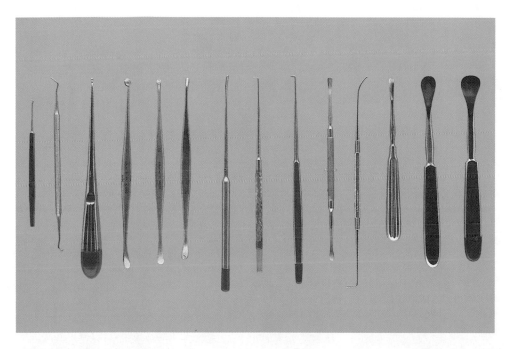

124-7 *Left to right:* 1 dura hook; 1 Woodson dura separator and packer, 7 inch; 1 Brun oval-cup curette, angled, 3-0; 3 Penfield dissectors, #1, #2, and #3, 7¼ inch; 1 Penfield dissector, #4, 8 inch; 1 Adson dura hook, sharp; 1 nerve hook, dull, flat; 1 Freer elevator; 1 Kistner probe; 1 Adson periosteal elevator (joker), curved, blunt, 6¾ inch; 1 Hoen periosteal elevator, narrow; 1 Hoen periosteal elevator, wide.

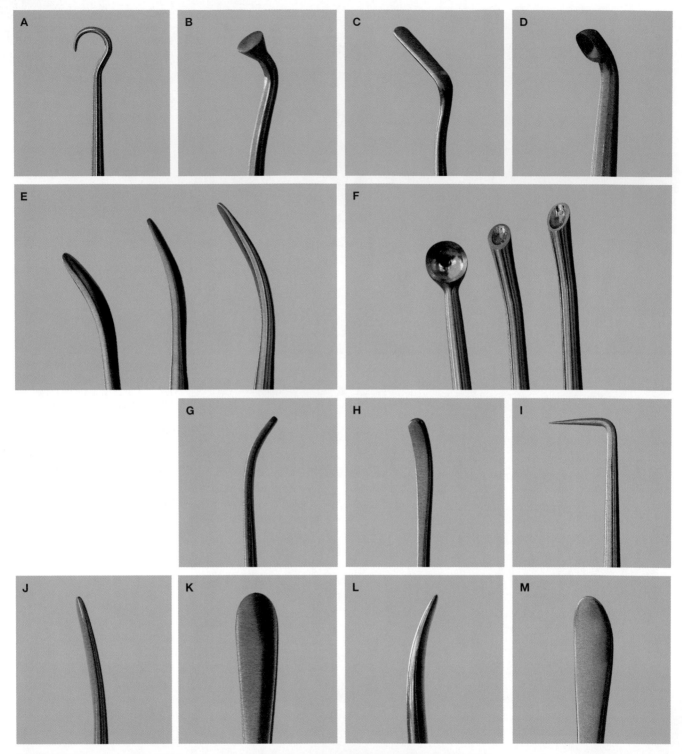

124-8 *Left to right:* Tips: **A**, Frazier dura hook, 5 inch; Woodson dura separator and packer, double-ended, 7 inch; **B**, packer end; **C**, separator end; **D**, Brun oval-cup curette, angled, 3-0; Penfield dissectors, #1, #2, and #3; **E**, side view, dissector end; **F**, front view, spoon and wax-packer end; Penfield dissector #4, 8 inch; **G**, side view; **H**, front view; **I**, Adson dura hook, sharp, 8 inch; Freer double-ended elevator, 7¾ inch; **J**, side view; **K**, front view; Adson periosteal elevator (joker), curved, blunt, 6¾ inch; **L**, side view; **M**, front view.

Neurologic Bone Pan Instruments*

Possible instruments needed for the procedure include a neurologic soft tissue set.

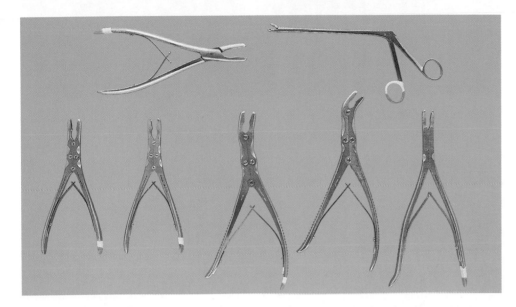

125-1 *Top, left to right:* 1 Adson rongeur; 1 cup rongeur, 6 mm. *Bottom, left to right:* 1 Ruskin double-action rongeur, small, straight; 1 Ruskin double-action rongeur, small, curved; 1 Leksell rongeur, side-curved; 1 Leksell rongeur, curved; 1 Smith-Petersen laminectomy rongeur.

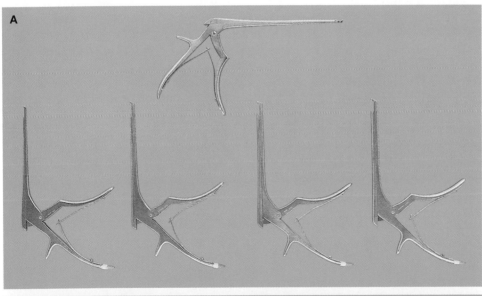

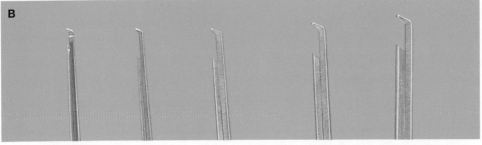

125-2 A, *Top:* 1 Kerrison rongeur, 45 degree, 1 mm. *Bottom, left to right:* 4 Kerrison rongeurs, 45 degree: 2, 3, 4, and 5 mm. **B,** *Left to right:* Tips: 5 Kerrison rongeurs, 45 degree, 1, 2, 3, 4, and 5 mm.

*Additional images are available on the Companion CD.

125-3 *Left to right:* 2 Senn retractors, side view and front view; 2 Army Navy retractors, side view and front view; 2 Green goiter retractors, side view and front view; 1 metal mallet. *Top to bottom, left to right:* 2 Weitlaner retractors, baby, angled; 2 Weitlaner retractors, small, angled.

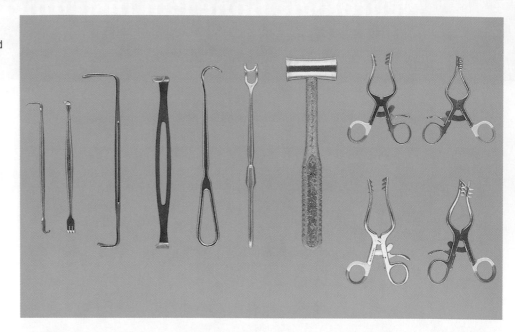

125-4 *Left to right:* 2 Weitlaner retractors, small; 2 Weitlaner retractors, medium; 2 Adson retractors, sharp, medium, angled.

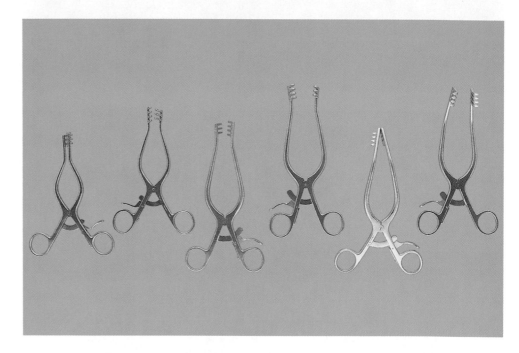

Possible instruments needed for the procedure include a neurologic soft tissue set.

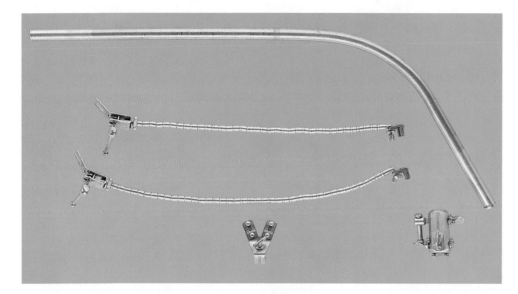

126-1 Leyla retractor: 1 fixation base for the 2 flexible arms, 2 flexible arms, square block, table brace.

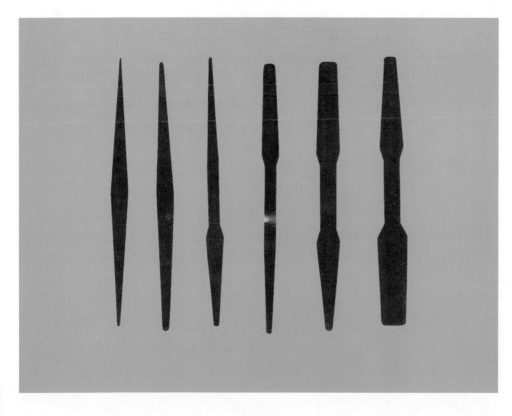

126-2 Tapered malleable brain retractors, which are often used with the Leyla retractor.

126-3 *Top to bottom, left to right:*
Greenberg Universal retractor: hand
rest with flexible bar to clamp;
2 primary bars; 1 long retractor arm.
Right side: 4 secondary bars.

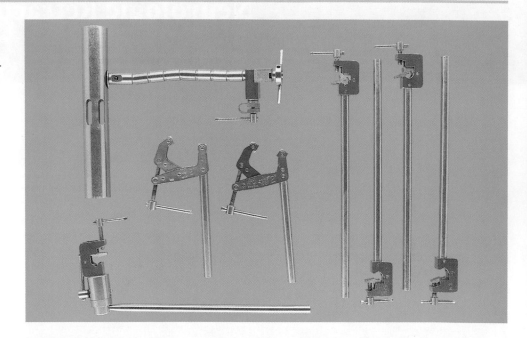

126-4 Greenberg Universal retractor,
continued: 2 flexible retractor bars,
long. *Middle, top to bottom:* 8 metal
brain spatulas, various widths; 10
plastic-coated blades, various widths.
Right: 2 flexible retractor bars, short.

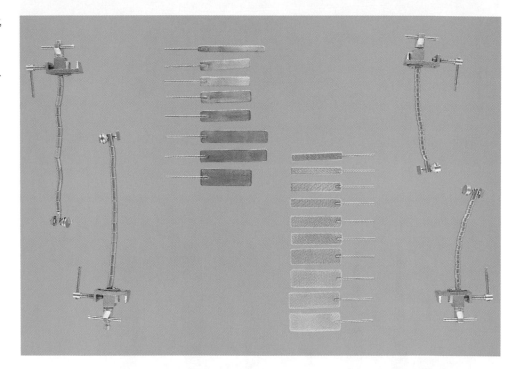

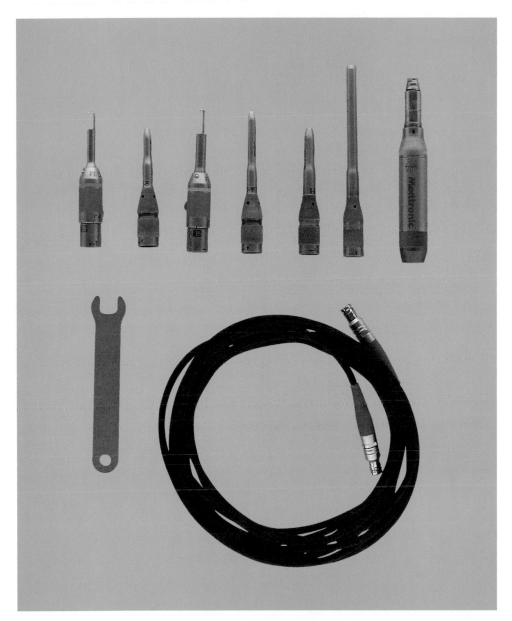

127-1 *Top, left to right:* attachments, 1, 8 Fr, 2, 10, 9, 14 Fr; and handpiece. *Bottom, left to right:* wrench; and power cord.

---

*Additional images are available on the Companion CD.

128-1 **A**, *Left to right:* 2 Beaver blade handles with insert, knurled; 1 microscissors, straight; 1 microscissors, curved; 1 micro–needle holder, straight; 1 micro–needle holder, curved; 1 micro–grasping forceps. **B**, *Left to right:* Tips: microscissors, straight; microscissors, curved; micro–needle holder, straight; micro–needle holder, curved; micro–grasping forceps.

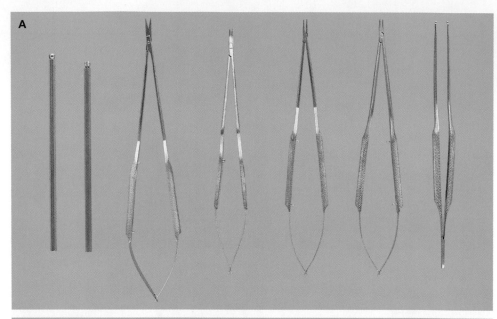

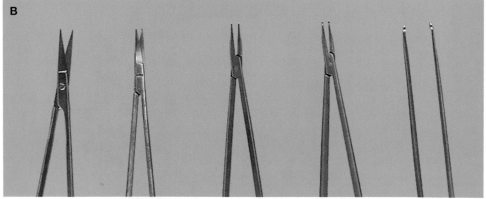

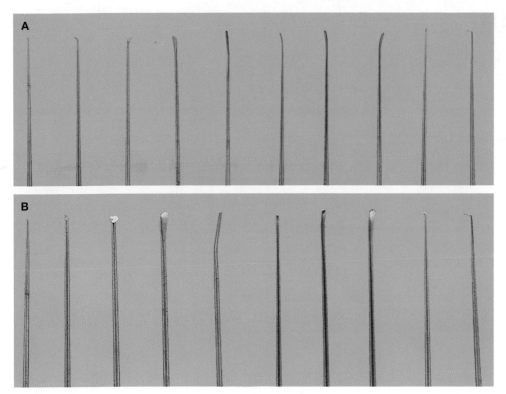

128-2 A, *Left to right:* 3 round microdissectors: 1, 2, and 3 mm; 2 general-purpose microelevators: curved and angled; 3 spatula microdissectors: small, medium, and large; 2 microhooks, 90 degree: semisharp and blunt. **B**, Tips: 3 round microdissectors: 1, 2, and 3 mm; 2 general-purpose microelevators: curved and angled; 3 spatula microdissectors: small, medium, and large; 2 microhooks, 90 degree: semisharp and blunt.

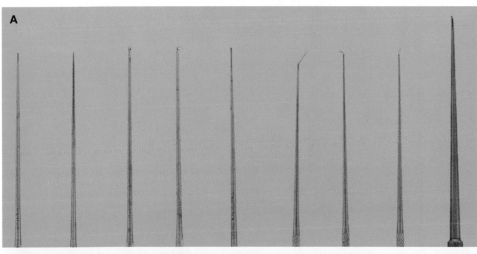

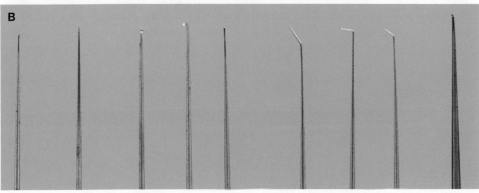

128-3 A, *Left to right:* 1 microhook, 45 degree, semisharp; 1 micro–needle point, straight; 2 microcurettes: straight and angled; 4 ball microdissectors: straight: 40 degree, 4 mm; 90 degree, 5 mm; 40 degree, 8 mm; 1 arachnoid microknife. **B**, Tips: microhook, 45 degree, semisharp; micro–needle point, straight; 2 microcurettes: straight and angled; 4 ball microdissectors: straight; 40 degree, 4 mm; 90 degree, 5 mm; 40 degree, 8 mm; arachnoid microknife.

128-4 *Left to right:* Enlarged Tips: 3 round microdissectors: 1, 2, and 3 mm; 1 general purpose microelevator, angled.

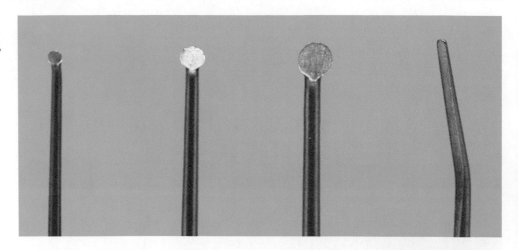

128-5 *Left to right:* Enlarged Tips: 4 spatula microdissectors: large, small, medium, and medium straight.

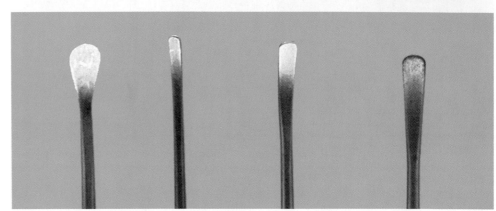

128-6 *Left to right:* Enlarged Tips: 2 microhooks, 90 degree: semisharp and blunt; 1 general-purpose microelevator, curved; 1 micro–needle point, straight.

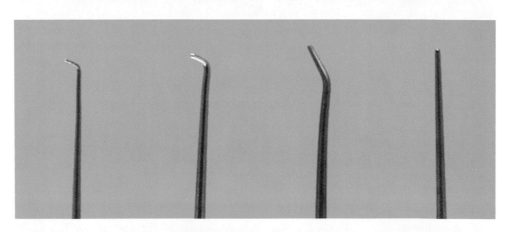

128-7 *Left to right:* Enlarged Tips: 2 microcurettes: straight and angled; 1 ball microdissector, 90-degree–angle tip.

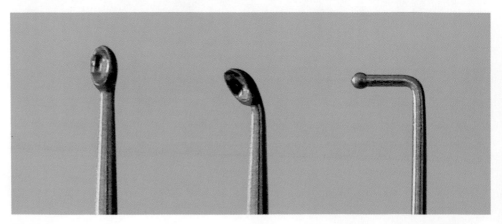

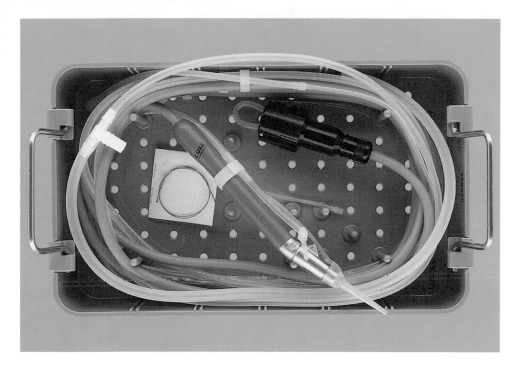

129-1 CUSA handpiece with attachments in tray.

Neurologic Shunt Instruments

130-1 *Top to bottom, left to right:*
2 Bard-Parker knife handles, #7;
2 Bard-Parker knife handles, #3;
2 Adson tissue forceps with teeth;
1 Cushing bipolar cautery forceps,
bayonet handle; 1 thumb-dressing
forceps without teeth, bayonet handle.
Bottom, left to right: 2 DeBakey
vascular Autraugrip tissue forceps,
short; 2 Cushing tissue forceps with
teeth (1 × 2); 2 DeBakey vascular
Autraugrip tissue forceps, medium;
12 Backhaus towel forceps, small;
4 Backhaus towel forceps; 4 tonsil
hemostatic forceps, short; 4 tonsil
hemostatic forceps, long; 6 Halsted
mosquito hemostatic forceps,
curved; 2 Allis tissue forceps; 4
Crile hemostatic forceps, curved;
1 iris scissors; 1 Stevens tenotomy
scissors; 1 Metzenbaum dissecting
scissors, 5 inch; 1 Metzenbaum
dissecting scissors, 7 inch; 1 Mayo
dissecting scissors, straight; 1
Webster needle holder, 4½ inch; 1
Sarot needle holder; 1 Ryder needle
holder; 2 Crile-Wood needle holders,
7 inch.

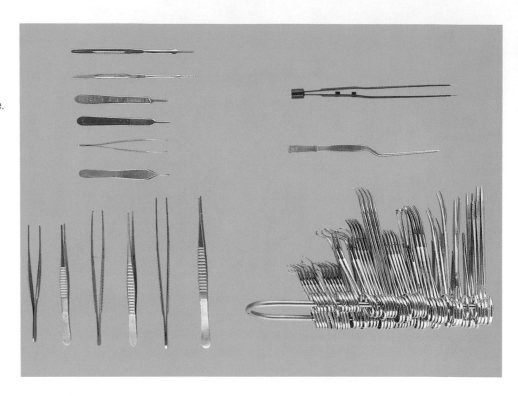

130-2 *Left to right:* Tips: **A**, Webster
needle holder, 4½ inch;
B, Sarot needle holder, 7⅛ inch;
C, Ryder needle holder, 7 inch;
D, Crile-Wood needle holder, 7 inch.

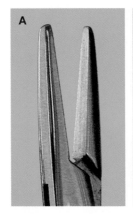 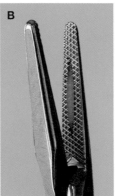 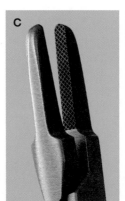 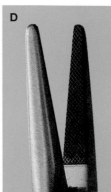

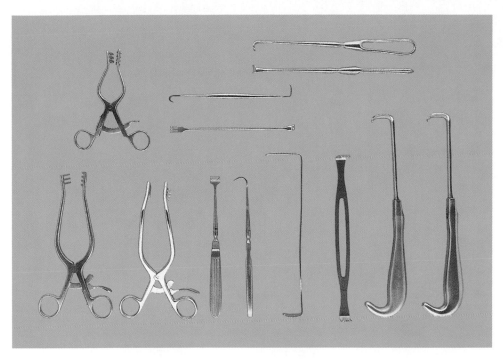

130-3 *Top, left to right:* 1 Weitlaner retractor, small, angled; 2 Senn retractors, side view and front view; 2 vein retractors, side view and front view. *Bottom, left to right:* 1 Weitlaner retractor, medium; 1 Adson retractor, angled; 2 Cushing vein and nerve retractors, front view and side view; 2 Army Navy retractors, side view and front view; 2 Richardson retractors, baby, side view.

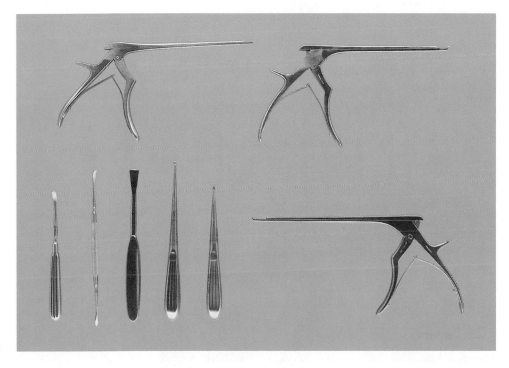

130-4 *Top, left to right:* 2 Kerrison rongeurs: 90 degree, 2 mm; 40 degree, 3 mm. *Bottom, left to right:* 1 Adson periosteal elevator (joker); 1 Freer elevator, double-ended; 1 Langenbeck periosteal elevator; 1 Brun curette, oval cup, #0, angled tip, 9 inch; 1 Brun curette, oval cup, #0, straight, 6¾ inch; 1 Kerrison rongeur, 40 degree, 2 mm.

130-5 *Top, left to right:* 5 ventricular needles with stylets, 3½ inch: 12, 14, 16, 18, and 20 gauge; 4 Frazier suction tubes: #3, #4, #6, and #8. *Middle, left to right:* 2 bulldog clips, straight, small; 2 Titus needles with stylets. *Bottom, left to right:* 1 hand drill handle; 1 drill bit; 1 Jarit tendon-pulling forceps, curved shaft, serrated jaws, 5 inch.

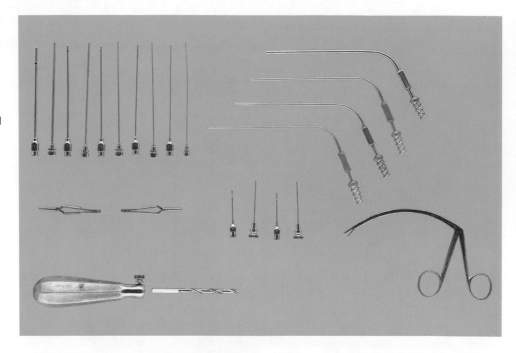

130-6 *Top left:* 2 Weitlaner retractors, angled, baby. *Middle, left to right:* 2 Jarit cross-action retractors, blunt prongs, 4 inch; 1 glass syringe with Luer-Lok, 10 ml; 1 Huber needle, 26 gauge; 1 Delta shunt tool; 1 metal ruler, 15 cm. *Bottom:* 1 Salmon passer, 14 inch, 2 parts.

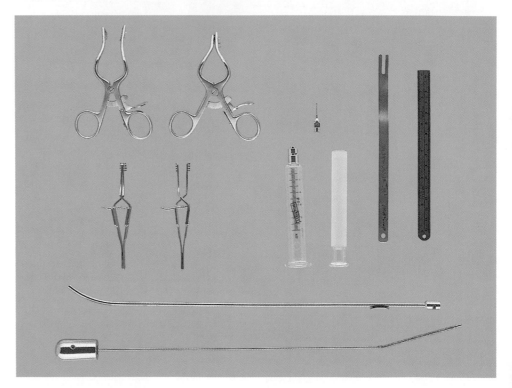

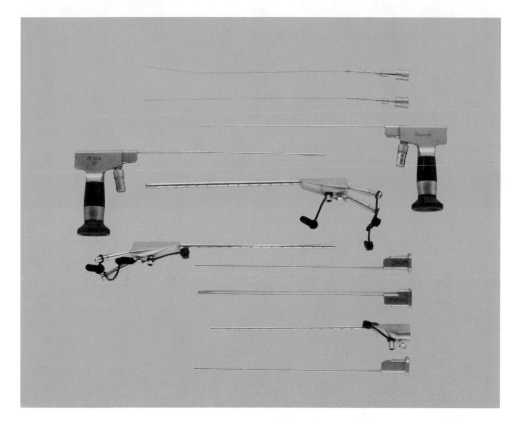

131-1 *Top to bottom:* 2 guide wires; 1 endoscope lens, 0 degrees × 2.7 mm; 1 endoscope lens, 30 degrees × 2.7 mm; 1 sheath, 6 mm; 1 sheath, 4.6 mm; 1 trocar, 4.6 mm; 1 trocar, 6 mm; 1 sheath (no working channel), 3.2 mm; and 1 trocar, 3.2 mm.

*Additional images are available on the Companion CD.

131-2 *Top to bottom in rack:*
2 microscissors, B/B, S/S; 1 biopsy
forceps; 1 fixation and dissecting
forceps; 1 surgical mircoforceps; and
2 suction tips.

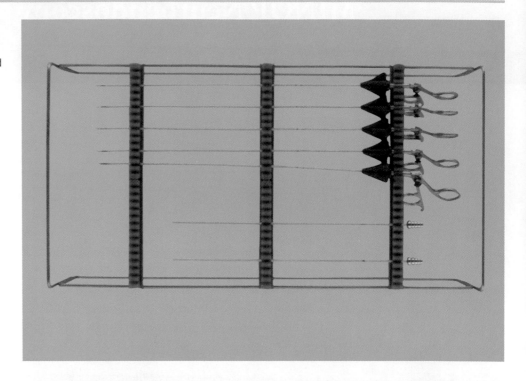

131-3 *Left to right:* 1 monopolar
cord; 1 hook electrode; 1 needle
electrode; 3 hook electrodes; and
1 blunt electrode. *Top to bottom:*
1 Silastic tubing; *in center of tubing:*
2 lightcord adapters; and 1 bipolar
cord. *Right:* 1 bipolar fork electrode.

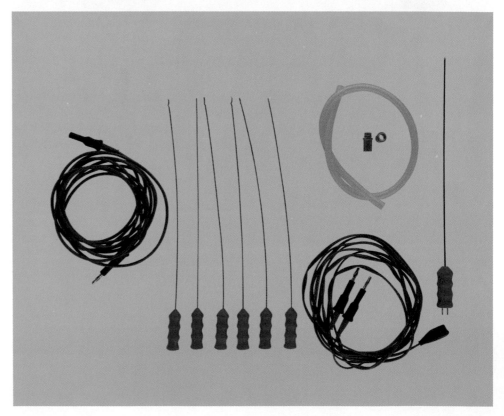

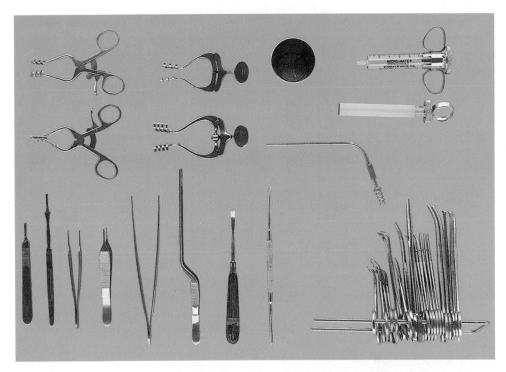

132-1 *Top, left to right:* 2 Weitlaner retractors, baby, front view and back view; 1 mastoid articulated retractor, 3 prong; 1 Jansen retractor, 4 prong; 1 metal medicine cup, 2 oz; 1 Frazier suction tube, 12 Fr; 1 Luer-Lok glass syringe with plunger and finger holds. *Bottom, left to right:* 1 Bard-Parker knife handle, #3; 1 Bard-Parker knife handle, #7; 2 Adson tissue forceps with teeth (1 × 2), front view and side view; 1 Cushing tissue forceps without teeth; 1 thumb-dressing forceps, bayonet shaft; 1 Adson periosteal elevator (joker), curved, blunt, 6¾ inch; 1 Freer elevator; 4 Backhaus towel forceps, small; 1 Backhaus towel forceps, regular; 1 iris scissors, curved; 1 Metzenbaum dissecting scissors, 5½ inch; 1 Mayo dissecting scissors, straight; 3 Halsted mosquito hemostatic forceps, curved; 3 Halsted mosquito hemostatic forceps, straight; 2 Mayo-Péan hemostatic forceps, curved, 6 inch; 2 Allis tissue forceps; 1 Mayo-Hegar needle holder, 6 inch.

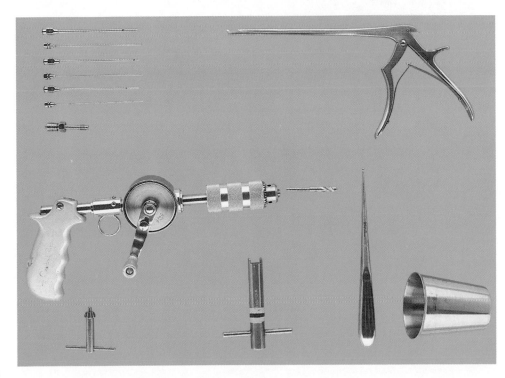

132-2 *Top, left to right:* 3 cone ventricular needles with stylets; 1 Richmond subarachnoid screw; 1 Spurling-Kerrison rongeur, 40-degree angle, 3 mm. *Bottom, left to right:* 1 hand drill with bit; 1 chuck key; 1 Richmond subarachnoid wrench (T handle); 1 Spratt (Brun) curette, 3-0, small angle; 1 metal medicine cup, 8 oz.

Yasargil Aneurysm Clips with Appliers

133-1 Yasargil aneurysm clips in marked tray.

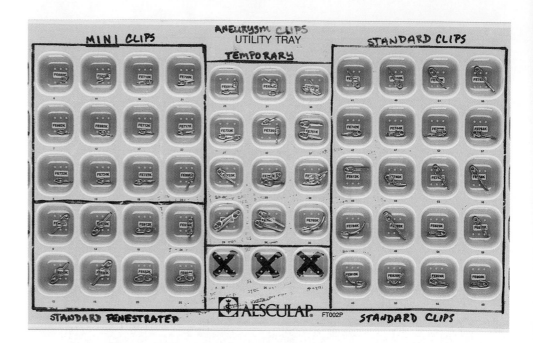

133-2 *Left, top to middle:* 1 Casper appliers, angled, standard; 1 Casper appliers, angled, mini. *Bottom:* 1 bayonet clip appliers, standard; 1 bayonet clip appliers, mini. *Right, top to middle:* 1 Titan-Vario clip appliers, standard; 1 Titan-Vario clip appliers, mini. *Middle:* 1 aneurysm clip, silver, permanent; 1 aneurysm clip, gold, temporary.

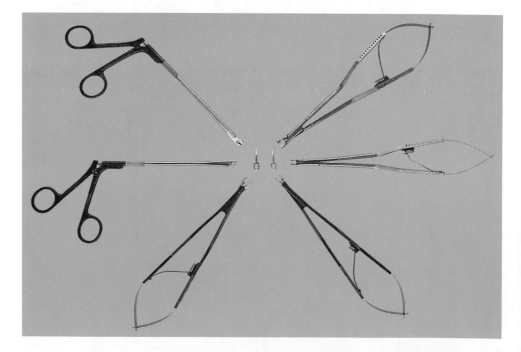

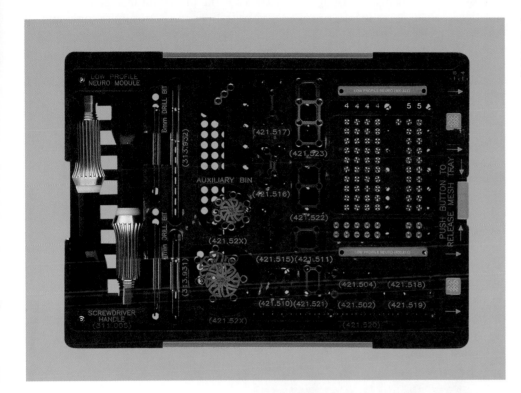

134-1 Synthes low-profile cranial plating set. *On left side:* 2 screwdriver handles and a variety of drill bits, 4 mm, 6 mm; *on right side:* 1.5 mm screws.

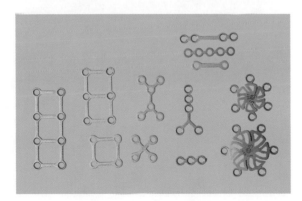

134-2 Variety of Synthes low-profile implant cranial plates; *on right side:* 2 bur-hole covers, 12 mm, 17 mm.

*Additional images are available on the Companion CD.

Laminectomy*

A laminectomy is an incision in the back to remove the lamina so as to expose the spinal column.

Possible instruments and equipment needed for the procedure include a neurologic soft-tissue set; an operating microscope for visualization; an electrosurgical unit; and an electric drill, bits, and burs.

A brief description of the procedure follows:

1. A Beckman-Adson retractor is used to expose the vertebrae.
2. A Hibbs retractor is used if deeper retraction is needed.
3. A Cobb elevator is used to remove periosteum from the laminae.
4. A Smith-Petersen rongeur is used to remove the spinous processes.
5. Cushing bayonet forceps with teeth are used to grasp the ligamentum flava.
6. A Bard-Parker scalpel handle #7 with #15 blade is used to incise close to the midline.
7. A Mellon curette is used to remove lateral gutter ligaments.
8. A Brun curette is used to define the laminae edges.
9. A Leksell rongeur is used to remove the laminae and expose the spinal cord.
10. An Adson blunt nerve hook is used to explore nerve roots and extradural space.
11. A Love retractor is used to protect nerves from injury.
12. A Cushing disk rongeur is used to remove disk material.

135-1 *Top, left to right:* 4 Cushing intervertebral disk rongeurs, 2 mm: straight, 6 inch; upbiting, 6 inch; straight, 6 inch; straight, 7 inch. *Bottom, left to right:* 1 Cushing intervertebral disk rongeur, 3 mm, 7 inch, upbiting; 1 Ferris Smith pituitary rongeur, 6 mm, 7 inch; 1 Cushing intervertebral disk rongeur, 4 mm, 7 inch.

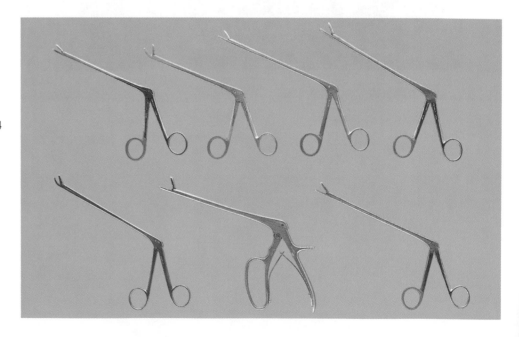

*Additional images are available on the Companion CD.

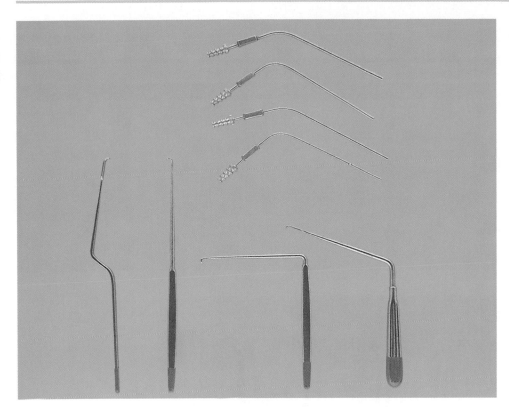

135-2 *Top to middle:* 4 Frazier suction tubes: 12, 10, 8, and 6 Fr. *Bottom, left to right:* 1 D'Errico nerve root retractor; 1 Love nerve retractor, straight; 1 Love nerve retractor, 90-degree angle; 1 Scoville nerve root retractor, angular.

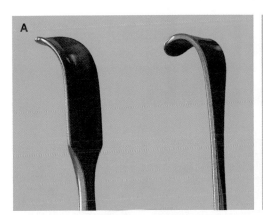
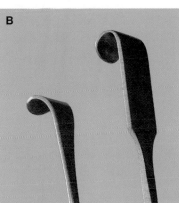

135-3 *Left to right:* Tips: **A**, D'Errico nerve root retractor, Love nerve root retractor, straight; **B**, Love nerve root retractor, 90-degree angle, Scoville nerve root retractor, angular.

135-4 A, *Left to right:* 4 Spurling-Kerrison rongeurs, 40 degree: 2, 3, 4, and 5 mm. **B,** *Left to right:* Tips: 4 Spurling-Kerrison rongeurs, 40 degree: 2, 3, 4, 5 mm.

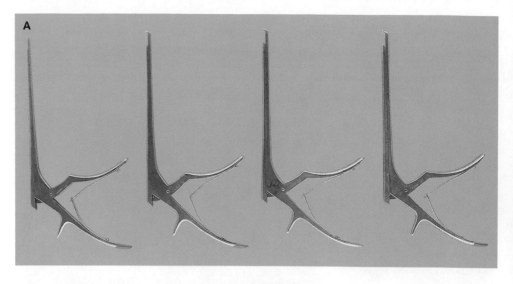

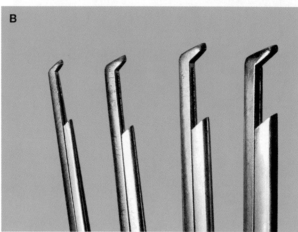

135-5 *Top:* 2 Adson cerebellar retractors, medium. *Bottom, left to right:* 2 Weitlaner retractors, straight, long; 2 Taylor spinal retractors: short, front view; long, side view; 2 Hibbs laminectomy retractors: narrow, front view; wide, side view.

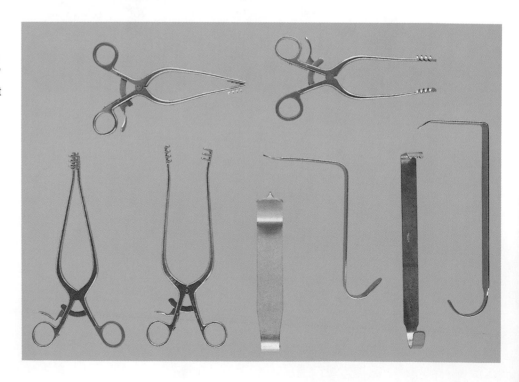

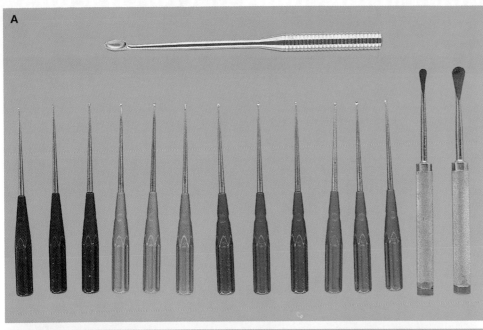

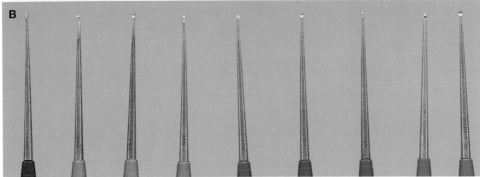

135-6 **A**, *Top:* 1 Mellon curette, long, large. *Bottom, left to right:* 3 curettes, size 4-0: reverse-angled, angled, and straight; 3 curettes, size 2-0: reverse-angled, angled, and straight; 3 curettes, size 3-0: reverse-angled, angled, and straight; 3 curettes, size 0: reverse-angled, angled, and straight; 1 Cobb spinal elevator, narrow; 1 Cobb spinal elevator, wide. **B**, *Left to right:* curette tips: 1 4-0, straight; 3 2-0: reverse-angled, angled, and straight; 3 3-0: reverse-angled, angled, and straight; 2 0: reverse-angled and straight.

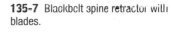

135-7 Blackbelt spine retractor with blades.

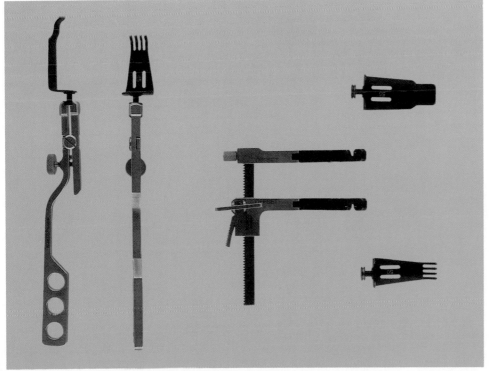

136-1 *Left to right:* Williams laminectomy microretractors: short blade, right-handed, back view; long blade, right-handed, front view; long blade, left-handed, front view.

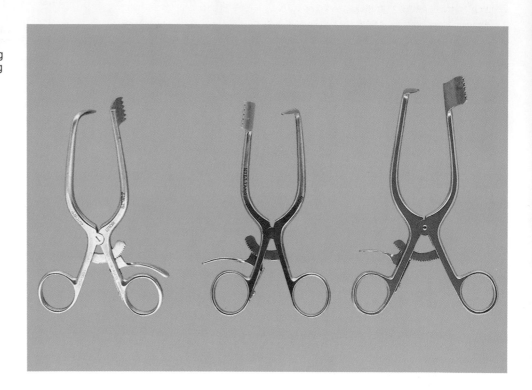

Anterior Cervical Fusion

Chapter

An anterior cervical fusion is performed to relieve pain and stabilize the neck by fusing the cervical vertebrae. The patient is placed in the supine position. Bone from the iliac crest or from a bone bank may be used for the fusion.

Possible instruments needed for the procedure include a neurologic soft-tissue set.

A brief description of the bone-retrieval procedure follows:

1. A Hudson brace is used to obtain bone from the iliac crest.
2. A Cloward dowel cutter is used to cut the bone to the appropriate size.

A brief description of the anterior cervical fusion procedure follows:

1. A Cloward cervical retractor with one long and one short blade is used to separate the carotid sheath, trachea, and esophagus.
2. A Ferris Smith pituitary rongeur is used to remove the disk.
3. A Cloward vertebra spreader is used to widen the space.
4. A Cloward double-ended impactor is used to seat the bone graft between the vertebrae.
5. ASIF plates and screws are used to stabilize the fusion.

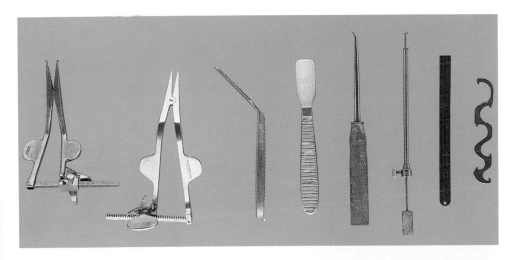

137-1 *Left to right:* 1 Cloward vertebra spreader, small; 1 Cloward vertebra spreader, medium; 2 Cloward blade retractors, modified, side view and front view; 1 osteophyte periosteal elevator; 1 depth gauge with set screw; 1 metal ruler; 1 spanner wrench.

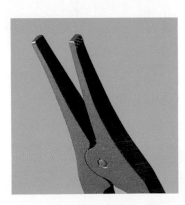

137-2 Tip of Cloward vertebra spreader.

137-3 *Top, left to right:* 6 sets of blunt cervical retractor blades, small to large. *Middle, left to right:* 1 Cloward cervical retractor handle, small; 1 Cloward cervical retractor handle, large. *Bottom, left to right:* 6 sets of 4-pronged cervical retractor blades, small to large.

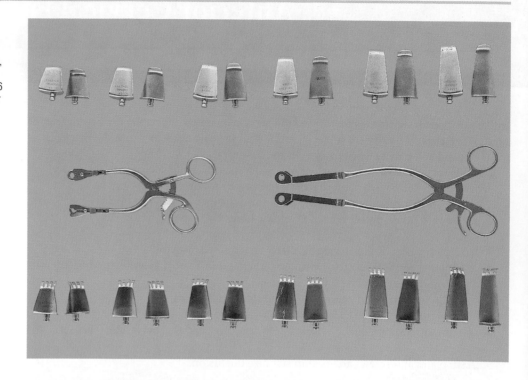

137-4 *Top, left to right:* 1 Hudson brace; 1 dowel ejector. *Bottom, left to right:* 1 dowel cutter shaft with removable threaded nut; 1 Cloward bone-graft double-ended impactor, $^{11}/_{14}$ mm; 1 Cloward drill shaft. *Middle, top to bottom:* 4 drill tips: 10, 12, 14, and 16 mm; 6 dowel cutters with center pins: 12 to 18 mm; 4 dowel cutters: 12, 14, 16, and 18 mm. *Bottom, right:* 1 dowel handle, cone tip with spring.

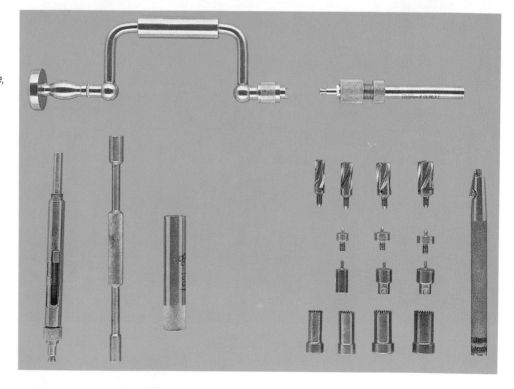

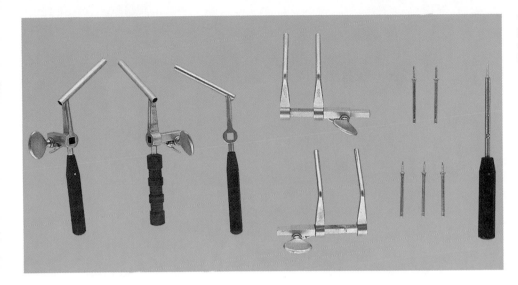

138-1 *Left to right:* 2 drill guides, left and right; 1 drill guide; 2 vertebra distractors, right and left; 5 distraction pins, 16 and 14 mm; 1 screwdriver.

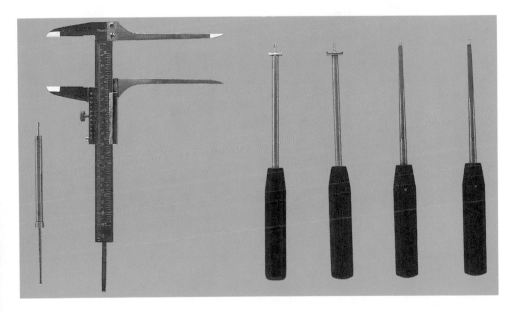

138-2 *Left to right:* 1 twist drill; 1 caliper; 1 vertebral-body dissector; 1 vertebral-body dissector, angled; 1 graft holder, small; 1 graft holder, standard.

138-3 *Left to right:* Speculum pattern with 4 blades, 3 front view and 1 side view; blade ejector; 3 bone tamps: 3, 5, and 8 mm.

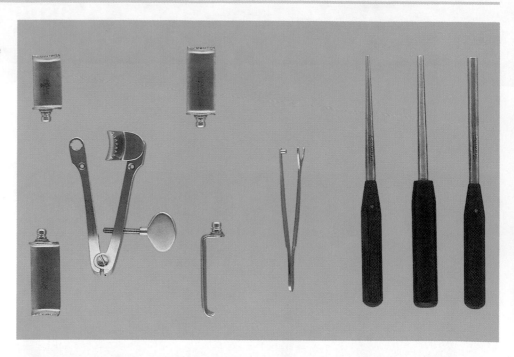

138-4 *Left to right:* Vertebra distractor with 5 pins of various sizes, 1 attached; Casper self-retaining retractor with 5 dull blades, 1 attached.

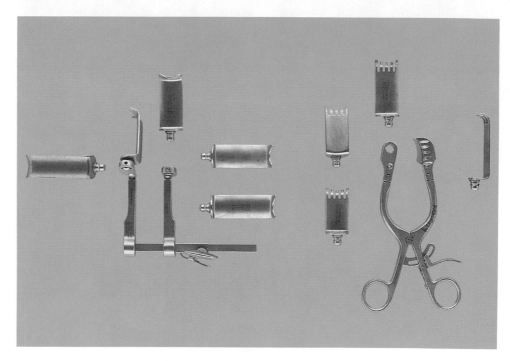

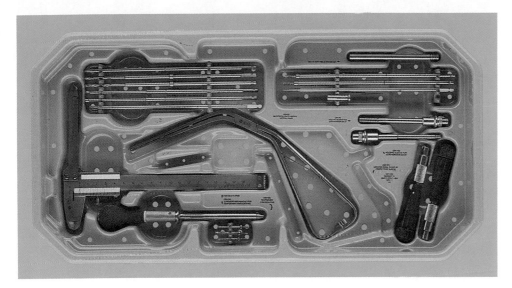

139-1 ASIF anterior cervical locking plating instruments in tray, with names marked, in case.

---

*Additional images are available on the Companion CD.

139-2 Drill guide with axillary bin, with names marked.

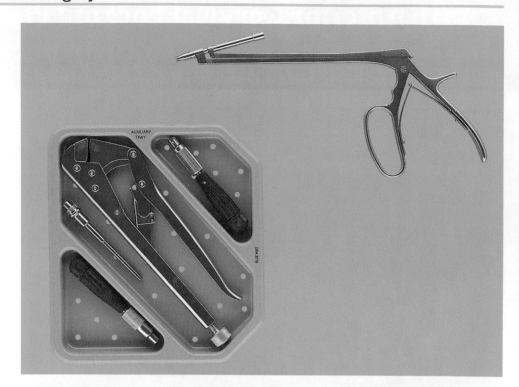

139-3 *Top, left to right:* 3 sizes of cervical plates taken out of trays. *Bottom, left to right:* 3 marked trays: 1 of screws and 2 of various sizes of cervical plates.

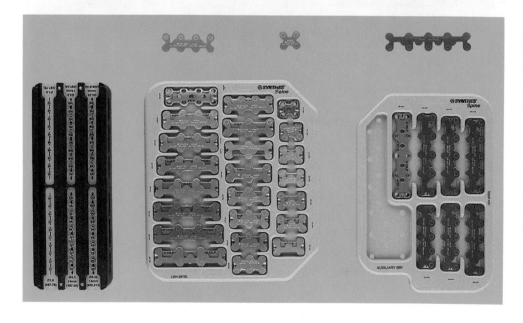

References

CHAPTER 1

American College of Chest Surgeons and American Association of Bronchology: consensus statement: prevention of flexible bronchoscopy-associated infections. *Chest* 128:1742-1755, 2005.

American Society for Gastroenterology Endoscopy and the Society for Infection Control and Hospital Epidemiology: multi-society guideline for reprocessing flexible gastrointestinal endoscopes. *American Journal of Infection Control* 31:309-315, 2003.

Association for the Advancement of Medical Instrumentation: *Guidelines for selection and use of rigid container systems for ethylene oxide sterilization and stream sterilization in healthcare facilities (ST33).* Arlington, VA: AAMI, 1996.

Association for the Advancement of Medical Instrumentation. *Steam sterilization and sterility in health care facilities (ST46).* Arlington, VA: AAMI, 2002.

Association of periOperative Registered Nurses: Recommended practice for care of instruments. In *Standards, recommended practices and guidelines*, pp. 555-563. Denver, AORN, 2006.

Broder B: Instrument knowledge: scoping out repairs. *Infection Control Today* 1:18-20, 2002.

Doderlein G: *Antique medical instruments.* Tuttlingen, Federal Republic of Germany: Aesculap, .

Descoteaux JG et al: Residual organic debris on processed surgical instruments. *AORN Journal* 63:23-25, 1995.

Hutchisson B, LeBlanc C: The truth and consequences of enzymatic detergents. *Gastroenterology Nursing* 28:372-376, 2005.

Knorr D, Heinz V: Development of nonthermal methods of microbial control. In Favero MS, Bond WW (eds): *Chemical disinfection of medical and surgical devices,* Philadelphia: Lippincott Williams and Wilkins, 2001.

Muscarella L: The benefits of ultrasonic cleaning. *Infection Control Today* 5:42-44, 2001.

Rutala W, Weber DJ: Creutzfeldt-Jakob disease: recommendations for disinfection and sterilization. *Clinical Infectious Diseases* 32:1348-1356, 2001.

RutalaShah S, Bernardo M: *Reusable surgical instruments: metallurgy and corrosion.* www.MedicalProductsSales.com, 26-27, 2000.

Skinner G: The history of surgical instruments. *Nursing Times* July, 28-30, 1984.

Smith L: Surgical instruments: quality on the cutting edge. www.MedicalProductsSales.com, 40-41, 2001.

Storz Instrument Company: *The care and handling of surgical instruments.* St. Louis: Storz Instrument Company.

CHAPTER 2-139

Bragg K, Van Balen N, Cook N: Home study program: future trends in minimally invasive surgery. *AORN Journal* 82:1005-1022, 2005.

Mosby's medical, nursing, and allied health dictionary, ed 7, St. Louis: Mosby, 2006.

Rothrock JC: *Alexander's care of the patient in surgery*, ed 13, St. Louis: Mosby, 2007.

Schultz R: *Inspecting surgical instruments: an illustrated guide.* International Association of Healthcare Central Service Material Management, 2005.

Index

Richmond subarachnoid screw, 321

Richmond subarachnoid wrench, 321

Right-cup forceps, 225

Ring curette, 223

Robotic instruments, 74-75

Rod
long bone, 169-170
spinal fusion with, 164-168

Rod cutter, 168

Root and splinter forceps, 248

Rosen knife, 224

Rosser crypt hook, 65, 66

Routurier lower third molar forceps, 248

Rowe disimpaction forceps, 242

Rumel tourniquet, 260

Ruskin double-action rongeur, 307

Ruskin-Liston bone-cutting forceps, 117, 118, 127

Ruskin rongeur, 117, 147

Russian tissue forceps, 27, 42, 247

Ryder needle holder, 113

S

Sagittal splitting osteotome, 245

Salmon passer, 318

Sarot bronchus clamp, 268

Sarot needle holder, 316

Satinsky neonatal vascular clamp, 296

Satinsky (vena cava) clamp, 101

Satterlee amputation saw, 183

Sauerbruch (rib) rongeur, 267

Saw, power, 120-123

Scalpel, harmonic, 69

Schepens orbital retractor, 208, 216

Schocket scleral depressor, 210

Schott eye speculum, 197

Schroeder uterine tenaculum forceps, 85, 89

Schroeder uterine vulsellum forceps, 85, 89

Scissors
in da Vinci Surgical System, 74-75
description of, 15-16
inspection of, 10
schedule for sharpening of, 11

Scott-McCracken elevator, 144

Scoville nerve root retractor, 325

Screw
ASIF standard, 151
dynamic hip, 153, 154
internal fixation with, 146-147
monoaxial, 189
polyaxial, 188

Seating chisel, 175, 176

Seldin periosteal elevator, 248

Semb gouging rongeur, 267

Semb ligature-carrying forceps, 279

Semb lung retractor, 267, 268

Senn-Kanavel retractor, 242

Senn retractor, 16, 43, 262

Septoplasty, 230-233

Serrefines, 217

Sheehy ossicle-holding forceps, 219

Sheets irrigating vectis, 199

Shell provisionals and acetabular instruments, 159

Shepard iris hook, 199, 200

Shoulder instruments, 140

Shoulder ligature carrier, 141

Sickle knife, 237

Sigmoidoscope, 64

Silber vasovasostomy clamp, 111

Silicone spatula retractor, 304

Sims uterine cuette, 82

Sims uterine sound, 82

Single-action rongeur, 248

Sinskey hook, reverse, 203

Sinskey iris hook, 194, 196, 200

Sinskey tying forceps, 199, 201

Sinus, surgery on, 236-240

Sinus curette, 237, 239

Sinus ostium seeker, 239

Sinus seeker, 237

Skin, 39

Skin expander, 253

Skin graft, 251-253

Skin hook, 16, 42

Skin stapler, 39

Slotted hammer, 176

Smith-Petersen laminectomy rongeur, 118, 156, 307

SMR. See Septoplasty

Snowden-Pencer dissecting forceps, 111

Snowden-Pencer fixation forceps, 111

Snowden-Pencer scissors, 25, 259

Soft tissue instrument set, 118-119

Spatula cautery, 48

Spatula retractor, 304

Spinal fusion, 164-168

Spratt (Brun) curette, 147

Spratt cureette, 119, 127

Spurling-Kerrison rongeur, 326

Stammberger antrum punch, 237, 238

Stapler
endoscopic circular, 61
linear, 61

Steinmann pin, 156

Stent grasper, 98

Steri Tite container, 22

Sterilization
methods of, 13
new techniques for, 1
preparation for, 12-14

Sterilization container system, 21-23

Sternal crimper, 273

Sternal saw, 276-277

Sternum knife, 276-277

Stevens tenotomy hook, 206

Stevens tenotomy scissors, 293

Stille-Horsley bone-cutting forceps, 183

Stille-Luer rongeur, 183

Storz microforceps, 95, 96

Straight-cup forceps, 225

Strauch vasovasostomy approximator, 111

Strully scissors, 255, 259, 304

Struyken nasal cutting forceps, 237

Stryker camera set, 22

Stryker cement gun, 138

Stryker cement restrictor inserter, 157

Stryker Mini 4200 Driver, 122

Stryker System 5, 120

Stryker TPS Ortho Power System, 123

Suction/irrigator system, 52

Suction tube, 19

Sullivan rectal retractor, 66

Surgery
cardiac, 269-273
eye muscle, 205-206
history of, 2
minimally invasive, 1, 44
orthognathic, 244-245
orthopedic, 116-117
pediatric, 184-190, 292
sinus, 236-240

Surgical instruments. See Instruments

Swanstrom grasper, 300

Switchblade scissors, 72

Swolin Teflon angled rod, 93

Synthes cannulated screw set, 177

Synthes chuck, 122

Synthes drill, 123

Synthes low-profile cranial plating set, 323

Synthes unreamed tibial nail, 173

Synthes unreamed tibial nail insertion and locking instruments, 174

T

T-handle femoral reamer, 157

T handle wrench, 167

T retractor, malleable, 266

Tan endoknife, 301

Tan spreader, 301

Tapered malleable brain retractor, 309

Taylor Spatial frame, 179

Taylor Spatial ring, 179

Taylor spinal retractor, 157, 326

Teflon Bardic plug, 285

Telescope
bariatric, 68
inspection of, 11

Telescope lens, 240

Tenaculum, 49

Terry scraper, 203

Texas Scottish Rite Hospital bending tray, 165

Texas Scottish Rite Hospital cross-link tray, 166

Texas Scottish Rite Hospital hook trials, 166

Texas Scottish Rite Hospital implant tray, 164

Texas Scottish Rite Hospital pediatric instrument tray, 165, 166

Texas Scottish Rite Hospital top tightening implant tray, 164

Texas Scottish Rite Hospital wrench tray, 167

Thomas uterine curette, 82

Thompson retractor, 36
Army, 34
blades for, 34, 35, 36
joints for, 36

Thoracic instruments, 266-268

Thoracoport, 264

Thoracoscopy, 263-265

Thorek scissors, 57

Thumb tissue forceps, 65, 104

Thornton fixation ring, 194, 196

Thorpe caliper, 208

Tibial alignment/resection instruments, 136

Tibial/femoral implant instruments, 137

Tissue protector, 170

Titan-Vario clip applier, 322

Titanium, instruments made from, 1, 2

Titanium 2.0-mm micro fixation system, 246

Titanium tying forceps, 96, 193

Titanium unreamed femoral nail instrument, 172

Titus needle, 318

Tonsil hemostatic forceps, 28, 38, 232

Tonsillectomy, 228-229

Tooth extraction set, 247-248

Total hip prosthesis (VerSys Hip System), 163

Total hip replacement, 155-162

Total knee prosthesis, 139

Total knee replacement, 133-138

Towel clamp, 17

Townley femur caliper, 156

Tracheal hook, 262

Tracheotomy set, 261-262

Transurethral resection of the prostate, 107-109

Triangular positioning plate, 176

Trilogy acetabular, 158

Trocar, for laparoscopy, 46

Trocar cannula, 245

Trousseau tracheal dilator, 262

Troutman-Barraquer forceps, 198

Troutman tier needle holder, 110

Trumpet-valve cannula, 91

TSRH. See Texas Scottish Rite Hospital implant tray

Tubal occlusion, laparoscopic, 90-92

TURP. See Transurethral resection of the prostate

Twist drill, 331

Tympanoplasty, 220-227

U

UltraCision 5-mm harmonic scalpel, 86

Ultrasonic irrigator, instrument cleaning with, 5

Universal femoral distractor set, 171

University of Minnesota cheek retractor, 242

Upper hand retractor, 32, 33

Upper incisor and cuspid forceps, 248

Ureteroplasty, 100-101

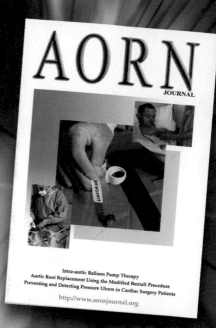